The Natural Health Bible
for Women

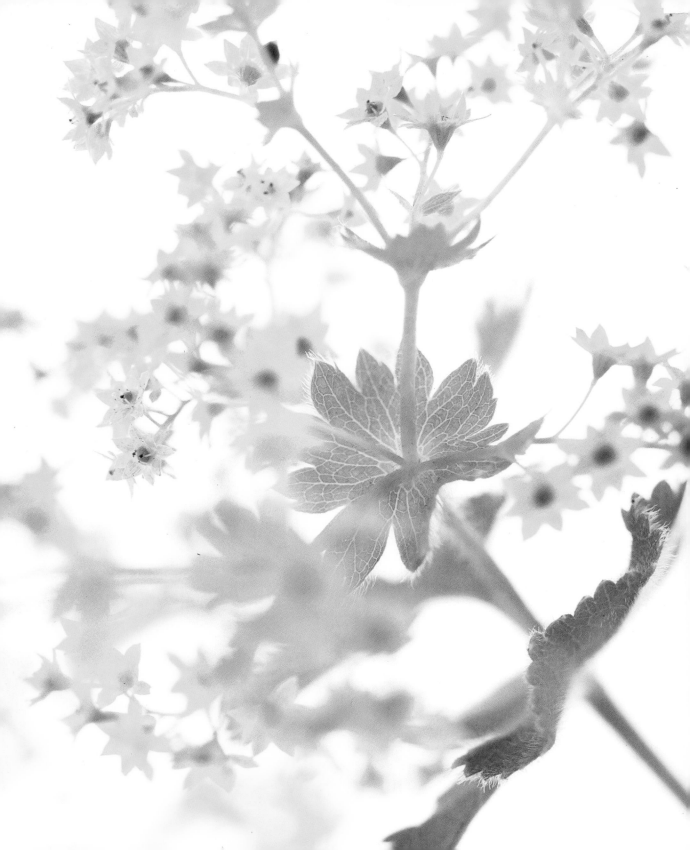

Marilyn Glenville, Ph.D.

The Natural Health Bible
for Women

The Complete Guide for Women of All Ages

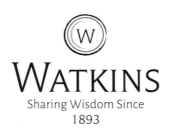

WATKINS
Sharing Wisdom Since
1893

To all my patients and readers over the years, whose inspiration and insights have made this book possible.

The Natural Health Bible for Women
Marilyn Glenville, Ph.D.

This edition published in the USA in 2017 by Watkins,
an imprint of Watkins Media Limited
19 Cecil Court, London WC2N 4EZ

enquiries@watkinspublishing.com

First published in the UK and USA in 2010 by Duncan Baird Publishers Ltd

Managing Editor: Grace Cheetham
Editor: Judy Barratt
Managing Designer: Suzanne Tuhrim
Picture Research: Annabel Evans
Commissioned artwork: Joanna Culley B.A. (Hons) MMAA RMIP (medical artwork);
  Mark Watkinson (pp.52 and 101),
Commissioned photography: Jules Selmes

Library of Congress Cataloging-in-Publication Data

Glenville, Marilyn.
  The natural health bible for women : the ultimate guide for women of all ages / Marilyn Glenville.
    p. cm.
  Includes bibliographical references and index.
  ISBN 978-1-84483-898-1
  1. Women--Health and hygiene. I. Title.
  RA778.G574 2010
  613'.04244--dc22

                          2009041174

ISBN: 978-1-78678-137-6

10 9 8 7 6 5 4 3 2 1

Typeset in Franklin Gothic and Scala
Color reproduction by Colourscan, Singapore
Printed in China

Notes:
1 tsp = 5ml
Never use clary sage essential oil within 12 hours of drinking any alcohol.

Acknowledgments

This is such a beautiful book visually that I wanted to thank everyone involved in helping to create it. So much work has gone on behind the scenes with me being just the tip of the iceberg. This is my first book with Watkins Media, and I would like to thank Grace Cheetham for giving me the opportunity to write it. Special thanks go to Judy Barratt, my editor, who has worked tirelessly to make sure that everything is in order and all the text fits correctly.

I would like to thank Theresa Cheung for her help with research, and all the people who worked on the wonderful photographs and illustrations.

I am also grateful to the team at the Tunbridge Wells Clinic, who work so efficiently and with such good humor while I am away writing. It is not always easy to put into words what everyone does, and often it is the little things that make such a difference and allow me the time to write. It is a privilege to thank Mel, Helen, Brenda, Sharon, Alex, Gayla, Marian, Wendy, Lee, Sophia, and Andree, who keep everything running smoothly. I would also like to thank my team of nutritionists at the clinics: Helen, Sharon, Lisa, and Alison, who take care of the patients while I am not there and work with such knowledge, passion, kindness, and care.

I want to express my appreciation to my medical colleagues, especially Dr. Yehudi Gordon, consultant gynecologist and obstetrician, who has such a passion for Integrated Medicine that he founded his clinic, Viveka, in London, based on its principles. It is a privilege to have worked at Viveka since its inception more than ten years ago and to see the wonderful results achieved there. This is the healthcare of the future.

My love to all my family: to my husband Kriss for running the business side of the clinics, so that I am free to do what I do best; and to my family: Matt, his wife Hannah, and daughter Katie; to Len and Chantell; and to my sister, Janet, and her husband Terry.

Publisher's acknowledgments: Watkins would like to thank Sarina from MOT Models for appearing in the commissioned photography and Justine Martin (make-up artist).

Contents

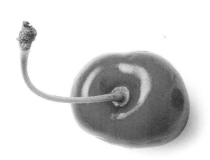
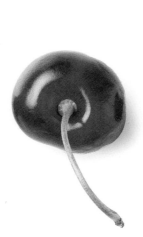
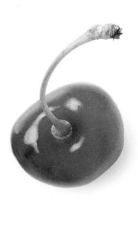

Foreword

I'm so pleased to have had the opportunity to write this book and to be able to share the information and knowledge I have gained over many years in the study and practice of nutritional medicine.

There are times in our lives when conventional medicine with surgery and drugs is vital, even life-saving. However, at other times a more natural approach can restore health and optimize well-being. Guiding you through the main health problems you might encounter as a woman, *The Natural Health Bible for Women* lets you know what choices are available, so you can take control of your health and make informed decisions about how best to take care of yourself. No matter what age or stage of life you're at, if you're interested in your health and want to know what options you have for your well-being, I've written this book for you.

Conventional vs natural

When you get symptoms, your body's usually trying to tell you that something's wrong. If you take medication, you'll suppress your symptoms but probably without treating the underlying cause. Natural medicine, on the other hand, works on all your body's systems to bring your body back into balance, relieving the symptoms but also treating the root of the problem. For example, women frequently come to my clinics with menstrual problems, such as irregular and absent periods. The medical approach is to put them on the contraceptive pill to "regulate" their cycles. However, for many, as soon as they come off the Pill, the problem returns because this approach hasn't addressed the underlying cause. After a few months following my natural guidelines, many women find that their periods regulate or reappear naturally and sustainably. This is because diet and herbal and other natural treat-

ments restore harmony (or homeostasis, a state of perfect balance) to the body, so that everything begins to work as it should.

In *The Natural Health Bible for Women*, I've given you essential information about both the medical and natural treatments available. I want you to be able to weigh the best options for you. It may be that you need to use a combination of both conventional and natural medicine, and this can be really effective. Or, it may be that you haven't realized that there's a wide array of natural treatments for women's health problems and that, at this stage, there's no need to take medication at all. *The Natural Health Bible for Women* shows you that there's a lot you can do to help resolve problems and to keep you in good health generally. It may take a bit of effort at first to adjust your diet and lifestyle but the benefits will be worth it. No matter how old you are, the sooner you start to make positive changes, the sooner you reap the benefits, now and in the long term.

ABOUT THIS BOOK

I've organized this book to give you a basic grounding in how your body and the natural remedies work, and then to give you detailed information on the most common conditions you may encounter during your life.

In the first chapter, I explain how all of your body systems are connected. Although conventional medicine tends to view your body as separate parts, you'll discover that there are many feedback loops that link each organ or system in your body with the others. I'll show you that by altering your underlying physiology (by eating well, changing your lifestyle, and using natural remedies), you set up a positive domino effect that gives your body the tools it needs to heal itself.

Chapter 2 of *The Natural Health Bible for Women* looks at the conditions I'm most often asked to treat in the clinic. I work top to toe through your body. For each particular health problem, I describe the symptoms, the possible causes, and how to go about getting an accurate diagnosis. I cover the conventional medical treatments you could be offered, how they work, and whether they're linked to any side-effects. Then, I look at the natural approach: how you can use your diet, food supplements, and herbal remedies to improve the condition. I also recommend other appropriate natural treatments, including homeopathy, acupuncture, aromatherapy, osteopathy, and yoga; and I've included lots of easy-to-follow self-help tips.

Chapters 3 and 4 look at fertility and menopause, respectively. As well as covering the various ups and downs of conception, pregnancy, and birth, Chapter 3 gives detailed information on both the conventional and natural approaches to fertility problems. This includes step-by-step guidance on my proven combination of diet and supplement, herbal and complementary treatments. If you're approaching menopause, in Chapter 4 the sections on HRT and my natural approach will help you to make an informed choice about how to deal with this important stage of your life. If you have a particular menopausal symptom (such as hot flashes or osteoporosis), look it up, and I hope you'll find all the advice you need to understand why it happens, what conventional medicine has to offer as treatment, and how to treat it naturally.

The final chapter is a general guide to well-being, with advice on how to optimize weight, boost immunity, and lower stress levels. This information is for you and all women at all stages of their lives.

When choosing supplements and herbs, it's crucial to use only those of the highest quality at the correct dosage for them to be effective. To help you to find the best, look at the Resources section on page 320.

The information contained in this book has come from more than 25 years' experience of working in clinics and using natural remedies—in particular, nutrition—to help women effectively. Nutrition is the foundation of your health: even if you have to use conventional medicine, you can still use the nutritional recommendations to keep you as healthy as possible.

I hope you find the information useful—for a few women it may even be life-changing. I'd love to hear about your experiences. My details are on page 320—please contact me with any questions or feedback.

HOW TO TAKE NATURAL REMEDIES

Unless instructed otherwise in the specific entries, please follow these general guidelines for taking the natural remedies:

- Take supplements on an ongoing basis until you notice a significant improvement in your symptoms (usually by three months), then take only a daily multi-vitamin and mineral together with omega-3 fatty acids and vitamin C as a good maintenance program.
- Take herbal remedies for three months, then, if you haven't noticed a significant improvement, consult a qualified herbal practitioner. If you're already taking medication, consult your doctor before taking any herbs.
- Take homeopathic remedies in a 30c potency for up to three days, then see a qualified homeopath if you feel they aren't working.
- In general, if you haven't noticed a significant difference after three months of using natural remedies, see a healthcare practitioner or call my clinic and speak to one of my nutritionists.

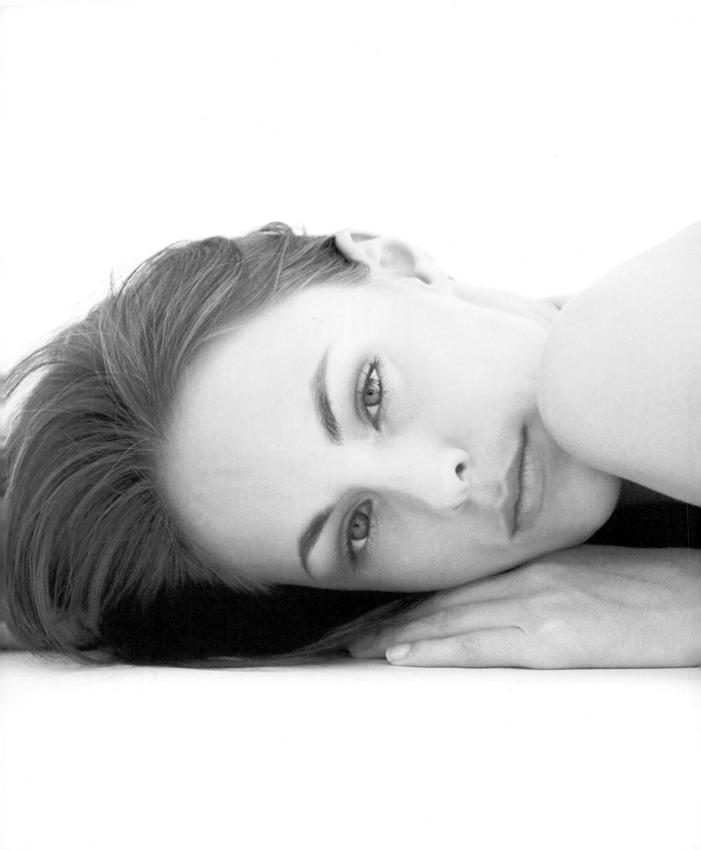

Introducing your body

1

A woman's body is an amazing machine. It's full of intricate systems that not only sustain life but may also create new life. Each of these systems must work with the others, in harmony, in order for the female body to function at its best.

We know more today about how a woman's body works than we have ever known before. Despite that, many women are still unaware of how their organs function or even where they are located. Even if we know something about our physiology, we rarely know much about our hormones. Many women I see have no idea of the staggering influence their hormones have, from birth, through puberty and pregnancy, to menopause, not only on their physical health, but on their emotional health, too. In fact, it's often not until we try for a baby, begin menopause, or just become ill that we really start to appreciate how each system in our body affects the others. Good health begins with a better understanding of how everything inside you fits together. Enjoy your voyage of discovery!

The female organs

The key to the workings of a woman's body lies in a small region around the pelvis. Here, all your reproductive organs sit together playing crucial roles in your fertility, hormones, and overall health.

THE OVARIES

A woman's main reproductive organs, the ovaries are about the size and shape of almonds, solid, and grayish-pink in color. They sit near the top of the pelvic bone. Each ovary is held in place by ligaments that anchor it to the uterus and pelvis. The ovaries contain ovarian follicles, little sacs in which eggs (known medically as oocytes) develop. The ovaries produce the hormones estrogen, progesterone, and testosterone (the "sex hormones") and are responsible for storing and releasing a woman's eggs—which, if fertilized by sperm, have the potential to become babies.

A baby girl is usually born with two ovaries, one on either side of the uterus. Some women are born with only one, while others may have an ovary surgically removed—perhaps because of a cyst, or after an ectopic pregnancy. (Both ovaries may have to be removed if you're at high risk of developing ovarian cancer; see box, p.89.) Although having one ovary may reduce the chances you have of becoming pregnant, many women with one ovary go on to have successful pregnancies.

At birth, the ovaries contain between one and two million immature eggs—amounting to a lifetime's supply. Although this number begins to diminish almost immediately (see p.188), the young eggs lie dormant within the ovary, inside the follicles, until puberty, when a cascade of hormones activates several changes in a girl's body and the reproductive system makes a dramatic swing into action.

After this, healthy ovaries begin to act in the way we probably all expect. Each month, about 20 immature eggs and their follicles begin to "ripen." As they do so, they move together towards the surface of the ovary. Usually, one follicle will mature fully, becoming dominant, while the others die away. The dominant follicle will literally "pop" or rupture on the surface of the ovary, releasing its egg into the Fallopian tube (see p.14). This is ovulation. Occasionally, more than one follicle will mature fully, releasing more than one egg. If two eggs are released and fertilized, then implant successfully in the uterus, the woman will be pregnant with non-identical twins (three eggs will bring non-identical triplets, and so on). (Identical twins are the result of a single egg "splitting" after fertilization.)

It's a myth that ovulation alternates monthly between ovaries. Every month, follicles on both ovaries start to mature eggs. The ovary that matures an egg first, gets to release it. The relative health of each ovary has some influence, but the winner could be the same ovary several months in a row, or it could be one then the other.

Throughout a woman's reproductive years, the ovaries also produce the sex hormones estrogen and progesterone, which control the menstrual cycle (see p.19). During the development of the ovarian follicle containing the egg, the ovary produces increasing amounts of estrogen. This is the main female hormone, and its primary job is to stimulate the body into building and maintaining the lining of the uterus. Estrogen also

EACH MONTH about 20 eggs begin to "ripen."

MAPPING THE FEMALE ORGANS

FRONT VIEW

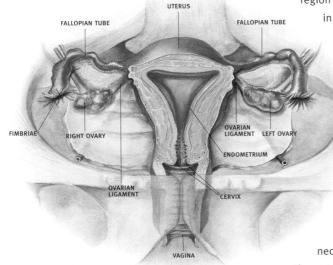

UTERUS

FALLOPIAN TUBE

FALLOPIAN TUBE

FIMBRIAE

RIGHT OVARY

OVARIAN LIGAMENT LEFT OVARY

ENDOMETRIUM

OVARIAN LIGAMENT

CERVIX

VAGINA

The female reproductive organs lie in the pelvic region in the lower abdomen. Each ovary is oval in shape and is attached to the uterus via a fibrous chord known as the ovarian ligament. Long, finger-like fronds, called fimbriae, at the ends of the Fallopian tubes, sweep over the ovaries to catch an egg as it's released, so it can begin its journey down the tubes towards the uterus. During the process of ovulation, the ovaries release the hormones estrogen and progesterone, which stimulate the uterus's lining (the endometrium) to thicken to receive a fertilized egg. At the neck of the uterus is a narrow passage called the cervix, which opens into the vagina.

SIDE VIEW

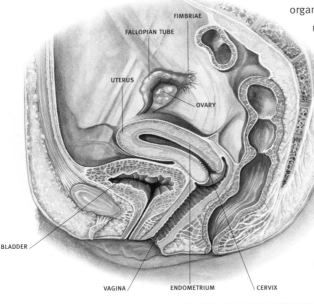

FIMBRIAE

FALLOPIAN TUBE

UTERUS

OVARY

BLADDER

VAGINA

ENDOMETRIUM

CERVIX

From the side, it's easy to see how the female organs sit among the other organs of the pelvic region. The vagina is angled slightly backward, probably to make intercourse easier, while in most women the uterus reaches forward over the top of the bladder, towards the stomach. In a few women (somewhere between ten and 20 percent worldwide), however, the uterus may be retroverted, meaning that it sits backward in the pelvic cavity, pointing towards the spine. This is not usually any cause for concern (for example, it's unlikely to have any effect on fertility), and is just another example of every woman's uniqueness.

maintains the health of your bones and your brain. After ovulation, the empty follicle (called the corpus luteum) produces the hormone progesterone, which stops the release of more eggs and prepares the uterus lining for implantation.

The ovaries also produce small amounts of testosterone (a male hormone), which, when released into the bloodstream, helps maintain bone and muscle strength and to boost libido.

THE FALLOPIAN TUBES

Named after the 16th-century Italian anatomist Gabriele Fallopio, who first discovered them, your two Fallopian tubes extend from the upper edges of the uterus towards the ovaries and are typically around 4in. in length. Amazingly, the tubes do not connect directly with the ovaries. Instead the end of each tube flares into a funnel shape with finger-like extensions—rather like tentacles—that reach towards the egg and catch it as it's released. Once the egg is caught, tiny hairs on the insides of the tubes, called cilia, along with mild muscular contractions, guide the unfertilized egg down the tube towards the uterus.

It can take three or four days for an egg to travel the length of a Fallopian tube, and it's during this time that a woman is at her most fertile—if sperm meet the traveling egg, fertilization may occur. To encourage the best conditions for fertilization, the mucous membrane that lines each Fallopian tube secretes a sticky fluid that helps keep the egg and sperm alive. This maximizes the chances of their meeting before the egg reaches the uterus. Bicarbonates (a salt solution) and lactic acid in the fluid enable the sperm to process oxygen, while glucose provides nourishment for both the sperm and the egg. If the sperm and egg meet, the fertilized egg remains in the Fallopian tube for up to seven days. During this time it develops tiny projections called chorionic villi that will help it implant in the uterus. If the egg and the sperm don't meet, the egg makes its way to the uterus anyway, where it's then expelled during a woman's monthly menstruation.

THE UTERUS

The uterus is situated low in the pelvis, hanging within the abdominal cavity between the bladder and the rectum. It's a hollow muscular organ, shaped somewhat like an inverted pear. The uterus is extremely small at birth, but develops during puberty so that, in an adult woman, it's about the size of a clenched fist—although it has the amazing ability to expand during pregnancy to accommodate a fully grown baby. (During menopause, the uterus atrophies, or shrinks, decreasing in size as a result of falling levels of estrogen in the body; see pp.246–8.)

Your uterus is made up of three layers: the endometrium, the myometrium, and the parametrium. The endometrium is the innermost layer, and we commonly call it the "lining of the uterus." It's a layer of mucous membranes, glands, and blood vessels that thickens after ovulation (to receive a fertilized egg) and during pregnancy (to cushion and nourish the growing fetus). You shed the thickened lining when you have your period (see p.19). The second layer, the myometrium, is a layer of muscle—in fact, it's one of the strongest muscles in your body, causing the powerful contractions during labor that push a baby out. Like the endometrium, this layer changes over the course of a month, becoming thickest and most engorged with blood vessels immediately after ovulation. If you're pregnant, by the time your baby is due, it will have expanded to fill almost your entire abdominal cavity. The outermost layer of your uterus is the parametrium, which consists of connective tissue that anchors the uterus in place.

For medical purposes, the uterus is divided into four parts. The first of these is the fundus. This is the top, domed part of your uterus, and on either side connects with your Fallopian tubes. If you are or have been pregnant, you'll know that the height of your fundus is one of the measurements your gynecologist or midwife will take regularly to assess the size of your growing baby. The second part of the uterus is known as the "body." This forms the widest section in the upper two-thirds of your uterus. The third part is only about a centimetre long and is the narrowing of the uterus, known as the isthmus. This leads into the fourth and lowest part—the cervix.

THE CERVIX

Sometimes known as the neck of the uterus, the cervix is cylindrical in shape and about 1in. long. It joins the uterus to the top of the vagina, enables menstrual blood to pass from the uterus into the vagina, and allows sperm to pass from the vagina into the uterus. The narrow opening of the cervix is called the os. The cervix also protects the uterus and a developing fetus from pathogens (such as invading bacteria) and plays a role in sexual pleasure. In short, the cervix is crucial for a woman's reproductive and sexual health.

Many women don't realize that every month, during the normal course of a menstrual cycle, the shape and position of the cervix changes. When the uterus sheds its lining during menstruation, the cervix widens to allow the release of blood. Once menstruation has ended, it lies low in the vaginal canal and feels firm like the rubber of a rubber ball. Then, as ovulation approaches, the cervix moves up towards the body of the uterus, softens and starts to open. This is one of the ways in which your amazing body makes it easier for sperm to enter your uterus in the hope that fertilization will occur. During childbirth the cervix can dilate up to 4in. to allow a baby to pass into the vagina and eventually out into the world.

Covering the cervix is a thin layer of cells called the epithelium. The epithelium cells are either squamous, which means they are flat and scaly, or columnar, which means they appear column-like.

One of the most influential anatomical features of your cervix is its lining. The cervical canal is lined with a smooth mucous membrane, which contains glands known as crypts. These constantly secrete a mucus that changes over the course of your monthly cycle. It's thick and sticky (infertile or hostile mucus) during the first half of the cycle (the follicular phase) to form a

stopper over the opening of the cervix into the vagina. This helps make the vagina an acid environment to kill off sperm. A few days before ovulation, the mucus becomes clear, wet and stretchy. This is fertile mucus that assists the sperm, forming channels that move them into the Fallopian tubes. After ovulation, the mucus becomes thick and sticky again to protect the cervix and uterus from bacteria—and from sperm.

THE VAGINA

A muscular tube that provides a passage between the uterus and the outside world, the vagina allows a penis in during intercourse, and menstrual blood and a baby out. The vagina is angled slightly backward inside the pelvis and contains three layers of tissue. The mucosa is a layer of mucous membranes on the surface that you can touch (similar to the lining of the mouth). The next layer is muscular wall, and the third layer is fibrous tissue that connects your vagina to your body. Normally about 4in. in length, the vagina has the most amazing muscles—they can stretch and lengthen the vaginal canal to allow the delivery of a baby weighing anything up to around 14lb.!

In its "virgin" state, before a woman has had intercourse, the vaginal opening is often partially covered by a thin membrane called the hymen, the tearing of which may cause slight bleeding (the hymen may tear as a result of inserting a tampon or strenuous exercise, as well as the first time a woman has sex). The walls of the vagina constantly produce secretions intended to optimize fertility, cleanse the vagina, and maintain a level of acidity that prevents infection. During intercourse, two glands in the vagina called "Bartholin" glands release moisture, which acts as a lubricant to make intercourse easier and more enjoyable for you and your partner. Sperm is alkaline and vaginal secretions change from acid to alkali around ovulation to provide the perfect environment for sperm to thrive. Sometimes the vagina can be so acidic that it becomes a hostile environment for sperm, and this can be one obstacle to successful natural conception.

The female hormones

At every stage of your life, from birth to death, your hormones play powerful roles. The most notable is that of your sex hormones, which trigger the changes that take place in your body over your lifetime.

Hormones are natural chemicals that trigger activity in different organs throughout your body. The body system responsible for producing your hormones is the endocrine system (see box, opposite). This consists of several glands, including the pituitary gland (which, for example, secretes growth hormones), the adrenal glands (you have two, and they control energy levels and the stress response), the thyroid gland (which influences metabolic rate and brain function), the thymus gland (which is essential in your immune response), and, of course, the glands of the reproductive system, most notably the ovaries in women and the testes in men. The pancreas, liver, and kidneys are all hormone-secreting parts of the endocrine system, too. In fact, as far as the human body's communication systems go, the endocrine system is second only to the nervous system.

In this book, estrogen is the hormone that probably features most frequently (although women are more prone than men to problems with thyroid hormones, too). Estrogen influences your reproductive system and the physical changes that take place during puberty and menopause. The best way to understand how estrogen and the other hormones affect your body is to take a journey through a woman's life.

CHILDHOOD

Between birth and puberty, the levels of estrogen in a girl's body remain quite low—girls have enough to differentiate their characteristic sexual organs but not enough to mature sexually.

At some point between the ages of eight and 11 (although sometimes earlier and sometimes later), a part of the brain called the hypothalamus begins to send signals to the pituitary gland, also in the brain, stimulating it to produce luteinizing hormone (LH) and follicle-stimulating hormone (FSH). These important hormones prompt a girl's ovaries to begin producing larger amounts of estrogen—and this heralds the start of puberty.

PUBERTY

No matter at what age it starts, the process of puberty takes around four years. During this time, the female sex hormones—estrogen and also progesterone—and the male sex hormones (also known as androgens), of which the hormone testosterone is the most well known, influence the development of what doctors call secondary sexual characteristics. Secreted by the ovaries, estrogen triggers the breasts to develop and the vagina to darken in color (to become a duller pink, rather than the bright red of childhood). The vaginal walls begin to thicken and produce white mucus. Estrogen also stimulates the distribution of body fat around the bottom, hips, and thighs—giving you your much-desired womanly, hourglass figure. Androgens, which are secreted by the ovaries and the adrenal glands, stimulate the growth of pubic and underarm hair, as well as growth in your muscles and bones, making them stronger and longer. And, while all this is going on and the activity of your sex hormones is in overdrive, your monthly periods begin.

YOUR ENDOCRINE SYSTEM

As we already know, the hormones released from your ovaries are not the only hormones that control your monthly cycle and affect your reproductive health, and your health in general. The glands of the endocrine system release many other hormones and, as you can see from the examples right, they are all dependent on each other. An imbalance in one hormonal system will have a knock-on effect on another. Your health relies upon the hormone balance within your body, so optimizing your reproductive health is not just about taking care of your reproductive organs, but taking care of the whole of you, too.

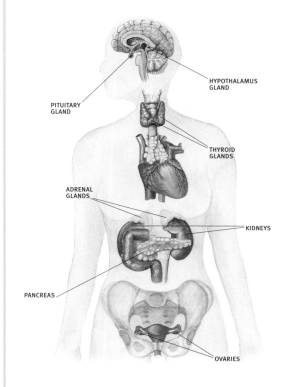

HYPOTHALAMUS GLAND

PITUITARY GLAND

THYROID GLANDS

ADRENAL GLANDS

KIDNEYS

PANCREAS

OVARIES

- Your pituitary gland releases three hormones known collectively as gonadotropins: FSH and LH (see opposite), and adrenocorticotrophic hormone (ACTH), which helps control the function of your adrenal glands. This gland also releases thyroid-stimulating hormone (TSH), which prompts your thyroid gland to release thyroid hormones (such as thyroxine), growth hormone, and prolactin (which stimulates milk production).

- Your thyroid gland controls your metabolism, which helps determine how fast you burn calories; and affects temperature. An underactive thyroid (see pp.58–61) can impact fertility.

- Your adrenal glands produce the stress hormones adrenaline and cortisol. These are released not only when you're under pressure, but also when your blood-sugar level drops too low. The hormones trigger your body to raise sugar levels by releasing its own sugar reserves. The adrenals also produce small quantities of sex hormones.

- Your pancreas secretes the hormone insulin, which controls levels of blood sugar. If your pancreas doesn't produce enough insulin, or produces it in very small amounts, you have type I diabetes and will need insulin by injection. If your pancreas produces enough or too much insulin but your body cannot use it properly, you have type II diabetes. If you have PCOS (polycystic ovary syndrome; see pp.83–7), your pancreas is often producing high amounts of insulin, which in turn causes your ovaries to produce excess testosterone. This will lead to "male" symptoms, such as excess hair, and also cause irregular periods or no menstrual cycles at all.

INTO ADULTHOOD

After the end of puberty, your bones mature (become strongest) and you reach your full height. This happens at about age 16 to 17 in girls. Although the sex hormones settle down, estrogen, progesterone, and the androgens, in particular, continue to operate in the body, playing a vital part in regulating your menstrual cycle (see opposite). Each hormone follows its own timetable, rising and falling at different points in your cycle, but all these sex hormones work together to keep your periods as regular as possible (roughly on a 27- to 33-day cycle, although the length of a regular cycle varies from woman to woman). That's why if you ever experience irregular periods (see p.94), you shouldn't ignore them—they are a sure sign that your sex hormones are not in optimal balance.

XENOESTROGENS

Produced by some plastics and pesticides, xenoestrogens are chemicals similar in structure to estrogen. They can confuse your body, sometimes causing early puberty, and may increase your risk of breast cancer. Reduce your exposure to xenoestrogens by following the hormone-balancing diet (see box, p.57). Also:

- Reduce your intake of food and drinks that come in plastic containers and avoid heating food in plastic containers (including putting hot or warm drinks in plastic bottles)
- Watch your weight—xenoestrogens are stored in body fat and overweight people tend to have higher concentrations
- Buy natural household cleaning products
- Use natural, organic toiletries, especially for products that you rub into your skin.

PREGNANCY

The dramatic hormonal changes of puberty pale into insignificance compared with the spectacular ones that occur during pregnancy. Once fertilization takes place, estrogen and progesterone levels remain raised at the end of your menstrual cycle (preventing a period), and the developing placenta produces a new hormone known as human chorionic gonadotrophin (HCG). This hormone stimulates the ovaries to produce even larger amounts of estrogen (to maintain the thickness of the uterus lining) and of progesterone (to prepare the uterus for successful, secure implantation and prevent your body from rejecting the embryo). HCG is the hormone detected by most pregnancy tests.

After three to four months, the well-established placenta takes over from the ovaries as the main producer of estrogen and progesterone. Large amounts of these hormones cause your uterus lining to thicken further and increase the blood supply to your uterus and breasts. They also encourage the muscles of your uterus to relax so it can expand for the growing baby. Eventually, these hormones stimulate contractions in labor and encourage the production of breast milk.

After pregnancy, hormone levels drop sharply. This drop encourages your uterus to shrink back nearly to its original size and your muscles to firm up again. It's also thought to be the reason why many mothers experience the "baby blues" (see box, p.229).

MENOPAUSE

Eventually, when your ovaries run out of eggs, your periods will stop altogether. This is called menopause (see pp.256–7). Between the ages of 35 and 50, a woman enters a phase called the perimenopausal years, when ovarian production of estrogen and progesterone begins to decline in preparation for menopause. During this time your periods may become irregular, or heavier or lighter than usual. These gradual hormonal changes may also affect other functions or aspects of your body, such as your sleep, memory, and body-fat distribution.

Your menstrual cycle

A healthy menstrual cycle is perhaps the best indicator you have of general good health. You can get to know your body more intimately by observing the changes that take place in it each month.

One common misconception many women have about their menstrual cycle is that they ovulate 14 days after menstruation starts. Actually, it's the other way round. The first half of the cycle may vary from woman to woman and cycle to cycle, but the second half tends to be typically the same length every month. In essence, ovulation usually occurs about 14 to 16 days before menstruation starts, not 14 days after it starts.

Poor diet, too much or too little exercise, lack of quality sleep, taking medication, being under stress, and poor health can all disrupt menstruation. However, on average, the process outlined in the box (right) lasts for 28 days, from the first day of bleeding in one cycle to the first day of bleeding in the next. However, it's possible to be healthy and to have normal cycles that are shorter or longer. It's also possible to have a period without ovulation and to ovulate more than once in a cycle. Nevertheless, whatever "regular" means for you, your menstrual cycle progresses according to the pattern set out in the box. Use this guide to get in tune with your body, to recognize the changes in yourself as you progress through the cycle, and to understand better what's going on inside you.

Every woman's cycle is unique to her, and unusual menstrual cycles are not always unhealthy. However, if your periods are irregular, I do recommend that you visit your doctor to have things checked out because irregularity could be a sign of hormonal imbalance or even illness. For example, one study found that women with very irregular menstrual cycles were more at risk of developing diabetes.

YOUR CYCLE—STEP BY STEP

- On day one of your period, the pituitary gland releases follicle-stimulating hormone (FSH). Although your period seems to signal the end of a cycle, it's actually the start of the next.
- FSH causes a number of egg-containing follicles to grow on the surface of the ovary.
- During the "follicular phase" of your cycle (before ovulation), the eggs inside the follicles mature. The ovaries produce higher levels of estrogen during this phase, too.
- As the estrogen levels from the ovary increase, FSH production decreases. At the same time, the pituitary gland releases luteinizing hormone (LH). In the cervix, acidic, hostile mucus becomes alkaline and fertile.
- Ovulation occurs when a follicle releases at least one mature egg into the Fallopian tube.
- You are now in the "luteal phase," the second half of your cycle. The corpus luteum (the structure left after the egg has been released), produces progesterone.
- If the egg is unfertilized, your body prepares for a period, which discharges the built-up uterus lining. Estrogen and progesterone levels drop, and your body begins a new cycle.

Knowing your fertility

The continuation of human life is one of evolution's primary goals, so your reproductive system is a crucial part of you. With practice, you can learn to detect when your body is at its most fertile.

All sorts of myths surround how female fertility works and what affects it. If you want to have a baby, there are two things it's crucial to understand: first, that a woman's fertility is influenced by age—the older you get, the less fertile you are (see pp.188–91); and, second, that a woman is fertile for only a few days every month. We cover age in detail later in the book, so here I want to tell you about Fertility Awareness—about reading the signs that tell you which are the few days in your cycle on which you can conceive.

YOUR THREE FERTILITY SIGNS

Over the course of a menstrual cycle, hormonal triggers cause changes in your body that provide signs you've ovulated. The following are every woman's top three fertile-time indicators. (Bear in mind an egg can live for only 24 hours once it's outside the ovary.)

"Fertile" cervical mucus

About three or four days before ovulation, your cervical mucus (see p.15) becomes clear and stretchy and there can be lots of it. This is "fertile" mucus. It makes your vagina an alkaline, "sperm-friendly" environment (becoming rather like male semen), it contains sugar, salt, and amino acids that help nourish the sperm, and it forms "canals" through which healthy sperm can easily swim. Amazingly, it also provides a filter that helps stop abnormal sperm from continuing their journey. In all, your fertile cervical mucus helps healthy sperm to survive inside your body for up to seven days, maximizing the chances of conception.

Testing your cervical mucus is easy to do (see box, opposite) and, most importantly, provides advance warning that ovulation is about to occur. This is true even when your menstrual cycle is irregular. The only time mucus-testing can be misleading is if you have a yeast infection, such as thrush, or other vaginal infection, because discharge from the infection may mask the true appearance of your cervical mucus.

Once you've identified that you have fertile mucus, if you want to conceive, you need to make the most of your fertility window. Have intercourse on the first day that you feel "wet," then as soon as the mucus becomes stickier and stretchier, make love every other day (a day's break can optimize your partner's sperm count).

Basal body temperature

If your cycles appear to be regular, taking your basal body temperature every day can indicate when you've ovulated, so that in subsequent cycles you know when to have intercourse. Your basal body temperature is your temperature when you're fully at rest—and you can measure it only in the morning, *before* you get up.

Once you've ovulated, your basal body temperature will rise by a few degrees (sometimes by only tenths of a degree)—it's this rise you're looking for. (Sometimes it will dip slightly immediately before ovulation, too.) If your cycles are approximately regular, counting from the first day of your last period, you should have a temperature rise between days 14 and 16. Having intercourse every day from about day 11 to about day 16 maximizes your chances of conception.

Plot your temperature readings on a graph (put temperature up the side and days along the bottom), counting the first day of your period as day one. Bear in mind that illness, lack of sleep, alcohol, and stress can all affect your basal body temperature, so it's probably best to combine the temperature method with mucus testing to optimize your chances of conceiving.

Cervical changes

Your cervix changes quite noticeably over the course of a menstrual cycle. If you haven't yet felt your cervix, it can take a few months' practice to feel how it changes.

First, empty your bladder and then wash your hands. Insert your right index finger into your vagina until you can feel your cervix. If this is just after your period has ended, your cervix will feel like the tip of a nose and be quite low down. At this point, your cervix is closed.

As ovulation gets closer, and your body's estrogen levels rise, your cervix opens and softens, so that it feels more like a pair of lips; it will also be quite high up. This rising and opening creates a kind of funnel effect to help the passage of the sperm into the uterus.

OVULATION TESTING

Ovulation kits can provide a more measured indicator of your fertility window. They measure the LH surge (see box, p.19) that occurs about 24 to 36 hours before you ovulate. The ovulation tester is a dip stick you place in your urine stream first thing in the morning. The indicator window shows when the stick detects a surge in LH. In order not to use sticks unnecessarily, you'll need to have a good idea of your cycle (taking temperature can be helpful for this). If you suffer from PCOS (see pp.83–7), ovulation kits tend to be ineffective.

YOUR CERVICAL MUCUS

The following is the simplest method for testing your cervical mucus.

1 The next time you go to the bathroom, use some white toilet paper to blot mucus from the mouth of your vagina. Is it clear, with the slipperiness of raw egg white?

2 Pull the mucus gently with your index finger to see if it stretches. If you can, remove it from the toilet paper. (If you can't, use your finger to remove more mucus from your vagina.)

3 See if you can stretch the mucus between your thumb and index finger up to several centimetres. If you can, this mucus is fertile. If, however, the mucus is dry and crumbly or sticky and not stretchy, then it is acidic and infertile.

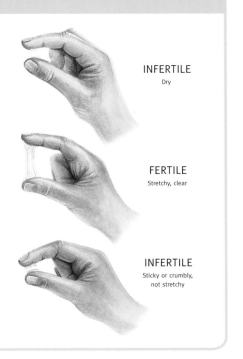

INFERTILE
Dry

FERTILE
Stretchy, clear

INFERTILE
Sticky or crumbly, not stretchy

THE ROLE OF NUTRITION

What you eat plays a crucial role in your health—a fact borne out time and again by medical research. The overriding principle is easy: The quality of what you put into your body affects the quality of you.

The food you eat is your body's fuel. This fuel is used to operate all your body's organs, whether they're intended to fire your nerve pathways, increase your circulation, or make a baby—among a host of other functions your organs perform. Your brain, heart, lungs, skin, ovaries, and every other part of you need hundreds of essential minerals and vitamins to work at optimal levels, and the better quality these nutrients are, the better-quality body systems you have.

All of us—male or female—need good food, but, for women, nutritional health can have dramatic effects on specific aspects of our physiology. We learned in the last section about how crucial hormonal balance is to your well-being. Well, what you eat can dramatically affect your endocrine system, influencing the amounts of hormone your body produces, as well as the quality of your hormones. I've discovered that nutrition provides a cornerstone treatment for almost all women's hormonal problems, including mood swings, weight problems, issues with menstruation, and infertility. In addition, a good diet can reduce your susceptibility to heart disease, osteoporosis, and arthritis—all of which can, in particular, affect women during menopause. Even without specific problems to treat, good nutrition is a must for any woman who simply wants to take care of herself, making her not only feel beautiful, but look beautiful, too (a poor diet will quickly show itself in the condition of your skin and hair).

However, with so much advice out there, it can be hard to know what exactly makes up a "balanced," healthy diet. My aim over the following pages is to simplify all the advice that's available. First, I want to show you the basics of good nutrition and help you understand what foods are made up of—the good and the bad—so you know what to look for and what to avoid. I'll talk about toxins, plant hormones, and the importance of drinking pure, clean water. And crucially, I'll give you my advice on supplementation— why I think it's important and how to make the most of the supplements you take. The ultimate aim is to provide you with all the knowledge you need to improve your diet so you can give your body all the nutrients it needs, not just to survive, but to thrive.

NUTRITIONAL MEDICINE

Food is a powerful therapy, and nutritional medicine is a system of healing based on the belief that food is medicine and that you can relieve many health conditions by making the right diet and supplement choices. Today, there's a vast amount of scientific evidence to prove the positive effects of certain foods and nutrients on preventing and treating illnesses, such as cancer. Nutritional medicine also benefits you if you don't have a specific illness but want to optimize your health.

If you follow the suggestions in this book and find that your health doesn't improve, you may want to see a nutritionist. There are a number of tests that can assess nutritional deficiencies and discover if allergies, intolerance, or other factors are at the root of any problems. A nutritionist (see p.320) can also work with you to make sure your diet is at an optimum and not aggravating your symptoms in any way.

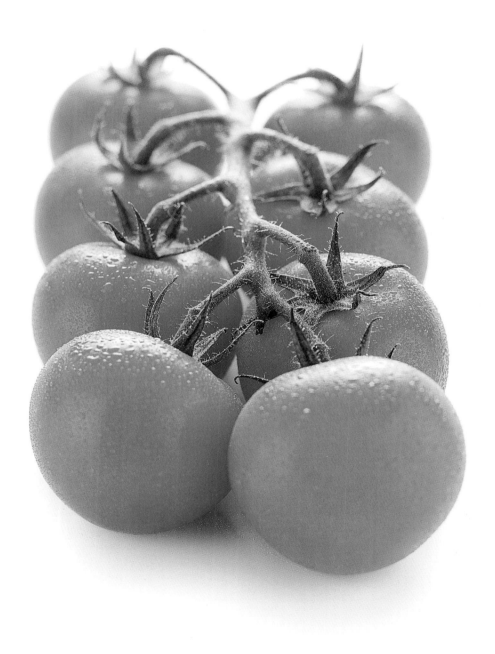

The basics of good nutrition

Look on the back of any packaged food and the list of ingredients can be mind-boggling. What are they all? Do you need them? If you do, how much do you need? And which are the ones you should avoid?

A woman's body relies upon a balanced diet for its well-being. In particular, you can achieve hormonal balance only by eating the right nutrients in the right quantities. As a basic principle, a balanced diet is made up of a combination of good-quality protein and essential fats, unrefined complex carbohydrates, and fiber, as well as plenty of vitamins and minerals. Over the following pages I'll give you a brief overview of what these are and what they do for you. Use the box opposite to guide you regarding how much of each type of food you should eat every day.

PROTEIN

Protein is one of the three most important nutrients for your body (the others are unrefined complex carbohydrates and essential fats; see below). This is because protein provides your body with amino acids. These nutrients build and repair cells in the skin, muscles, organs, and glands, and they help make hormones. There are eight amino acids we have to derive from food—these are known as essential amino acids and they're all found in "complete" proteins, such as meat, fish, poultry, eggs, milk, quinoa, and soy beans. "Incomplete proteins," found in beans, nuts and seeds, contain some, but not all, the essential amino acids.

Your diet should provide a combination of a few complete proteins and a wide variety of incomplete proteins to ensure you gain all eight essential amino acids. Equally important, though, is that all the protein you eat is of high quality—that is, unprocessed and as low in saturated fat as possible. I recommend that you don't get your protein from meat products, especially processed meats, such as sausages, as these are high in saturated fat and additives. Instead, opt for soy beans, peas, nuts, seeds, quinoa, eggs, and fish. By mixing and matching your non-meat sources of protein, you'll obtain all the essential amino acids your body needs in order to thrive at optimal levels. Dairy products also provide good-quality protein, but they can be high in saturated fat. Try to find organic (see p.30) dairy products and eat them only in moderation—for example, one small container (around 6oz.) organic yogurt or approximately 1½oz. (¼ cup) organic cheese.

Protein deficiency is rarely a problem in affluent societies—in fact, we often have too much protein. This in turn makes our systems too acidic (a healthy body should be slightly alkaline; see box, p.272). Your body corrects this imbalance by taking calcium, which neutralizes acidity, from your bones and teeth. However, using up your calcium reserves to restore alkalinity can make your bones more brittle, increasing your susceptibility to fractures and even to osteoporosis. As a general rule, the higher your protein intake, the more calcium you'll lose. Interestingly, however, this correlation applies only when the protein is derived from animal sources. Research shows that no matter how much vegetable protein you eat (such as from tofu, nuts, and seeds), you'll not deplete your calcium reserves.

CARBOHYDRATE

Your body's most important source of energy is carbohydrate. This includes both sugars and starches. One way or another, all forms of carbohydrate end up being broken down into glucose (your body's fuel), but it's the speed with which this breakdown happens that's crucial to your health.

The amount of sustained energy you derive from your food depends upon whether the carbohydrates you eat are "simple" or "complex." Simple carbohydrates include, for example, fruit and fruit juices, honey, white and brown sugar, and the glucose that's added to sports drinks. The energy effect of these foods is fast and unsustainable. Complex carbohydrates give you greater, longer-lasting energy because your body digests them more slowly. These come in the form of grains (including wheat, rye, oats, rice, and so on), beans and peas (including lentils, kidney beans, and soy beans), and vegetables. Complex carbohydrates can be refined or unrefined. A source of unrefined

carbohydrate has had no goodness stripped from it. So, for example, the grains you eat will be made up of the seed and husk, and they'll contain many essential nutrients, such as vitamins B and E and the minerals magnesium, selenium, and zinc, as well as fiber and other valuable nutrients such as flavonoids, oligosaccharides, and phytoestrogens. These have all been shown to promote good health in women. Complex carbohydrates, and in particular whole grains, are better for you because they regulate blood sugar, lower cholesterol, and balance hormones. On top of all that, whole grains encourage better digestion, helping your body assimilate more efficiently all the other nutrients in the food you eat. Good examples of whole grains include amaranth, barley, brown rice, corn, millet, oats, rye, and wholewheat. Aim for at least one serving of whole grains with each meal (see diagram, below).

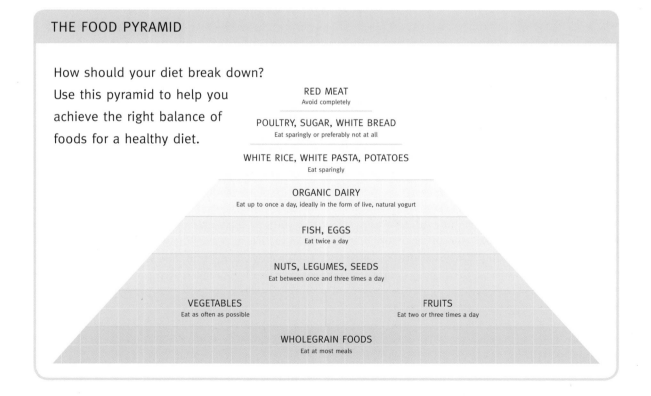

THE FOOD PYRAMID

How should your diet break down? Use this pyramid to help you achieve the right balance of foods for a healthy diet.

RED MEAT
Avoid completely

POULTRY, SUGAR, WHITE BREAD
Eat sparingly or preferably not at all

WHITE RICE, WHITE PASTA, POTATOES
Eat sparingly

ORGANIC DAIRY
Eat up to once a day, ideally in the form of live, natural yogurt

FISH, EGGS
Eat twice a day

NUTS, LEGUMES, SEEDS
Eat between once and three times a day

VEGETABLES
Eat as often as possible

FRUITS
Eat two or three times a day

WHOLEGRAIN FOODS
Eat at most meals

FATS

"Fat" tends to be a dirty word in the vocabulary of most women, and many of us, especially those of us who are watching our weight, go to great lengths to avoid eating it. However, as with carbohydrates, there are good fats and bad fats. Your body needs good fats to ensure that, among other things, your hormones work properly and your heart and skin are healthy. Broadly, bad fats are saturated fats (such as those in red meat and processed foods) and good fats are unsaturated fats, of which some are essential fatty acids (EFAs).

Saturated fats

These block your body's ability to absorb essential fats (see below), and it's known that the more saturated fat a woman eats, the higher the levels of estrogen in her blood, leading to hormone imbalance. Also, saturated fats can increase your risk of heart disease by raising your body's cholesterol level and clogging up your arteries. They also encourage your body to produce unhealthy prostaglandins that can trigger pain and swelling in your body, and contribute to period pain, endometriosis-related cramps, and the spread of endometrial tissue (see pp.118–124).

To avoid saturated fats in your diet, cut out all red meat and keep your consumption of dairy products, butter, and palm oil to a minimum. You can help counter the negative hormonal effects of the saturated fats that you do consume by taking a probiotic supplement (see box, p.33), which can help control levels of estrogen in your gut (see opposite).

I make one exception to the saturated-fat rule and that's butter. Although butter is high in saturated fat, the alternative—margarine—often contains hydrogenated vegetable oil. The process of hydrogenation makes fat more solid and easy to spread, but it also turns the harmless unsaturated fats of vegetable oil into trans fats, which are more deadly than saturated fats and have been linked to causing heart attacks. So, I recommend that instead of hydrogenated margarine, you use organic butter, but only in moderation.

Unsaturated fats

A healthy diet needs to include unsaturated fats, which come in two forms—monounsaturated and polyunsaturated. Monounsaturated fats (also known as omega-9 fats) are fatty acids that research shows lower levels of bad (LDL) cholesterol in the blood and raise good (HDL) cholesterol (see pp.286–8). Polyunsaturated fats comprise two EFAs: omega-6 and omega-3. (EFAs are those fats the body can't manufacture for itself, so we have to get them from food.)

In my clinic, I've found that most women have too much omega-6 and not enough omega-3 fats, even to the point at which they may be deficient in omega-3. Found in oily fish and certain nuts and seeds such as flax seeds, walnuts, and pumpkin seeds, omega-3 fats are important for your circulation and cardiovascular health, boosting your immunity and moisturizing your skin cells to keep them soft and supple. They also act as an anti-inflammatory to help relieve painful joints and the pain of arthritis.

Omega-6 fats, found in avocados and evening primrose and borage oil, and in nuts and seeds, can also reduce inflammation and improve the flow of blood through your circulatory system. So, if they have these good effects, how can we have too much? Unfortunately—and paradoxically—the body can convert omega-6 fats into substances that can increase blood clotting and produce yet more inflammation. These substances are called prostaglandins, and they can be "good" (derived from omega-3 fats) and "bad" (derived from omega-6 fats). The "good" prostaglandins are anti-inflammatory and anti-clotting, whereas the "bad" ones can create more inflammation and pain in the body, increasing the likelihood that you will, for example, suffer from period pains.

Sadly, the Western diet is often severely lacking in EFAs, so try to eat foods rich in them every day. Good sources include leafy green vegetables such as kale and cabbage; nuts; seeds; flax seed oil; hemp seed oil; and oily fish, such as salmon, herring, sardines, and mackerel. Fresh tuna is also a rich source of EFAs and,

CARE WITH COOKING OILS

Depending on what oils you buy and how you cook and store them, oils can change from being healthy to unhealthy. Free radicals, marauding cells that run riot through your body causing disease and premature aging, form when an oil is heated to a high temperature, if it is left in the sunlight, or if you keep reheating it. Buy only organic, cold-pressed, unrefined vegetable oils (such as extra-virgin olive oil). Always use olive oil in cooking because it's a monounsaturated oil and has less chance of creating free-radical damage. If, during cooking, the oil starts to smoke, you have a visible sign that you're damaging it, which means that it's time to turn down the heat. Once you've used a batch of oil, discard it and don't be tempted to use it again. For the safest forms of cooking, try other methods, such as steaming and baking, instead of frying.

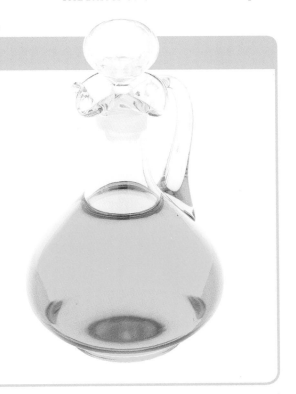

Above: Olive oil

although there are concerns about the mercury levels in some fish, I believe that the benefits of eating fresh tuna far outweigh any concerns.

Another way to make sure you're getting enough EFAs is by supplementation. However, avoid cod liver oils, which tend to be high in toxins and mercury (which the fish accumulate in their livers while in the sea) and instead buy fish-oil capsules from companies that check their fish-oil supplements for contamination. If you prefer not to take fish oil, you can get omega-3 fatty acids from flax seed oil capsules.

FIBER

Fiber ensures that your bowel movements are regular and your stools are healthy, reducing bloating and flatulence. A fiber-rich diet is also a weight-loss essential because it boosts digestion and increases feelings of fullness after a meal. However, fiber has another very important benefit for women: It helps control levels of estrogen in the body. As "old" estrogen (that is, the estrogen that your body has finished with) enters your gut, fiber helps "bind" it so that it's excreted out of the body with a bowel movement. Without that binding effect, your body reabsorbs the "old" estrogen into your circulatory system, creating a condition called "estrogen dominance"—an imbalance of too much estrogen. Breast cancer, endometriosis and fibroids are all conditions associated with high estrogen levels.

People with vegetarian diets naturally have a higher intake of vegetables than meat-eaters, with a greater fiber content. In these women, any estrogen that has done its job (so to speak) is excreted from the body, instead of being recirculated. As a result, vegetarians and those women whose diets contain only a little meat excrete 30 percent more "unwanted" estrogen than women who eat a lot of meat.

THE BENEFITS OF LEGUMES

Peas and beans (such as chickpeas) belong to a family of vegetables called legumes. They're a major source of complex carbohydrate and provide inexpensive, low-fat fiber, protein, and minerals, making them essential in any healthy-eating plan. Chickpeas support adrenal function and are rich sources of protein, EFAs, and iron. Protein- and iron-rich lentils are good for your heart and kidneys, and soy beans are a powerhouse of nutrients such as protein, EFAs, and lecithin (a brain food). In addition, soy acts as a phytoestrogen (see p.31), or "natural" source of estrogen, which is invaluable for women coming up to menopause. Try to eat legumes twice a day. Experiment with all the different types in stews and salads or on their own as a snack. Try aduki beans, black-eyed peas, mung beans, edamame beans, or kidney, lima, borlotti, or cannellini beans.

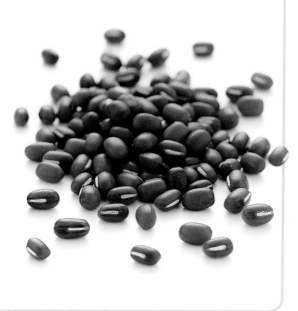

Above: Aduki beans

As with fats and carbohydrates, there are two main categories of fiber: soluble and insoluble. Soluble fiber is found inside the structure of vegetables, fruits, oats and beans. It comes in several forms, one of which is beta glucan (found in oats), a binding agent for cholesterol. The beta glucan removes cholesterol, as well as fats and carcinogens, from your food, depositing them in your stools. Insoluble fiber, found in whole grains and nuts, is the kind known as "roughage" and helps with good bowel movements. It binds with water to bulk out stools, making them easier to eliminate.

ANTIOXIDANTS

Among the most important nutrients in your diet, antioxidants protect your body against damage by free radicals—nasty substances produced by simple bodily functions, such as breathing, as well as by lifestyle factors such as smoking, fried food, pollution, and UV rays from the sun. Free radicals can wreak havoc in your body's cells, making you more vulnerable to heart disease, weight gain, cancer, and premature aging. Fortunately, you can find a wealth of protective antioxidants in foods that are rich in vitamins A, C, and E (the "ACE" foods) and beta-carotene; the minerals selenium and zinc; and the compound lycopene (most famously found in tomatoes). Excellent sources include orange, yellow, red, and purple fruits and vegetables (for example, mangoes, red grapes, eggplants, carrots, peppers, and pumpkins), leafy greens, berries, sweet potatoes, avocados, nuts, seeds, and fish.

SUGAR

For a number of good reasons, added sugar has no place in a healthy diet. It's a refined food and so does not provide any nutritional value, only unhealthy, "empty" calories. As your body quickly digests refined foods, sugar hits your bloodstream fast, causing an immediate energy boost—however, this is soon followed by an energy slump (and often a craving for something else that's sweet). In addition, the more sugar (glucose) there is in your bloodstream, the more insulin your pancreas releases to help your body use the sugar for energy. The long-term effects of the blood-sugar roller coaster can be serious. If your pancreas is constantly called upon to produce insulin to lower glucose levels, it becomes tired. As a result, the regulatory mechanisms in your body start to malfunction. One of two things can then happen. Either your pancreas can't produce enough insulin to do the job of moving glucose from your blood into your cells; or it does produce enough—or even too much—insulin, but your body has become lazy (a condition known as "insulin resistance") and can't properly use all the insulin the pancreas has produced. In either scenario, you end up with too much glucose in your blood, a condition known as hyperglycemia (high blood sugar). This is often the first step on the road to full-blown diabetes, so it's crucial to keep your blood-sugar levels balanced during the day (see box, below).

There are other problems with fluctuating blood-sugar levels, too. When the sugar isn't burned off as energy, your body stores it as fat, which contributes to excess estrogen in the body (with all the problems this brings) and weight gain.

In all, sugary foods, and sugar itself, can cause mood swings (including irritability, aggression, and even depression), reduced sex drive, night waking (often with a pounding heart), hormone imbalance, and weight problems.

HOW TO MAINTAIN BLOOD-SUGAR BALANCE

The following are my top tips on how to balance your blood-sugar levels so that your body receives a constant supply of fuel throughout the day.

- There's an important truth in the adage "breakfast like a king." Always eat a good breakfast, which sets up your energy levels for the day. However, avoid packaged cereals. Instead, make your own oatmeal using oats, which you can sweeten with a little fruit or pure fruit puree.
- Eat small, frequent meals, no more than three hours apart.

That energy dip that you may get in the mid-afternoon is a drop in your blood-sugar levels. You can avoid it if you eat little and often—but stick to slow-releasing snacks and foods to avoid a roller coaster.
- Eat unrefined complex carbohydrates, such as wholewheat bread or pasta, brown rice, millet, oats, or rye, with every meal. If you aren't sure how refined something is, consider how close it is to its natural state: the closer, the less refined. Think brown instead of white. Avoid cakes,

cookies, and pastries, all of which include highly refined white flour.
- Even fruit sugar can cause havoc in your system. Dilute juice 50/50 with filtered water.
- Avoid anything that contains stimulants, including tea, coffee, chocolate, and canned drinks that contain caffeine and high amounts of sugar. Smoking (although not a dietary stimulant) is also to be avoided.
- Take the sugar bowl off the table and avoid high-sugar foods—again, chocolate, candy, cookies, and pastries.

An organic future

Making the most of your diet isn't just about choosing foods that are rich in the right nutrients, it's also about making sure that the foods you eat are of the best quality.

In this world of increasing toxicity, the best-quality foods are organic because they expose your body to fewer man-made chemicals—many of which play havoc with your hormones—than non-organic foods.

The media constantly provides us with food "fads," but eating organic is not a fad. Only by buying and consuming organic produce can you be certain that what you eat is nutritious, free from artificial chemicals (which have been linked to cancer, hyperactivity, insomnia, birth defects, anxiety, asthma, and allergies), and grown without chemical pesticides and fertilizers, as well as without genetic modification (the notorious "GM foods").

Best of all, there's plenty of research to prove that organic food is more nutrient-rich than non-organic food. Research from Denmark and Germany shows that "Organic crops ... have a measurably higher level of vitamins, and that this can benefit people who eat them. By contrast, intensive farming is devitalizing our food." Organic produce is believed to have higher levels of nutrients because it's grown in naturally nutrient-rich soil and allowed to ripen naturally in the sun (which concentrates its nutritional content).

Whenever you can, eat local organic produce. The longer it takes for produce to get from the soil, tree, or bush to your stomach, the more nutrient-depleted it will be. Take green beans: It takes only three days for these nutrient-rich vegetables to lose 58 percent of their vitamin-C content once they've been harvested.

EATING ORGANIC is a crucial way to safeguard health.

Eating not only organic, but fresh, locally produced organic food is probably the best thing you can do for your overall nutritional health.

As well as fruits and vegetables, it's important to eat organic animal foods whenever you can. So buy organic free-range eggs to ensure they come from chickens fed a natural, chemical-free diet. Buy organic dairy products, such as yogurt and cheese, but eat these foods in moderation. Ideally you should avoid meat (organic or not) as much as you can, but if you do eat it, you should definitely choose organic so the meat is not pumped full of hormones and antibiotics, which can upset your own delicate hormone balance. If you're eating poultry, choose organic free-range. Buy wild or organic fish, which will have been fed a natural diet and is not "enhanced" with artificial chemicals (for example, farmed salmon is often colored to make the flesh pinker).

Many people don't buy organic foods because of the expense. However, even small changes can have a dramatic affect on your health. If you can't stretch to a fully organic diet, choose organic for the foods you eat most—if you eat lots of grapes, choose organic grapes; if pasta is your staple, choose organic pasta, and so on. For every fruit and vegetable that you don't buy organic, wash the foods thoroughly before eating them and, if you can, peel them. Limit your exposure to any single chemical residue by eating a wide range of non-organic fruits, vegetables, and whole grains.

Phytoestrogens

The prefix "phyto" means "plant"—phytoestrogens are estrogen-like substances found naturally in plant foods. These foods can have a significant hormone-balancing effect on a woman's body.

Phytoestrogens can help protect against breast cancer (which is often associated with too much estrogen) and reduce menopausal symptoms, such as hot flashes (which are linked to not having enough estrogen). In countries such as Japan, where women eat a soy-based diet, breast cancer rates are much lower than in other countries, and the average age of menopause is 55, compared with 51 in the West.

Phytoestrogens may contain compounds that can inhibit uterine cancer, fibroids, and osteoporosis, and they can help reduce cholesterol levels, improving your cardiovascular system and protecting your heart.

The form of phytoestrogens that has the most positive effect on hormone balance is isoflavones. In nature, isoflavones protect the plant from microbes that might cause disease. Members of the bean family (including soy beans, lentils, and chickpeas) provide the main dietary source of these important nutrients. Grains, vegetables, and seeds such as flax seeds also contain phytoestrogens, but these come in the form of lignans. Although lignans are beneficial, they don't have such a strong hormone-balancing effect as isoflavones. Try to eat one serving of isoflavone-rich food daily (about 2oz.), to give around 1½oz. isoflavones. Or, take 1 tsp. flax seeds per day.

THE SOY MYTHS

Concerns about food abound, and among the most common are those relating to levels of aluminum in soy, which have been linked to Alzheimer's disease. However, most of the negative research on soy has focused on soy protein isolates—a part of the soy plant—but not the whole soy bean and raw soy, which can affect thyroid function.

Soy protein isolates are highly refined forms of soy. An alkaline solution is used to remove the fiber from the soy bean, and the remaining soy is put into an aluminum tank with an acid wash. This removes the soy bean's carbohydrate, leaving mainly the protein part of the bean. Dried and powdered, this is then used in many different foods.

I strongly urge you to read food labels and avoid foods that contain soy isolates or genetically modified soy products. Always eat soy in its natural form, choosing products such as miso, tofu, edamame beans (fresh soy beans), and organic soy milks that are made from whole beans. Be aware that some seemingly healthy foods, such as tofu and soy milk, can be made with isolates. Check the labels of each brand until you find one that's isolate-free.

VARIETY IS KEY

Remember, also, that a healthy diet is a varied diet. Although scientists have concentrated on soy as a provider of beneficial phytoestrogens, there are also other good sources. These include all the legumes (such as lentils, chickpeas, and kidney beans), as well as garlic, celery, flax seeds, sesame seeds, sunflower seeds, grains (such as rice and oats), certain fruits, leafy green or cruciferous vegetables (such as broccoli, cabbage, and Brussels sprouts), alfalfa, mung beans, and herbs (such as sage, fennel, and parsley).

Supplements

In an ideal world, a diet rich in healthy foods would give your body all the nutrients it needs. However, modern farming and agricultural methods make that ideal virtually impossible to achieve.

Even small nutritional deficiencies in the body (called "trace" deficiencies) are enough to upset the fine balance of your body systems. For this reason, I strongly advise everyone to take supplements.

FOOD FROM SOURCE TO TABLE

Most of us do our food shopping in supermarkets, so even if we buy the right foods, it's often hard to know if those foods are fresh and nutritious. The problems begin at source. All plants extract nutrients from the soil as they grow. But this means the plants are only as good as the richness of the soil. Traditional farming methods meant that fields were periodically "rested," giving the soil time to replenish its stocks of nutrients. Overfarming means that this rarely happens, leaving fewer nutrients to feed our food. Instead of nutrients, we add pesticides. The result is soil that's not very nutrient-rich at all. Once harvested, many plants go through a stage of processing, further depleting their nutrient-content. For example, the milling process removes 80 percent of zinc from wheat (although it ensures a longer shelf life).

USING SUPPLEMENTS

In my opinion, everyone can benefit from taking supplements. Do remember, though, that they're just what the name suggests—supplements. They're never a substitute for a healthy diet, so don't imagine that you can stock up on junk food and fast food and then take supplements to counter the effects of your bad diet. Unfortunately, it doesn't work like that.

In each of the sections in parts 2 to 5, I give detailed information on how to tailor your supplement plan to your specific needs. However, as a general plan (a supplement routine to get into every day), take a good essential fatty acid (EFA) supplement, such as omega-3 fish oil containing 700mg EPA and 500mg DHA. You need only take two of these capsules per day to get the correct amount. In addition, your daily routine should include a good probiotic (see box, opposite) and a good-quality multi-vitamin and mineral supplement. When choosing a multi-vitamin and mineral supplement (a "multi"), don't be impressed by a long list of vitamins and minerals on the packaging. Yes, you want lots of nutrients, but it's the amounts of each vitamin and mineral that are the most important things to consider. Some multi-vitamin and mineral supplements look as though they contain a good combination of nutrients, but the amounts of each nutrient are so low, it's hardly worth taking the supplement at all. Compare the brands available and choose the one that has the highest levels of nutrients. The staff in specialized health-food stores will be able to advise you if you're unsure.

Apart from the nutrient levels in a multi, make sure you find one that's designed for your age and stage of life. For example, if you're trying to get pregnant, find a multi that's aimed at boosting fertility. If you're going

> SUPPLEMENTS should aid a healthy diet, not replace it.

PROBIOTICS

By increasing the growth of "healthy" bacteria (also known as flora) in your body, probiotics can boost your digestion and improve the transit time of a bowel movement through your body. This is important for hormone balance because the longer waste material stays in your body, the more likely it is that "old" hormones and also harmful toxins will be reabsorbed back into your system, potentially causing illness.

Acting as a first line of defence to prevent an overgrowth of unhealthy bacteria in your gut, which can cause illness, probiotics are also important for a robust immune system. Nutritionists especially recommend taking a probiotic supplement if you suffer from a fungal condition, such as yeast overgrowth (see pp.144–5).

Probiotics are present in foods such as yogurt with active cultures, fermented milk, and some fermented soy products, such as miso, tempeh, and tamari (wheat-free soy sauce). You can also get them as capsules and powders. In your general supplement plan (which you follow every day), take a probiotic that contains a minimum of ten billion viable organisms per capsule.

through menopause, find one that will help balance your hormones. I use a number of different supplement companies in my clinics, and I choose only the best. If you're unsure, talk to someone at a specialized health-food store or look at a good resource online to find a selection of supplements you can trust.

THE BEST SUPPLEMENTS

In order to make the most of your supplements, you need to make sure your body can absorb them as easily as possible—and this means buying supplements that are of good quality.

To give you some pointers as to what makes a good supplement, look at the form of the minerals listed on the container. If the minerals are listed as chlorides, sulphates, carbonates, or oxides (for example, magnesium oxide or calcium carbonate), your body will find these difficult to absorb. This, in turn, means that you will need higher amounts in your supplement in order to get the benefit. If, on the other hand, the minerals are in the forms of citrates, ascorbates, or polynicotinates, your body will absorb them more easily and, as a result, will get better use from them—and you'll need smaller amounts.

Take capsules instead of tablets. In order to make a tablet, companies use binders and bulking agents. Your body has to break these down (an extremely difficult job in the case of some tablets) in order to obtain the benefits of the supplement. A capsule is usually filled with only the essential nutrients—your body only has to "melt" the capsule in order to release the nutrients. I recommend that you choose vegetable capsules instead of bovine gelatin; and you can get fish-oil supplements in fish-oil gelatin.

WHEN TO TAKE SUPPLEMENTS

Generally, it's an advantage to take your supplements with food so they can be broken down with your food as you eat. Also, if you pick a meal of the day (perhaps breakfast) at which to take supplements, you're more likely to get into the habit of taking them. However, there are some supplements that should be taken away from meal- or snacktimes, so always read the label.

Essential water

Without water, your brain can't send messages to your cells, your stomach can't break down your food, and your body can't metabolize your fat reserves or detoxify properly. Water is essential to life.

Water is also essential for anti-aging: it keeps your skin supple, and it helps maintain your circulation.

WATER AND VITALITY

You are between 60 and 70 percent water. If it had to, your body could function on very minimal amounts of food, and even no food at all, for several weeks. However, deprive it of water and things could go wrong very quickly. This is because:

• Water is crucial for digestion. If you don't drink enough water between meals and snacks, the flow of your saliva slows down, making digestion less efficient. When this happens, your body is unable to absorb nutrients properly.

• Every day, your body excretes up to 2 quarts of water through your skin, urine, lungs, and gut in order to eliminate toxins—the less water you drink, the more toxins will accumulate in your body.

• Without enough water in your body, your blood volume decreases, which starves your cells of vital oxygen and nutrients, and it also means your cells can't create new tissue to repair any damage. Altogether, these effects can leave you feeling weak and tired and put you at an increased risk of illness.

I recommend you drink around six glasses of water a day. Coffee and tea (see box, opposite) and alcohol don't count towards these six glasses, as these drinks are actually dehydrating and increase your body's overall water requirements. Unhealthy drinks, such as cordials and carbonated drinks, also don't count. Only drinks that come in the form of pure water, herbal teas or diluted fruit juice can count towards your six-a-day. I like to start my day with a cup of warm water with a slice of lemon.

WHAT IS PURE WATER?

We're very lucky to have water on tap. However, the water supply piped to your home may not be as pure as you think. All the water that comes through your taps has traveled through the ground, collecting pesticides and other chemicals, and through piping that may deposit heavy metals such as lead and arsenic.

Although people often think that bottled mineral water is the healthiest option, I'm more in favor of water that's filtered from your tap. You can use either a pitcher filter or one plumbed into your sink.

Bottled mineral water that comes in a glass bottle is the next-best choice. However, take the time to read the labels on the water you buy—some contains high levels of sodium (salt), which you should avoid. Don't buy water that comes packaged in a plastic bottle. Estrogen-like chemicals in the plastic can leach in and contaminate it. Drinking this water can create a hormone imbalance in your body.

HEADACHES, FATIGUE, dizziness, poor concentration, and bloating are all symptoms of dehydration.

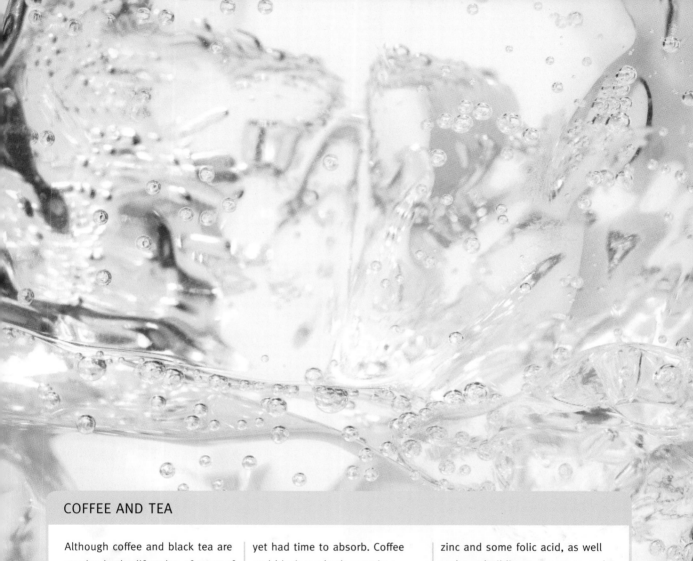

COFFEE AND TEA

Although coffee and black tea are staples in the lifestyles of most of us, neither has much of a place in the diet of a healthy woman.

Because water is so essential to your well-being, as a general rule you need to avoid anything that has a diuretic effect on your body. Diuretics increase the flow of urine (water) out of you. Along with this water, you lose essential nutrients that your body hasn't

yet had time to absorb. Coffee and black tea both contain a diuretic in the form of the stimulant caffeine. But decaf isn't necessarily any better for you. The decaffeination process uses chemicals to remove the caffeine, and coffee still contains two other stimulants (theobromine and theophylline), anyway.

Caffeinated tea can have some health benefits. It contains some

zinc and some folic acid, as well as bone-building manganese and potassium, and flavonoids, which are good antioxidants (see p.28).

I recommend you try to eliminate coffee entirely from your diet, but at worst have only one cup of organic coffee a day. Then, instead of drinking black tea, switch to green tea (the health benefits of green tea outweigh its caffeine content) or herbal tea.

THE ROLE OF LIFESTYLE

Drinking too much alcohol and smoking can damage your body, while how much exercise you get affects the health of your heart, and your fertility, weight, and mood. A good lifestyle is crucial to good health.

Your lifestyle is how you live every day—the habits that determine whether or not you optimize your health. In this section, I'm going to introduce you to the good as well as the bad choices you can make in your life. But I shall start by going right back to basics and looking at how well you sleep (which in turn affects how well you feel when you wake).

We all have a daily rhythm (known as the circadian rhythm), and by tuning into this natural rhythm, you can maximize your use of your waking hours. In other words, you can achieve more personally and profession-ally, cope better with stress, and feel more energized and positive. Then, when it comes to bedtime, you'll sleep more peacefully and restfully, resulting in a positive sleep–wake cycle. Never under-estimate the power of good sleep—without it, you sim-ply can't have a healthy lifestyle.

Of course, sleep isn't the only factor that influences whether or not you live a healthy life. We've already talked about the importance of nutrition, and it's com-mon knowledge that regular exercise has wonderful, health-promoting effects on your body's systems, keep-ing everything in optimum balance, so that you both feel and look great. Then there are the temptations life throws at us—the most common of which are your choices whether or not to smoke and how much alco-hol you drink. Few people live a life of absolute purity,

EXERCISING THREE or four times a week lowers your risk of death from coronary heart disease by 40 percent.

but it's important to understand how negative lifestyle factors can detrimentally impact your health—so that you can start to make good lifestyle choices.

Overall, the aim of this section of the book is to show you two things. First, how by understanding your body's rhythms better, you can turn bad lifestyle choices into good ones. And, second, how you can boost the good to ensure that your body is as fit and healthy as it possibly can be. Just making a few simple lifestyle changes (such as getting as little as 20 to 30 minutes exercise a day, or cutting back on your alcohol consumption) has been proven time and again not just to protect your health now, but also to reduce your risk of getting sick in the future from typical women's health problems, such as heart disease (see pp.286–91) and osteoporosis (see pp.271–7). Best of all, there are no age restrictions on the suggestions I've made—from puberty to meno-pause and beyond, you can benefit from the advice in this section.

On a personal note, suggesting how women can make adjustments to their lifestyle is one of my favorite aspects of treatment—because it's so simple and because it merely guides you back into a more natural state of living, which can have only beneficial effects on your health. It's all part of the aim to put your body back into a state of homeostasis, or perfect harmony.

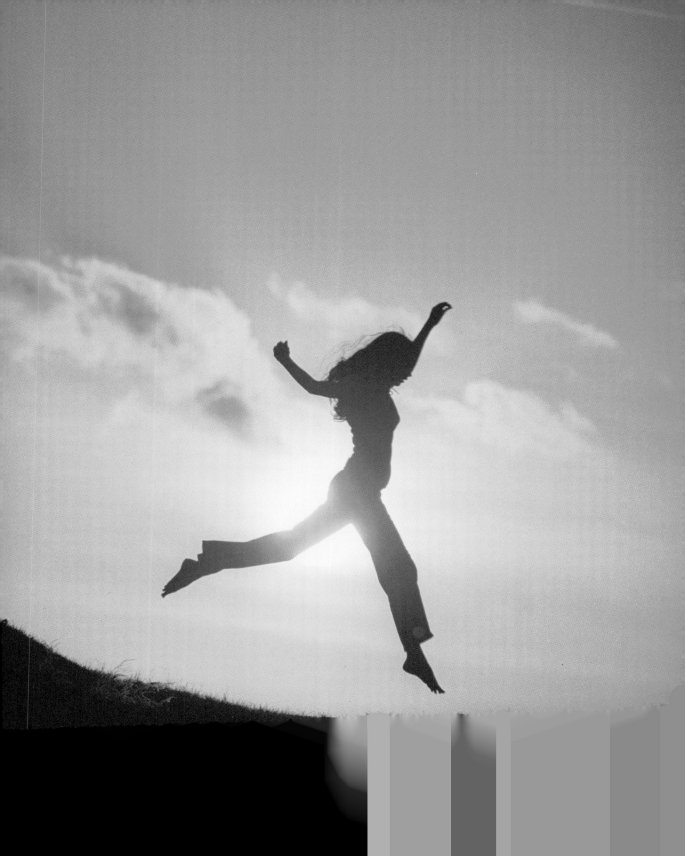

Waking and sleeping

During your waking hours, whether you're at a desk or taking care of children; or whether you're seeing friends or getting some "me time," your body is on the go. You need sleep in order to restore.

After all the busy-ness of the day, when finally you sleep, if you're like many of the women I see, you'll often sleep fitfully—your mind is busy processing the day, your body is too full of caffeine, and sometimes alcohol or nicotine, to sleep deeply. A healthy lifestyle begins with healthy waking hours and healthy sleep.

Your sleep–wake cycle is known as a circadian rhythm, and it lasts for approximately 24 hours. In some people, this rhythm is slightly faster—they will tend to wake up early and go to bed early (you may hear them called "larks"). In others the opposite is true—the rhythm is slightly slower, and they sleep late and go to bed late (they're often called "owls"). Slight variations in the 24-hour cycle aren't problematic—they're simply another indication of your individuality. Understanding your sleep–wake cycle, tuning into it, and trying to live by it as much as is practicable is the key to a healthier lifestyle—most importantly, it'll ensure you're getting the right amount of sleep to function optimally during the day (see box, opposite).

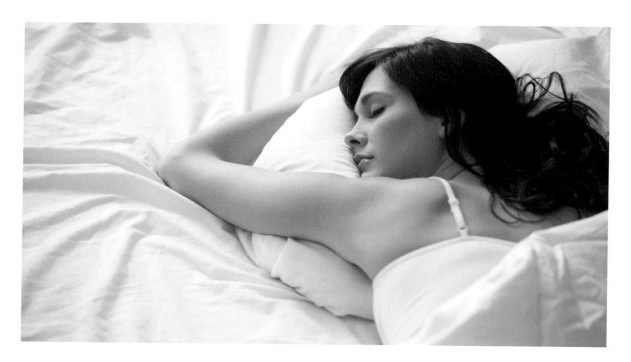

There are all sorts of ways in which modern living upsets the body's natural, daily rhythm. One of the greatest culprits is stress. Modern life is full of stressors—from little things such as traffic jams to life-changing things such as moving to a new house. While you can probably take steps to minimize stress in your life, you won't ever eradicate it. Instead, you have to give your body the chance to deal with stress effectively. I cover coping with stress later in the book (see pp.309–11). If you suffer from sleep problems, I urge you to read that section and follow its guidelines.

Try to end each day with a going-to-bed routine that enables you to "let go" of the day's stresses. This may be a simple visualization in which you imagine freeing yourself from stress; or it may be a more active metaphor for letting go—perhaps washing your face before bedtime and imagining that the stress of the day is flowing away with the water. One of my favorite ways to relax is to add a few drops of bergamot or lavender aromatherapy oils to a warm bath just before bedtime, and to soak in the bath for 20 minutes or so. A cup of chamomile tea or the herbal remedies valerian or passionflower can encourage relaxation, too.

Steer clear of caffeine in all its guises—ideally all day, but if you find this difficult, drink your cups of coffee or tea in the morning only. Nicotine and alcohol (see pp.42 and 43) are stimulants, too—and although you might think that a nightcap lulls you to sleep, it actually damages the quality of that sleep.

Although you don't have to plan your day around making sure your night is wholesome, do be aware that certain activities during the day will help improve your sleep. Regular exercise (even as little as 20 minutes a day) can have a beneficial effect. Aim simply to raise your heart rate a little and so raise your temperature (incidentally, falling temperature brings sleep more easily). Mid-afternoon is the best time to exercise, so perhaps take the stairs at work instead of the elevator, or have a brisk walk around the block. Do what you can in the time you have available.

THE RIGHT AMOUNT OF SLEEP

In 2009, Carnegie Mellon University in Pittsburgh published results of a sleep study showing that people who slept seven hours a night were three times more susceptible to a cold virus than those who got eight hours. The results confirmed the theory that how much you sleep has dramatic effects on your immunity.

Too little sleep can also result in weight gain. Chronic sleep deprivation (in which you never get a good night's sleep) can make you feel hungrier than normal and affect the way your body processes and stores carbohydrate. It may also take the enjoyment out of life and result in irritability, impatience, inability to concentrate, and loss of memory. In addition, sleep disorders have been linked to high blood pressure (hypertension), increased stress hormone levels, irregular heartbeat, and even cancer.

And there's more. Most cells of your body are renewed during sleep, so if you don't get enough you'll age faster—there really is such a thing as beauty sleep.

However, before you take to your bed, note that extended bouts of sleep aren't the answer. A number of people find that if they "sleep in" on weekends they feel groggy and can even wake up with a headache. The answer lies in going to bed earlier and rising at the same time each day. In all, aim for around eight hours of sleep a night.

Staying fit

I can't emphasize enough how important exercise is for women of any age. From improved mood to a reduced risk of diabetes, exercise has many benefits, including lots specifically related to female health.

Exercise has a positive effect on your bowels, helping them detoxify waste products efficiently, including excess hormones; and it speeds up your metabolism, helping you burn calories faster. Because exercise helps with the removal of excess hormones, it's even more important to exercise regularly if you suffer from problems caused by a hormone imbalance, such as fibroids and endometriosis. In one study of 220,000 women, all types of exercise cut the risk of breast cancer (according to another study, by 58 percent), even housework!

Exercise is absolutely essential for healthy, strong bones because placing demands on your bones, in particular through weight-bearing exercise, encourages them to maintain their density, in turn helping to reduce the risks associated with osteoporosis (see pp.271–7). We know from research that the lowest risk of hip fracture is seen in women who are active for at least 24 hours a week, although only four hours a week can have a significant effect, reducing the incidence of hip fracture by up to 44 percent. Exercise boosts circulation, optimizes blood pressure, and increases your body's levels of killer T-cells to boost immunity, too.

However, there is such as thing as too much exercise. Although exercise helps balance hormones, too much can stop women having periods at all. This is because the body needs certain levels of fat, a certain amount of energy, and not too much stress for periods to occur. If it perceives that fat and energy levels are

THE PSYCHOLOGICAL BENEFITS OF EXERCISE

The following are the psychological benefits of regular exercise, no matter what your age. They're available to all of us for as little as a few hours a week.

- EXERCISE OPTIMIZES ENERGY
  Because it improves the air-flow through your lungs, exercise increases your body's overall oxygen supply. This has the mental effect of making you feel revitalized and rejuvenated.

- EXERCISE REDUCES STRESS
  Exercise uses up adrenaline (the stress hormone) and creates endorphins (the feel-good hormones).

- EXERCISE IMPROVES ALERTNESS
  It does this by increasing the supply of oxygenated blood to your brain and boosting neurotransmitters.

- EXERCISE BOOSTS SELF-ESTEEM
  Feeling great as a result of exercising can improve body confidence, mood, and libido.

low, or that a lot of stress is being placed on the system, your body shunts you into survival mode. Periods stop because your body thinks it would be unhealthy for you to become pregnant at this time. Lack of periods can have a serious knock-on effect, increasing your risk of developing osteoporosis.

But how much exercise is too much? Well, it's hard to generalize, but most of the women I see would be fine to exercise gently for one or two hours a day— much more would be overdoing it. Above all, though, listen to your body and if you feel tired, if you're under-weight, or if your periods become erratic when they've otherwise been regular, maybe it's time to slow down.

EXERCISE FOR WEIGHT LOSS

Because it helps build calorie-burning muscles and speeds up your metabolism (which is fat-burning), exercise simply has to be an essential part of any weight-loss program. But if you want to lose weight, you need to exercise in the right way.

Studies show that the best way to lose weight with aerobic exercise is to exercise with gentle intensity for sustained periods of time. Your body can mobilize fat only in the presence of oxygen—so if you're exercising so hard you can't talk, your oxygen supplies are low and you aren't actually using fat as an energy source because the lactic acid in your system prevents this from hap-pening. So go for a jog rather than a sprint. Think about extending the time you're running rather than the rate at which you run—run more slowly but for longer. The same goes for all other kinds of aerobic exercise. Build up time, not speed, to lose more fat.

It's important to do non-aerobic exercise, too, because this strengthens and tones your muscles, and the more muscle you have, the more fat you'll burn— even when you aren't working out.

The best fat-loss exercise program combines daily 30- to 45-minute aerobic workouts, such as brisk walk-ing, light jogging, or swimming, with three or four half-hour sessions a week of weight-training or toning exercises to increase your muscle strength.

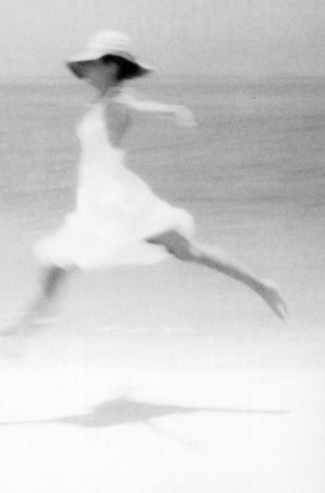

Smoking

The negative effects of nicotine on general health are well known, but it's important for women to know how smoking affects reproductive health in particular, and how they can quit successfully.

Recent studies show that a woman who smokes 20 or more cigarettes a day is likely on average to die seven years earlier than a woman who doesn't smoke. My firm belief is that the only things smoking will help you lose are your cash and your good health.

Smoking increases your risk of lung cancer and heart disease and lowers your immunity. The chemicals and toxins in cigarette smoke can dramatically lower your estrogen levels, with significant effects.

The first of these is infertility: components in cigarette smoke have been shown to interfere with the ability of cells in the ovary to make estrogen, causing a woman's eggs to be more prone to genetic abnormalities. The second is premature menopause. Smoking appears to accelerate the rate at which a woman loses her eggs, hampering reproductive function and potentially advancing menopause. The third is an increased risk of osteoporosis, and the fourth a doubled risk of developing abnormal cervical cell changes.

The final knock-on effect of smoking is the rate of miscarriage. If you smoke while you're pregnant, every time you inhale the contents of a cigarette, all the toxins pass directly into your baby's blood supply. Even if it doesn't result in miscarriage, smoking during pregnancy results in low-birth-weight babies and has been linked to several malformities in the fetus.

That's a lot of bad news—for you, your partner, and even any unborn children. But if you're a smoker there's plenty of hope. Studies show that if you stop smoking, your risks of developing smoking-related illnesses reduce with every day, week, month, and year that you're a non-smoker. Although you'll never be able to replace the eggs you may have lost through smoking, your amazing body will nourish and strengthen damaged cells in your lungs, heart, and anywhere else. The positive effects on your circulation and blood pressure begin from the moment you quit. In ten years, your risk of lung cancer will have returned to that of a non-smoker and, in 15 years, your risk of heart attack will have returned to that of a non-smoker, too.

HOW TO QUIT

What works for you will depend entirely upon the nature of your own addiction and your commitment to quitting. If you smoke to control your weight, try something weight-loss-centered like replacing the cigarette with a stick of celery. It sounds ridiculous, but celery has all sorts of valuable nutrients, including vitamins C and K, and folate (which is essential for reproductive health). It'll fill a hunger gap and has almost zero calories. Holding it and munching on it will give your hands and mouth something to do until your cigarette craving has passed. Eventually, you'll break the habit and the addiction, without gaining weight.

You may find that nicotine replacement therapy, such as patches or gum, will work for you (but remember that these still contain harmful nicotine, so you still need to deal with your addiction). However, I've seen some of the best results in smokers who try hypnotherapy. Acupuncture can be effective, too, and I'll cover this, as well as aromatherapy and homeopathy, in more detail in the following section of the book.

Alcohol and your body

Most of us know about the effects of alcohol on the liver in both men and women, but very few of the women I see have a sense of how alcohol affects other aspects of a woman's body.

Your physiology means that it takes smaller amounts of alcohol to affect you than it does a man. Also, estrogen enhances alcohol absorption, so your own hormones increase the effects of alcohol on your system.

If you suffer from any estrogen-specific problems, such as fibroids or endometriosis, eliminate alcohol from your lifestyle. Estrogen boosts alcohol absorption, but the alcohol increases the body's production of estrogen, too, creating a vicious cycle of imbalance.

According to the famous Framingham Study, which has been running for more than 50 years at Boston University, too much alcohol can increase bone loss and fractures, both of which have implications for osteoporosis. If you're trying for a baby, drinking alcohol can reduce your fertility by half—and, if you do conceive, it can increase the rate of miscarriage.

So, my advice is: If you're generally healthy, save drinking mainly for the weekends or special occasions and, when you do drink, make one or two glasses of wine or beer your limit. But if you have any known hormonal or other problems, cut out alcohol altogether. If you want to gain the benefits of the heart-boosting resveratrol in grape skins, you don't need to drink red wine—red grape juice does exactly the same job.

ALCOHOL AND YOUR LIVER

Lying on the right hand side of the body, the liver cleans your system of toxins, waste products and excess, and "old" hormones.

But this isn't all your clever liver does. It also helps optimize the function of your thyroid, secretes bile, and helps manage weight through its ability to break down fat and metabolize carbohydrates from your food. It makes little sense, then, to overindulge in anything that might cause your liver damage.

Alcohol is a "hepatoxin"—a toxin to your liver. The liver produces enzymes to break down alcohol into other substances that your body excretes through your urine and lungs. But some of these substances can be more toxic than the alcohol itself. In addition, free radicals, which are produced naturally as the liver breaks down alcohol, may also damage liver cells.

To boost your liver health, eat plenty of B-vitamins (found, for example, in sweet potatoes, bananas, and lentils), which help the liver process excess hormones, and take milk thistle (*Silybum marianum*), an herb that helps the liver regenerate. Take a tincture (1 tsp., twice daily) or a supplement (200–400mg, daily).

THE ROLE OF NATURAL THERAPIES

In conventional (allopathic) medicine, the tradition has been to treat the symptoms of a disease, or to cure the "piece" of you that isn't functioning properly. Natural therapies take a more holistic view.

Many natural therapies are based on the idea that illness happens when the body's systems are out of balance; natural therapies aim to restore that balance.

All my advice for specific health problems is designed to balance your body (create a state of homeostasis), so that every system works at the optimum level. I want to encourage you to help yourself and to enhance your body's innate process of self-healing. My aim is to give you the tools to create a tailor-made program that fits your particular needs.

To that end, many of the practices introduced in this section have an element of self-help about them. You can learn yoga, meditation, and some aspects of aromatherapy, reflexology, and massage at home and practice them on yourself. However, one rule for self-practice is to always follow my guidelines and remember that although the processes may be natural, they're acting on your body in potent ways. Listen to your body at all times and seek help from a registered practitioner if you're ever unsure about what you're doing.

When you visit a natural therapist—as you will have to for acupuncture and osteopathy—your treatment will be tailored specifically to you and is likely to vary from woman to woman. Many women also find that one particular therapy works better for them than others, or that a combination of different natural therapies, such as massage combined with aromatherapy, or meditation combined with homeopathy, can enhance the healing process to the best effect. It's important to find both what you enjoy and what works optimally for you. The natural therapy experience can be hugely reassuring for many women because it recognizes that someone who's in poor health needs more than a quick-fix cure. A practitioner should take plenty of time to uncover the causes of imbalances in your body and to plan your treatment. He or she works like a detective, fitting together the symptoms and other clues, such as lifestyle and diet, to help you find the areas of your life that could be affecting your health.

INDIVIDUAL CARE

If you do decide to try a natural therapy, whether or not it succeeds or fails will depend largely on your commitment to it. For example, if you decide to take an herbal remedy, it won't be able to heal your body unless you combine it with positive diet and lifestyle changes that protect your current and future health. I frequently recommend natural therapies, but I always recommend them alongside a healthy diet and lifestyle. In addition, don't expect improvements overnight. You're retraining your body to heal itself, and this may take time.

The recommendations offered in this book are known to help with particular health problems. However, you may well find that you need to modify your treatment plan a little to make sure you address your specific symptoms. If this is the case, I strongly advise you to see a qualified practitioner in the relevant field for more individual help.

NATURAL THERAPIES help your body to heal itself.

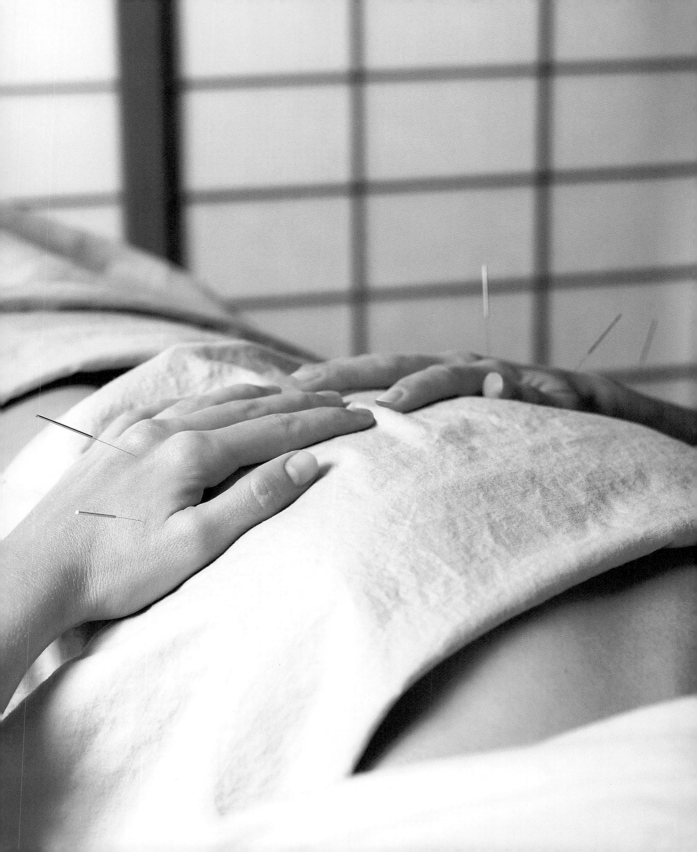

Herbs and homeopathy

For centuries, nature has provided us with medicines. In the case of herbs, the remedy comes directly from the plant, while homeopathy captures the energy of the natural substance in digestible form.

HERBS

Today, up to 70 percent of pharmaceutical drugs originate from herbs. When you use an herb for healing, you benefit not only from its active healing agents but from its modifying agents, too. The herb modifies its own actions and reactions, often eradicating side-effects. If you take only the active ingredient in pharmaceutical form, you may have to take another medicine in order to overcome the side-effects of the drug.

When you buy herbal remedies, you may see the phrase "standardized extract" on the labels. This process usually standardizes the herb to only one ingredient, so my advice is to avoid standardized remedies and instead use only those that make no mention of standardized extracts at all, having a label saying "whole herb," or mentioning only the name of the herb itself.

HOW TO TAKE HERBAL REMEDIES

Take remedies made from organic herbs and in tincture form, where possible. Place a small amount of the tincture (usually 1 tsp.) in a little water and drink it. The next-best choice is whole organic herbs in vegetarian capsules. Always read the label of any herbal remedy before you take it; if you're in any doubt, consult a qualified practitioner. Many herbs are not suitable during pregnancy or breastfeeding.

HOMEOPATHY

The guiding principle of homeopathy is that "like cures like." Minute doses of substances that, in a healthy person, would produce effects similar to those occurring in the disease, in a sick person stimulate the body's own healing powers, effecting a remedy.

Homeopathic remedies are made by a process called succussion. The active substance, which is often taken from plants but can come from any organic matter, is diluted tens or hundreds of times and violently shaken to leave its energetic imprint on the liquid. A remedy with a potency of 6c has been diluted six hundred times; of 6x, sixty times, and so on. The more dilute the remedy, the stronger its action. Many scientists believe that homeopathy works by placebo effect, saying that the "cure" is the result of positive thinking. This doesn't explain the positive effects of homeopathy on animals.

On the other hand, many scientific studies show that homeopathy can help treat hormone imbalance, fibroids, endometriosis, irregular periods, and unexplained infertility, among other problems. My experience tells me that homeopathy is a highly effective treatment for many women's conditions, especially when administered correctly according to advice from a registered homeopath. He or she can provide treatment geared to your constitution and symptoms after taking a detailed history of every aspect of your health, from how you sleep to your bowel movements.

Homeopathic remedies are harmless, non-addictive and suitable for women of all ages and at all stages of life, including pregnancy.

Acupuncture

Widely practiced as part of Traditional Chinese Medicine (TCM), acupuncture is a practitioner-led therapy that works to free up a vital force, called *qi,* in the body.

Qi (also spelled *chi*) regulates your spiritual, emotional, mental, and physical balance as it flows through your body along channels called meridians. When your *qi* gets blocked, imbalances and disharmony are said to occur, leading to poor health or even disease.

According to TCM, there are more than 2,000 acupuncture points (sometimes abbreviated to acupoints) on the human body, each of which stimulates one or more of the meridians. Inserting an acupuncture needle into these points stimulates the flow of *qi* along the relevant meridians, aiming to unblock and balance energy-flow and so restore good health.

Many women who come into my clinic are put off acupuncture because it uses needles. Typically, an acupuncturist will insert needles that are 1/10 to 2/5in. deep, although occasionally deeper. The needles are very fine, and the insertion is quite painless—the process is not at all like having an ordinary injection or a blood test.

The World Health Organization calls acupuncture "a clinical procedure of considerable value" and lists it as appropriate for many genito-urinary and reproductive problems, including infertility, premenstrual syndrome (PMS), irregular periods, and (in men) impotence. Scientific trials have shown it to be effective for women's hormone disorders, infrequent periods, and lack of ovulation. I, too, have found that acupuncture is particularly beneficial for women's health problems and that it works extremely well alongside nutritional medicine. It's also a therapy that you can use safely at all times—including during pregnancy—when you are in the expert hands of a qualified practitioner.

ACUPUNCTURE originated in China more than 2,000 years ago.

VISITING A PRACTITIONER

On your first visit, a good practitioner (who should have had at least three years of training) will spend quite a long time asking you about your medical history and your habits, likes, and dislikes. He or she may also look at your tongue and take your pulse. Only once the practitioner has a full picture of your history, your unique symptoms, and your constitution, will he or she recommend a course of treatment. This will be individually geared to you, and may last anything from four weeks to three months.

If you decide to go ahead with the treatment, you might find that the original symptoms of the disease worsen for a few days, or that you experience side-effects (often including changes in appetite or irregular sleep, bowel, or urination patterns). These adverse effects will soon pass, and merely indicate that the treatment is working, so do bear with it. Many women find acupuncture sessions deeply relaxing. It's common to experience mild disorientation immediately following a treatment, so make sure you have someone to drive you home and arrange to take the rest of the day off work, if need be.

Aromatherapy and massage

Smell and touch are two of our most potent senses and have been used to beneficial healing effect for hundreds of years. Aromatherapy and massage can work on both physical and emotional levels.

AROMATHERAPY

Every plant has a fragrance locked within its essential oil, which may come from its flowers, leaves, twigs, stems, or bark. By extracting the essential oil, usually through a process of steam distillation, we can capture this fragrance to use it therapeutically.

Smelling an essential oil triggers nerve pathways from the nose to the brain to bring about certain effects on the mind and body. By burning an essential oil in an oil burner, or by simply adding a few drops of oil to a tissue to periodically inhale, certain essential oils can lift mood, ease anxiety, and even relieve depression. Aromatherapy is particularly useful to treat PMS, to help improve mood, and regulate hormones.

When essential oils are used in massage or added to bath water, you benefit not only from their scent but also by absorbing them through your skin into your bloodstream. The oils can have beneficial effects on your body's organs, tissues, and glands. For example, try lavender for cellulite and marigold (calendula) for varicose veins; and try sandalwood if you're suffering from cystitis. Period pains may respond to rosemary, and a lack of periods to rose. If you're going through menopause, Roman chamomile and clary sage can help relieve hot flashes and night sweats.

HEALING TOUCH

Massage is a bodywork technique that uses stroking, kneading, and pressing to work on the body's muscles, ligaments, and tendons. It can be extremely beneficial for relaxing muscles and can help lift the mood.

The gentle manipulation techniques used in massage help keep your lymphatic and circulatory systems flowing freely. Efficient circulation is essential for good health, nourishing all your cells; while your lymph is an essential part of your immunity, helping to flush toxins and waste from your body.

I think one of the most amazing things about massage is how it highlights the interconnectedness of

HOW TO USE ESSENTIAL OILS

With the exception of tea tree oil and lavender oil, essential oils must be diluted in a carrier oil, such as sweet almond, before coming into direct contact with your skin. As a general rule, use a maximum of 15 drops of essential oil (or combination of essential oils) per 30ml (6 tsp.) of carrier oil. However, some essential oils are more potent than others and will need to be more dilute before you apply them, so always check the labels. You can use drops of essential oil directly in the bath, without a carrier oil. For a basic, relaxing body massage, use a blend such as lavender, neroli, and rose oil in a carrier oil. Pregnancy is an exceptional time for your body: Check with an aromatherapist before using any essential oils when you're pregnant.

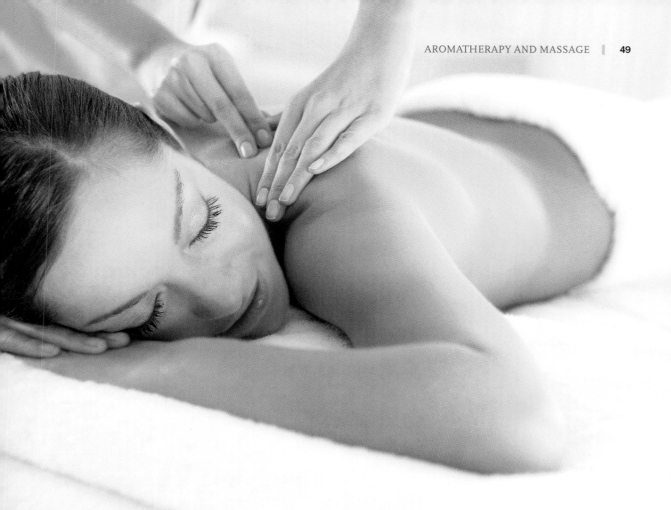

the body. Everything about us is connected—by energy channels, our circulation, and a staggeringly complex nervous system—so that stimulating one part with massage can "refer" the therapeutic benefits to a completely different area. For example, massage therapists will often massage the legs in order to ease back pain—and vice versa.

Having a massage

Although some forms of massage can be painful (for example, when the practitioner kneads very tight muscles), most massage is entirely painless and may be relaxing or stimulating, depending on which massage technique you use. In the therapeutic sections of the book, I've included lots of beneficial self-massage to help you manage your conditions at home. However, nothing can really beat a professional massage, which will target specific areas of your body to ease aches, pains, and health problems according to your needs.

If you have a professional massage, talk through what you're comfortable with—if you're nervous about having a full-body massage the first time round, break yourself in gently and go for a head massage or one for the head, neck, and shoulders. Everyone reacts differently to massage, and you may come away feeling energized or slightly tired (and either response may last through the following day). These reactions are perfectly normal, but listen to your body and don't plan anything too strenuous for immediately after a massage. Most of all enjoy it and feel pampered!

Yoga and meditation

Yoga originated in India at least 7,000 years ago. A system of training for body, mind, and spirit, it aims to stimulate and balance the flow of life-force energy, known as *prana*, around the "subtle" body.

YOGA

The Sanskrit word *yoga* means "to join or merge," and the practice of yoga aims to create balance between body, mind, and spirit. To achieve this, yoga teaches sequences of postures (*asanas*), as well as breathing, relaxation, and meditation techniques. Practiced regularly, yoga can increase flexibility and circulation, relieve stress, and encourage peace of mind.

According to the international research organization the Yoga Biomedical Trust, evidence shows that yoga helps overcome infertility and menstrual problems, possibly by a combination of increasing blood flow to the reproductive organs and relieving stress, which can help balance female hormones. It's also thought to improve blood flow generally to the organs of the body and to be good for the heart. Several studies show that yoga can help balance hormones, relieve digestive disorders, and improve posture, strength, endurance, energy, immunity, sleep, and breathing. It's no wonder that the practice is still gaining in popularity, thousands of years after its conception.

Practicing yoga

The most wonderful thing about yoga is that no matter what your age or lifestyle, there's a type to suit you. Visit your local yoga center and experiment until you find your perfect style. For example, if you're new to yoga or recovering from an illness, it may be best to try a gentle style, such as Sivananda yoga (which often includes a resting pose after each *asana*); or if you prefer something more dynamic, you might choose ashtanga yoga. Whichever style you go for, it's often a good idea to have some guidance from a teacher at the beginning because he or she will show you how to hold the postures correctly and perhaps even tailor a program to your ability and level of fitness. Once you've mastered the basics, yoga is easy to practice by yourself, so I've included several simple but effective postures throughout the book for you to do at home.

One very important part of yoga practice, and available to us all, is *pranayama*—or breathing exercises. This is a sort of science of breath control. Practitioners believe that different methods of breathing affect the body by influencing the flow of *prana*. *Pranayama* also helps yoga practitioners prepare for another important aspect of yoga practice—meditation.

DISCOVERING MEDITATION

The term meditation refers to a number of techniques intended to focus or control the mind so you can find a state of inner contentment—similar to the kind of feeling you get when you're totally absorbed in what you're doing and have lost track of time. Although its roots lie in yoga and esoteric religions, and to some people meditation might seem "alternative" or somehow intangible, in actual fact there are traditions of meditation in almost all cultures across the globe, and it can be a powerful tool for people from all walks of life.

YOGA HELPS balance the female hormones.

Many people who practice meditation regularly say it eases stress and encourages relaxation and feelings of calmness and positivity. It also helps reduce blood pressure and improve circulation. One study in 2003 found that meditation could boost parts of the brain and enhance the immune system. Other research shows that it can ease a host of stress-related problems, including chronic pain, headaches, anxiety, PMS, sleep disorders—and even infertility because the stress of infertility can interfere with the release of the hormones that regulate ovulation.

Tips for successful meditation

Among the best meditation practices are simply to focus on your breathing (see box, below) or to relax every part of your body in turn. Alternatively, you might decide to turn your attention to a certain word or phrase that you keep in your mind's eye—it could be "peace" or "calm"—or you might hold an image of a serene or happy place in your mind to focus upon. You could have an actual visual focus—a candle flame, a flower, or a mandala (a geometric diagram, used in Buddhism). The point is to focus your attention, let go of stressful thoughts, and find a state of inner peace.

The best time to meditate is first thing in the morning or just before you go to bed at night, and at least two hours after a meal. If you're new to meditation, start by practicing in short, regular sessions—say ten to 20 minutes a day—which you build up gradually, until you're able to meditate, without losing your focus, for approximately an hour. Try to differentiate your meditation time by going to a particular room, or perhaps by simply imagining that you're inside a bubble that blocks out all distraction. You might even decide that you need to go to a meditation class at first. The important thing is to switch your mind into a different state from the busy, frantic state of the normal day. Sit in a comfortable position that will enable you to keep still (don't lie down as you might fall asleep) and keep your spine straight.

A SIMPLE MEDITATION ON THE BREATH

If you're new to meditation—or even if you aren't!—use this exercise to get you started. Try to practice it for five minutes, twice a day, every day. When you feel confident, extend the sessions by five minutes every other day until you are doing around 20 minutes twice a day. You can make the meditation more personal, too—rather than your breath, choose a word or a phrase as your focus, or a positive image that you hold in your mind's eye.

1 Find a quiet place where you know you won't be distracted, and turn off your phones. Sit on the floor, or use a chair if it's more comfortable (but keep your feet flat on the floor). Close your eyes.

2 Gently and slowly begin to take deep breaths. Breathe in through your nose for a slow count of three and out through your mouth for a slow count of three. Continue to do this until the long, slow breaths feel completely natural and rhythmical.

3 Now concentrate on the flow of air past your nostrils as you breathe in and against your lips as you breathe out. As thoughts come into your mind, don't ignore them—instead, simply observe them and then let them go. This may seem hard at first, but the technique will get easier with practice.

Reflexology

An energy-based practice, reflexology involves stimulating, massaging, and holding points on the feet (and sometimes hands) to stimulate energy flow through the body and promote self-healing.

Reflexologists believe the body is divided into ten vertical zones or channels, five on the left and five on the right. Each zone runs from the head to the reflex areas on the hands and feet. By applying pressure to the reflex points, you can stimulate energy flow through the corresponding body part and release an energy blockage in any part of the zone. For example, stimulating a reflex point on the foot that corresponds to the ovaries may release blocked vital energy in the pituitary gland. The more energy pathways that you open up, the more efficiently the body works and the greater the chance for restoring harmony, or homeostasis, to every body system.

HAVING A REFLEXOLOGY MASSAGE

Like many other natural health practices, reflexology is easy to practice yourself at home but is best from a practitioner, who can treat your unique symptoms. The treatment itself will typically involve working all the areas on the right foot and then all the areas on the left. After a treatment, you may experience sweating, diarrhea, and increased urination for a few days. These are good signs that your body's elimination systems are flushing out toxins. You may also feel temporarily lethargic or tearful. A few people may experience cold-like symptoms, flatulence, a skin rash, or increased energy—all part of the natural healing process.

THE REFLEXOLOGY POINTS OF THE FEET

This diagram shows the reflex points of the feet. During a reflexology massage, you or a practitioner will stimulate the area corresponding to your area of weakness or ill health. This helps release the energy blockage (which could be elsewhere in the body) that is causing the imbalance, thus encouraging your body to self-heal.

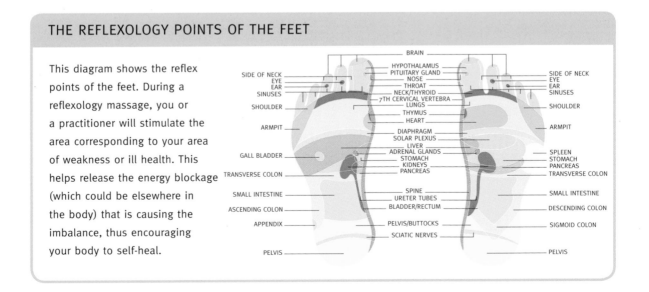

Osteopathy

Originating in the 19th century in the USA, osteopathy is a natural therapy in which a practitioner manipulates the musculo-skeletal system in order to treat imbalance in the body and disease.

A common misconception about osteopathy is that it treats diseases that are bone-related. Despite its name (*osteo* meaning "bones"), osteopathy is a system of whole-person well-being.

According to the principles of osteopathy, any misalignment of your spine and skeleton can impair the circulation of blood and lymph around your body and cause your organs to function less efficiently. If a practitioner can correct these misalignments, blood can flow smoothly to your organs, your nervous system can send messages effectively, your lymphatic system can keep your immune system functioning properly (allowing toxins to be eliminated safely and efficiently), digestion and respiration can improve, pain and discomfort can abate, and a state of balance (homeostasis) can return throughout your entire body. Tense muscles are thought to be particularly damaging to the health of your body because when muscles contract they impede the flow of blood and lymph.

VISITING AN OSTEOPATH

When you visit an osteopath, he or she will be trained to "feel" problems or disruptions in your muscles, bones, and ligaments. As with many other natural therapies, you'll be asked for your medical history and will need to talk about your lifestyle habits. This is so the osteopath can gain a full sense of your well-being. He or she may ask you to move in certain ways in order to gain a sense of where problems in your musculo-skeletal system might lie. The osteopath then uses a range of techniques, including manipulation, massage, and stretching, to improve the flexibility and range of movement in your joints. He or she will apply greater pressure to joints that are misaligned. This will set blood and lymph flowing freely, and so restore harmony throughout your nervous and musculo-skeletal systems, as well as through all your body's organs.

As well as stress-related disorders, asthma, ear infections, and swelling, pain and inflammation in the joints, osteopaths successfully treat "female" conditions, such as hormonal imbalances, period pain, menstrual irregularities, some types of infertility, and a number of pregnancy and birth-related health conditions. Osteopathy is suitable for all ages and stages of life, and it's not usually necessary to consult your doctor before embarking on a course of osteopathic treatment.

There's also a subtle form of osteopathic treatment called cranial osteopathy. This is suitable for all ages but has been found to be particularly helpful for babies, children, and pregnant women. Cranial osteopathy aims to release tensions and stresses in the body by picking up very slight muscular disruptions and movements—these are known as the Cranial Rhythm. By using gentle techniques to restore the normal Cranial Rhythm, the practitioner can help your body get back into balance and good health.

OSTEOPATHS use touch to manipulate the body and restore balance.

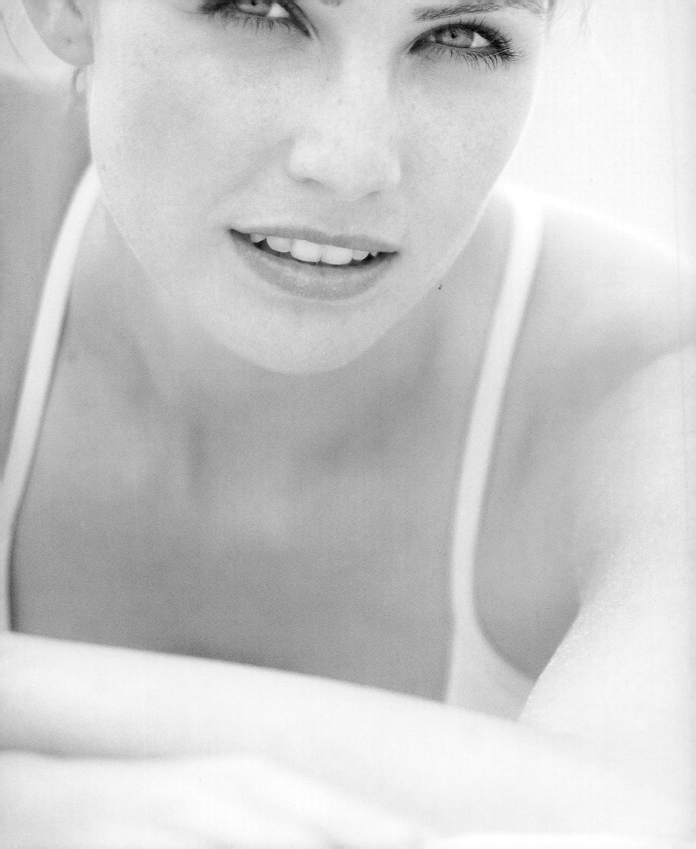

General body systems 2

As you already know, your body is a complex, intricate machine. Keeping it healthy requires a delicate balance of the right nutrition, the right lifestyle, and the right healthcare. However, from time to time, things do go wrong.

In this chapter, I'm going to look at each of the main female organs and the most common problems you may encounter with them as you pass the various milestones in your life. The thyroid, breasts, all the reproductive organs, and even the legs are tackled here. I cover such topics as an overactive or underactive thyroid, breast pain, ovarian cysts, all aspects of the menstrual cycle (including period pain, fibroids, and endometriosis), cervical tests, cystitis, and varicose veins—to name a few. This chapter provides the heart of your natural health bible, the core that will enable you to take care of yourself in the most sensitive and effective ways available— both at home and under the guidance of conventional healthcare professionals.

THYROID, ADRENALS, AND HORMONAL BALANCE

All the hormones in your body are secreted by the glands of your endocrine system (see p.17). Two of the most significant endocrine glands are the thyroid and the adrenals.

As we've already seen, many women's health concerns find their roots in hormonal imbalance. Problems such as osteoporosis, menstrual issues, PMS, menopausal symptoms, weight gain, blood-sugar imbalances, mood swings, and breast discomfort can all stem from some kind of dysfunction in your hormone system. Often, this dysfunction begins in your thyroid and adrenal glands, which produce and regulate your hormones. One positive thing you can do to optimize the health of these glands is to follow a hormone-balancing diet (see box, opposite). You'll find that throughout this book, and most importantly in this section, references to my hormone-balancing diet appear again and again. This is because I believe it's the fundamental key to success in your quest to find hormonal balance in your body, and as a result to overcoming many of the "women's" problems you might face.

WHERE ARE YOUR THYROID AND ADRENAL GLANDS?

Your thyroid gland lies at the front of your neck. It's a large butterfly-shaped gland that secretes thyroxine. This hormone has a powerful influence on nearly every tissue in your body because it regulates your metabolism (the speed at which you burn food to make energy).

> BALANCE IS KEY for your hormonal health, and natural therapies can help you achieve it.

The thyroid gland itself is controlled and regulated by your hypothalamus and your pituitary gland, both located in your brain.

You have two adrenal glands, one lying at the top of each kidney. Each adrenal gland consists of a medulla (the center of the gland) surrounded by a cortex. In all, the cortex makes up about 80 percent of the gland. Your adrenals make adrenaline (the so-called "stress hormone") and noradrenaline, as well as steroid hormones that influence the effectiveness of your immune system.

FEMALE SUSCEPTIBILITY

Over the following pages, you'll find information on how to overcome an over- or underactive thyroid and how to treat adrenal problems. Although these conditions can affect men, too, they tend to be more common in women. Statistics vary, but generally women are thought to be between five and eight times more likely to suffer from a thyroid problem than men (see p.62). A woman's risk of developing thyroid problems increases with age and family history. Views differ as to why adrenal problems tend to be more common in women. Some experts put this down simply to the fact that more women are likely to come forward with adrenal fatigue, while others believe it's to do with women's susceptibility to imbalances in estrogen.

THE HORMONE-BALANCING DIET

A healthy diet naturally balances your hormones. This is my hormone-balancing diet, which is your key to overcoming any kind of hormone-related problem.

- Make sure you eat at least five servings of fruit and vegetables a day—with the emphasis on more vegetables than fruit. In particular, increase your intake of cruciferous vegetables, such as broccoli, Brussels sprouts, cabbage, and cauliflower, because they are high in indole-3-carbinols, which help prevent your body from absorbing toxic forms of estrogen (see p.18).

- Have at least three helpings of phytoestrogens (see p.31) each day. Opt for legumes such as soy, chickpeas, lentils, and so on, and flax seeds. Phytoestrogens reduce the toxic estrogens in your body and stimulate your liver to produce sex-hormone-binding globulin (SHBG; see p.78), which controls how much estrogen and testosterone circulates in your blood.

- Eat whole grains. Change from white rice to brown rice, white bread to wholegrain bread and opt for other whole grains, such as oats, rye, and so on.

- Up your fiber intake. The fiber naturally contained in whole grains, fruits, and vegetables helps prevent your body from absorbing estrogenic chemicals (such as from plastics and pesticides) and encourages the swift elimination of toxins and old hormones out of your bowels.

- Keep up the "good" fats. Eat a portion of oil-rich foods, including oily fish, nuts, seeds, and cold-pressed vegetable oils, every day. They help balance your hormones by encouraging your cells to respond to hormonal triggers more effectively.

- Reduce the "bad" fats—that is, saturated fats, found in animal foods such as red meat, dairy, and so on because they are more likely to contain xenoestrogens, and they block your body's ability to absorb essential fatty acids ("good" fats). Foods high in saturated fat also encourage the body to produce "bad" prostaglandins, hormone-like substances that cause imbalance.

- Eliminate sugar from your diet as much as possible. Sugar encourages weight (fat) gain, and fat cells manufacture estrogen, creating an estrogen overload in your body.

- Drink plenty of healthy fluids—six to eight glasses a day—to help flush "old" hormones from your body. Make sure the water you drink is mineral water or filtered, as the chlorine and fluoride in tap water can block iodine receptors in the thyroid gland, causing hormonal imbalance.

- Cut out "bad" fluids. Reduce your caffeine intake and also how much alcohol you drink. Alcohol places an extra toil on your liver, making it harder for your body to eliminate "old," toxic hormones circulating in your system.

- Choose organic food as much as your budget allows because it helps reduce your exposure to harmful xenoestrogens and other toxins.

- Read food labels and try to avoid foods containing preservatives, additives, and artificial sweeteners. To keep your hormones in balance your food needs to be as natural as possible.

Underactive thyroid

Your body burns food rather like a car burns fuel. Just as the accelerator regulates how much fuel gets to the engine of the car, so your thyroid regulates how quickly your body uses food.

Because of its function as a fuel regulator, your thyroid gland is responsible for maintaining your energy levels and regulating your weight. It performs these functions by secreting the hormones thyroxine (also called T4) and triidothyronine (also called T3). These are the hormones that tell your body how fast to burn calories. Most T3 is converted from T4 (itself an inactive hormone), and the production of both T3 and T4 is regulated by another hormone called TSH (thyroid-stimulating hormone or thyrotrophin), which is made in the pituitary gland in the brain (see box, p.17).

With the right amount of thyroid hormones, your body burns fuel at the optimum rate, and you'll have plenty of energy. You'll also have a constant body temperature and a regular heart rate and menstrual cycle. When you have too little T4 in your blood, your thyroid gland is said to be underactive—a condition known as hypothyroidism. This can happen as a result of an auto-immune disorder, a congenital abnormality in the thyroid gland (present at birth), or a nutritional iodine deficiency (the body needs iodine to manufacture thyroid hormones). Alternatively, if your pituitary under-produces TSH, your thyroid isn't stimulated to create T4, and this can be another cause. Left untreated, hypothyroidism puts you at risk of diabetes, high blood pressure, emphysema, arthritis, depression, migraine, and carpal tunnel syndrome (a condition in which you experience pain, tingling, or numbness in the wrist). Answer the questions in the box (right) and I urge you to see your doctor immediately if you suspect that an underactive thyroid may be affecting you.

HYPOTHYROIDISM CHECKLIST

A poor diet, stress, inactivity, smoking, antibody attack (see p.62), and certain drugs can all influence the functioning of your thyroid. There are certain symptoms that may indicate an underactive thyroid condition when they appear together. If four or more of the following apply to you, visit your doctor right away.

- [ ] Have you put on weight despite keeping to your eating and exercise patterns?
- [ ] Do you often feel cold, even when the weather is warm?
- [ ] Do you suffer from constipation?
- [ ] Is your mood low?
- [ ] Do you suffer from irregular periods?
- [ ] Is your hair thinner and drier than before?
- [ ] Do you suffer from fatigue?
- [ ] Does your skin feel much drier than usual?

DIAGNOSIS

Blood test If you ticked the boxes in at least four of the questions in the checklist (opposite), you should ask your doctor to test you for an underactive thyroid. Normal levels of TSH and T4 in your blood indicate your thyroid is working properly. If your results are borderline normal (only just within the normal range), your doctor will take into account your symptoms when deciding whether or not you should be treated for an underactive thyroid.

Basal body temperature If your blood test comes back normal but you continue to have all the symptoms of an underactive thyroid, I would suggest you take your temperature over the course of three days. This is because if the problem doesn't lie with your thyroid itself but with the cells in your body that are supposed to latch on to your thyroid hormones, you don't have a full-blown thyroid problem. However, you may have a slow metabolism, which can show up as a low body temperature.

For accurate measurements, use an electronic thermometer. During your menstrual cycle, your temperature rises after ovulation, which will affect your reading. Take your temperature on the second, third, and fourth days of your menstrual cycle to avoid this anomaly. On the first day, note the reading for that day, even before you get up. This is your basal body temperature, which is your body temperature when you're resting. Over the following two mornings, take your basal body temperature in exactly the same way, first thing in the morning. If you find that your average basal body temperature is below 97.6°F, your thyroid could be sluggish. (If your temperature is much lower than this, ask your doctor to repeat your blood test, as this suggests your thyroid is underactive.)

CONVENTIONAL TREATMENTS

If a blood test reveals an underactive thyroid, your doctor is likely to offer you the standard treatment for hypothyroidism, which is the drug thyroxine. It may take a few months for your doctor to establish the correct dosage—he or she will test and, around three months later, retest for hormone levels in your blood until the balance is right. After that, you'll be asked to repeat the blood test at regular intervals (usually six monthly to a year) to make sure that the dosage doesn't need to alter in any way.

If your doctor does prescribe thyroxine, be sure to avoid taking iron supplements, and any vitamin and mineral supplements containing iron, at the same time of day that you take the thyroxine. This is because iron seems to bind to the thyroxine so that the body can't use it. Natural sources of iron don't trigger problems with thyroxine medication, so you can still keep eating plenty of iron-rich foods, such as leafy green vegetables and dried fruit.

YOUR DIET

Other than following the hormone-balancing guidelines on page 57, it's important to stock up on iodine-rich foods—in particular seaweed (which also has anti-cancer benefits and the ability to reduce cholesterol and improve fat metabolism in the body), as well as cod, prawns and tuna. Iodine is an essential component of the thyroid hormones, and deficiency has been

AVOID GOITROGENS

Goitrogens are foods that can hinder the uptake of iodine in the blood, which can then make an underactive thyroid worse. In their raw state cabbage, turnips, soy, peanuts, and pine nuts are all classed as goitrogens. However, after cooking, the problem disappears, so you needn't avoid these foods altogether. If you suffer from hypothyroidism, you can benefit from all their healthy properties, but only once they're cooked.

directly linked to hypothyroidism because it hampers the body's production of T4 (see p.58). When the pituitary gland recognizes that levels of T4 are low in the blood, it produces more TSH. If your TSH levels stay too high for too long, the thyroid gland can become enlarged to produce a goitre.

SUPPLEMENTS

Take good-quality supplements (see p.320) to help ensure you're optimizing your thyroid function.

- MANGANESE (5mg, daily) This is an important mineral for healthy thyroid function because it's needed for the efficient production of T4.

- SELENIUM (100μg, daily) Selenium is a vital component of the enzyme that helps trigger the creation of the thyroid hormone T3, so it's essential that your levels of this mineral (found naturally in the soil, and also in shellfish and Brazil nuts) are optimum.

- OMEGA-3 FATTY ACIDS (1,000mg fish oil containing at least 700mg EPA and 500mg DHA, daily)

Essential fats are crucial for healthy thyroid function because they help keep cells more fluid, which means that they are more sensitive to thyroid hormones and respond more effectively. (Take flax seed capsules if you're vegetarian.)

- TYROSINE (200mg, daily) This amino acid plays an important role in the healthy functioning of the thyroid gland, improving metabolism and suppressing appetite.

NATURAL TREATMENTS

Homeopathy Take Arsenicum 30c twice daily for up to five days, then wait two months and ask your doctor to assess the levels of thyroid hormone in your blood. If there's no improvement, consult a registered homeopath. Arsenicum is believed to help improve the thyroid's ability to manufacture hormones.

Acupuncture You may find this therapy helpful if you have an underactive thyroid *and* thyroid antibodies that show your immune system is attacking your thyroid cells. An acupuncturist will use moxibustion (burning the herb mugwort near your skin) to reduce the levels of thyroid antibodies and try to help recover proper thyroid function.

Traditional Chinese Medicine A study at the Shanghai Medical University treated 32 patients with

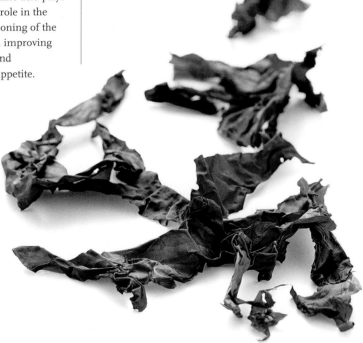

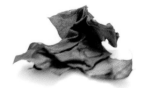

hypothyroidism for a year with a Chinese herbal preparation to stimulate the kidney meridian (see p.47). The clinical symptoms of hypothyroidism were said to be markedly improved compared with a control group. You'll need to visit a qualified practitioner to see if this treatment could work for you.

Aromatherapy Geranium essential oil is thought to help balance the thyroid hormones. Place 5 drops of the oil in your bath and soak in it for 20 minutes. Try to do this every day. Alternatively, you could dilute 5 drops of the oil in 2 tsp. sweet almond oil and massage it into your skin in any way you find soothing.

SELF-HELP
De-stress your life Stress (along with high levels of inactivity and smoking) can encourage thyroid underactivity because stress raises your body's blood levels of

the hormone cortisol, which in turn reduces levels of T3, slowing your metabolism right down.

If there are high levels of cortisol in your body, your muscles will begin to break down to provide fuel (in the form of glucose) to your brain. The less muscle you have, the slower your metabolism (and equally, the more muscle you have the faster your metabolism, which is why exercise is so important for general good health). To make matters worse, high cortisol levels inhibit the production of TSH from the pituitary gland, so the thyroid fails to be stimulated to produce T4. So, if you suffer from an underactive thyroid, relaxation time is essential. Take time out to do the things you love—whether that's reading, walking, painting, or simply sitting and watching the world go by. Make relaxation an important part of your daily life. Schedule it in if need be, and make sure you stick to it. You could also try the exercise, below.

ENTER A PLACE OF PEACE

If you suffer from an underactive thyroid, regular relaxation should be a core part of your lifestyle. Practice this relaxation routine every day—it need take only a few minutes, if that's all you have. Sit comfortably in a quiet place where you'll be undisturbed.

1 Close your eyes and take a couple of slow, deep breaths. Let your mind take you anywhere you like but make sure you feel peaceful, comfortable, and relaxed. It might be somewhere you've been, such as a sandy beach or a field of flowers, or somewhere imaginary, such as an enchanted wood.

2 In your mind's eye, conjure up the place as vividly as possible. Use all your senses. Notice the color of your surroundings, the sounds near

and far, and the smells. What is the air like? Is it warm and comforting against your skin? Or does it feel cool and refreshing? Try to capture even the tiniest details until you feel completely absorbed in your space.

If you feel negative thoughts or interference from outside creeping in, acknowledge the distraction and then let it go—it has no place here. Remain in your peaceful haven for as long as you feel comfortable.

Opposite: Dulse seaweed (see Your Diet, p.59)

Overactive thyroid

If your thyroid gland produces too much thyroid hormone, you're said to have an overactive thyroid, a condition known as hyperthyroidism. It means that your body systems go into overdrive.

Although hyperthyroidism can occur in men, it's much more of a problem for women, with women aged between 25 and 50 being most at risk. Some sources suggest that in the USA around one in 1,000 women are diagnosed with hyperthyroidism every year.

SYMPTOMS

Symptoms of the condition can include: rapid heart rate and palpitations, shortness of breath, goitre (swelling of the thyroid gland), increased perspiration, shakiness, anxiety, increased appetite accompanied by weight loss, insomnia, swollen, reddened and bulging eyes, and occasionally raised, thickened skin over the shins, backs of the feet, back, hands, or even face.

If you suspect you have symptoms of hyperthyroidism, consult a doctor right away. By accelerating your metabolism, the condition places an extra strain on your heart, in the long term potentially increasing your risk of heart failure. It can also interfere with your menstrual cycle and has been linked to infertility.

CAUSES

The most common cause of an overactive thyroid is Graves' disease, which affects mostly young and middle-aged women. The triggers for Graves' disease are unclear (although stress and heredity may play a part), but the disease itself is thought to be an autoimmune condition in which the immune system launches an antibody attack on the thyroid gland. This causes the thyroid to overproduce the hormone T4 (see p.58), leading to an increased metabolic rate.

DIAGNOSIS

Blood test In order to diagnose an overactive thyroid, your doctor will perform a blood test. This test measures your blood levels of thyroid-stimulating hormone (TSH). In hyperthyroidism, you would expect these levels to be lower than normal as your body attempts to reduce the rate at which your thyroid gland produces the hormone T4.

CONVENTIONAL TREATMENTS

If your doctor diagnoses hyperthyroidism, he or she will try to reduce your body's levels of T4. There are several ways in which this can be done. The treatment you're offered will depend on what your doctor thinks is causing your particular problem.

Medication Anti-thyroid drugs, such as methimazole and propylthiouracil in the USA and carbimazole in the UK, dampen the action of your thyroid gland by blocking the production of thyroid hormones. Your doctor will try to find levels of medication that keep your thyroid gland functioning at a "normal" rate.

Intervention Your doctor may recommend that you have part of your thyroid gland removed. This procedure usually involves taking pills containing radioactive iodine. Your thyroid gland takes up iodine in your system to produce thyroid hormone, but, as it does so, the radioactivity in the medication destroys some of the thyroid cells. The result is that the thyroid shrinks and, so, produces less hormone. Note that this treatment can make some of the symptoms of Graves' disease temporarily worse, especially swelling in the eyes.

Alternatively, your doctor may advise surgery to remove a nodule or a large part of your thyroid gland; or you may have a procedure called thyroid arterial embolization, in which the blood supply to your thyroid is blocked to disable its hormone-producing capabilities. All these are permanent solutions: You'll need to take thyroid hormones in drug form for the rest of your life to do the work of your lost thyroid gland.

YOUR DIET
Your thyroid is one of the most important regulators your body has, and so it's crucial that your doctor manages any problem with it. However, nutrition can provide wonderful complementary care. Try to eat more foods that naturally suppress thyroid function, in particular raw cruciferous vegetables, such as cabbage, radish, cauliflower, and arugula. These foods help block the thyroid's uptake of iodine, which it needs in order to make T4 and T3. However, keep your doctor and/or nutritionist informed of any increase in these thyroid-suppressing foods in your diet, especially if you're on medication, as the foods' action may interfere with the dosage of any drugs you're given.

Cut down on dairy products because they can provide a high level of iodine in your system, and avoid caffeine-containing drinks, such as coffee, tea, and sodas. Caffeine stimulates the action of your thyroid gland (and you need to suppress it).

SUPPLEMENTS
Hyperthyroidism puts your body under great strain, so a good-quality multi-vitamin and mineral supplement (see p.320) is essential for optimizing all your body's functions. Take one that includes as many of the nutrients below as possible, then top up to the following levels.

- **B-COMPLEX (containing 25mg of each B-vitamin, daily)** All the B-vitamins are crucial for healthy thyroid function because your body uses them in the production of T4 and T3.

- **VITAMIN C with bioflavonoids (500mg twice daily, as magnesium ascorbate, in addition to the amount in your multi)** This important vitamin will give your thyroid a further much-needed antioxidant boost.

- **VITAMIN E (400–600iu, daily)** This is another important antioxidant to help fight free-radical damage in your body.

- **CALCIUM (700mg, daily)** This mineral is a co-factor for many metabolic processes and is essential for healthy thyroid function.

- **MAGNESIUM (200–600mg, daily)** Like calcium, magnesium is essential for healthy thyroid function and studies show that hyperthyroidism may cause magnesium deficiency, making supplementation essential.

- **BROMELAIN (250–500mg three times daily, between meals)** This enzyme is found in the stem of pineapples and can help ease inflammation in your body. (If your thyroid gland is inflamed it can produce too much thyroid hormone.)

- **CO-ENZYME Q10 (60mg, daily)** Research has shown that as levels of thyroid hormones in your body increase, so your body's levels of co-enzyme Q10 decrease. Co-enzyme Q10 is a powerful antioxidant. It's thought that having an overactive thyroid can increase free-radical damage (see p.28) in your body and antioxidants help offset these effects.

- **L-CARNITINE (500mg, daily)** Research has shown that this amino acid can reduce the activity of the thyroid hormones and reduce some of the symptoms of hyperthyroidism, including palpitations, sleeplessness, and anxiety or nervousness.

- **OMEGA-3 FATTY ACIDS (1,000mg fish oil containing at least 700mg EPA and 500mg DHA, daily)** Omega-3 or essential fatty acids can help reduce thyroid swelling as they help the body to make beneficial substances called prostaglandins, which have an anti-inflammatory effect on the body.

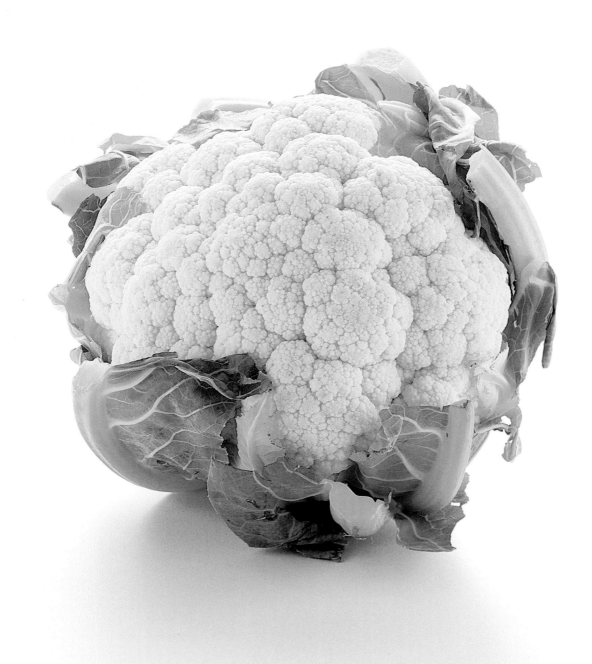

HERBS

You can take herbs to help normalize your thyroid function if your problem is mild and as long as you tell your doctor. Don't take herbs if you're already on anti-thyroid medication.

■ BUGLEWEED (*Lycopus virginicus*) This herb can help regulate an overactive thyroid by decreasing the production of thyroid hormones. Take it as a tincture (1 tsp. twice daily in a little water).

■ LEMON BALM (*Melissa officinalis*) Try using this herb as a tea because it has anti-thyroid and calming effects on your body. Steep 2 tbsp. dried lemon balm in 1 cup boiling water for ten minutes. Strain, cool, and drink. Take one cup like this, three times a day.

■ MOTHERWORT (*Leonurus cardiaca*) If one of your symptoms is a rapid heartbeat (as it often is with hyperthyroidism), motherwort will have a regulating action on your heart. Use 1–2 tsp. dried motherwort in 1 cup boiling water. Steep for ten minutes, cool, then drink. Take two or three cups like this, daily. If you prefer, you can use motherwort tincture instead of the tea. Take 1 tsp. in a little water, twice daily. (Note: consult your doctor before taking motherwort if you already take medicine to slow your heartbeat.)

OTHER NATURAL TREATMENTS

Homeopathy A qualified homeopath will usually prescribe some or all of the following remedies, all of which have a good track record against thyroid disorders. The normal dosage is 30c every hour for ten dosages (so a maximum of ten hours).
• Belladonna for flushed face and bulging eyes
• Iodine for weight loss and anxiety
• Lycopus for a pounding heart
• Nat mur for the weight loss

Acupuncture Acupuncturists consider hyperthyroidism to be caused by an imbalance of too much yang (masculine, dark) energy in the body. A practitioner will suggest a series of acupuncture sessions to try to bring this energy back into balance. I have seen good rates of success with hyperthyroidism clients who have consulted an acupuncturist, so this treatment is definitely worth considering.

Massage A gentle self-massage to the neck, shoulders, and chest area, or a general body massage from a practitioner, can help calm down the body, easing symptoms of hyperthyroidism. Use long, gentle strokes and always stroke towards your heart. Try using the essential oils (diluted in a carrier oil) suggested right.

Aromatherapy Lavender and marjoram essential oils will help calm your overactive body systems and encourage more restful sleep. Add 5 drops of each oil to a bedtime bath and rest in the water for 20 minutes or so. Alternatively, sprinkle 5 drops of each essential oil on your pillow to inhale as you sleep.

SELF-HELP

Avoid stimulants This means you need to avoid all caffeine, alcohol, and nicotine, but you should also avoid doing any strenuous exercise (gentle exercise is fine, though), which has an energizing action on your body. Steer clear of saunas and hot tubs, too. All these activities add heat to your body and put yet more strain on your thyroid gland to regulate your temperature.

Relax Keep your cool! An hour a day dedicated to relaxation will encourage your body to calm down, and this in turn will encourage your thyroid gland to slow down. You can use the relaxation exercise in the box on page 61 if you like. Otherwise, find a quiet activity that is fully absorbing (perhaps reading a book, painting, or listening to a favorite piece of music) and schedule time at the end of the day for this activity alone. Warn anyone you live with that this is time for you and they should leave you undisturbed.

Adrenal problems

Your two adrenal glands influence your blood-sugar levels and your sexual development, but they're most well known for making adrenaline and cortisol, two of the main stress hormones.

I see more and more women with problems relating to their adrenal function, and I have come to the conclusion that this trend is a byproduct of the way we live today—in a state of constant stress, but without the means to burn off all the extra stress hormones.

ADRENAL DISORDERS

Adrenal exhaustion

When your adrenal glands are under constant pressure, they become tired and overworked, leading to what is known as adrenal exhaustion. As well as being terrible for the adrenal glands themselves, exhaustion affects other body systems, too. Exhausted adrenals can't maintain blood-sugar balance, regulate the levels of salt and water in your body, or trigger proper carbohydrate metabolism or secretion of sex hormones. The malfunction causes depression, moodiness, and anxiety, as well as tiredness, hunger, sugar cravings, headaches, PMS, low blood pressure and blood sugar, low body temperature, dry or thin skin, poor memory and concentration, hair loss, poor resistance to infection, muscular pains, insomnia, and inflammation.

If your diet is low in protein or too high in carbohydrates, or if you suffer from severe allergies, chronic infections, insufficient sleep, or toxicity, or if you exercise excessively or have had surgery or an injury, these factors will also place a strain on your adrenals.

Overactive adrenals

It makes sense that through overuse your adrenals may become exhausted. However, a less common reaction is for your adrenals to go into overdrive. Under normal circumstances, your adrenal glands pump out cortisol first thing in the morning to give you the energy to get up. As the day goes on, the glands gradually release less cortisol until levels dip to their lowest at around midnight. If your adrenals are overactive, your cortisol levels remain high at bedtime, resulting in sleep problems. This puts additional stress on your adrenal glands, resulting in fatigue, weight gain (especially around the waist), diabetes, and mood swings.

Too much or too little hormone

As well as exhaustion and overactivity, the adrenal glands are subject to two syndromes. When the adrenal cortex (see box, opposite) produces too little cortisol (known as hypofunction), you may develop Addison's disease. Symptoms include weight loss, muscle weakness, fatigue, low blood pressure, hyperpigmentation (darkening of the skin), nausea, diarrhea, mood swings, dizziness, and depression. If the cortex produces too much cortisol (known as hyperfunction), you may develop Cushing's syndrome. Many of the symptoms of Cushing's syndrome are similar to those of people suffering from extreme stress, including weight gain (especially around the middle), depression, insomnia, and lack of sex drive, high blood pressure, insulin resistance, diabetes, and irregular periods.

Both Addison's disease and Cushing's syndrome are serious conditions that require medication, probably for the rest of your life. It's essential that if you suspect you have either one, you see your doctor right away.

ABOUT YOUR ADRENAL GLANDS

The adrenal glands lie directly above your kidneys (giving them their alternative name of supradrenal glands), one on each side of the body. They are separated from your kidneys by a layer of fat. Each gland itself is made up of two sections. The inner, smaller section is the medulla, which is made of nerve cells and is responsible for producing and regulating levels of the stress hormone adrenaline in your body. The larger, outer section is called the adrenal cortex and is responsible for producing steroid hormones (primarily cortisol, the stress hormone that stimulates the breakdown of protein and fat) and androgens (male hormones), which encourage the development of sexual characteristics at puberty. Women who produce too much androgen from the adrenal glands may suffer from excessive facial hair and a lack of periods. The adrenal cortex also produces aldosterone, a hormone that regulates salt–water balance in the body, and DHEA, a starting block for testosterone and estrogen.

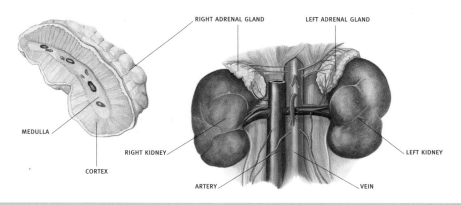

RIGHT ADRENAL GLAND — LEFT ADRENAL GLAND — MEDULLA — RIGHT KIDNEY — CORTEX — ARTERY — VEIN — LEFT KIDNEY

DIAGNOSIS

Adrenal stress test The best way to diagnose a problem with your adrenal glands is by an adrenal stress test, which you can perform at home and then send off for analysis. Using a home kit (available from many doctors or by mail; see p.320), you simply collect four saliva samples over the course of the day. The lab undertaking the analysis will look for how the levels of cortisol in your saliva change during the day (it should be high in the morning and gradually drop off), as well as measuring levels of DHEA (another adrenal hormone; see box, above). If the results show that cortisol is either too high or too low at any of the four points during the day, you can use both your diet and supplementation to help correct this.

Blood test If your doctor offers you a blood test as a first step to diagnosis, ask about the saliva test instead. In my experience, blood tests are designed to pick up only extreme cases of adrenal problems, such as Addison's disease or Cushing's syndrome, thereby missing milder adrenal dysfunction. However, for Addison's or Cushing's a blood test is essential to measure levels of sodium, potassium, and cortisol in your blood. The results indicate to your doctor whether or not you have a serious problem with your adrenals.

CONVENTIONAL TREATMENTS

When problems with your adrenal glands are extreme, for example, if you have Addison's disease or Cushing's syndrome, your doctor will prescribe you medication that attempts to regulate the function of your adrenal glands, including giving you corticosteroids (for Addison's disease) or hormone inhibitors (for Cushing's syndrome). In extreme cases, he or she may advise surgery or radiation therapy on your adrenal glands. Cases of adrenal exhaustion or overactivity that are not a result of Addison's disease or Cushing's syndrome are typically left to resolve themselves.

YOUR DIET

The first, and most important, step you can take to try to relieve the burden on your adrenal glands is to resolve any imbalance in your blood-sugar levels. Ensure that you eat regularly, which means little and often (at least every three hours). However, this doesn't mean that you should reach for sugary snacks. Instead, feast on snacks such as whole grains, nuts, and seeds, which release energy slowly, keeping your blood sugar as stable as possible. Avoid alcohol and other stimulants as these can trigger the release of cortisol and play havoc with your blood-sugar levels. Eat low-GI foods, avoid starchy carbohydrates after 6pm, and eat a little quality protein with every meal and snack. The latter is important because protein slows down the rate at which your body processes carbohydrates, keeping your blood-sugar levels stable.

SUPPLEMENTS

- B-COMPLEX (containing 25mg B1, B2, B3, and B6; 50mg B5 and 25µg B12; daily) Your body uses vitamin B5 to make adrenaline and cortisol. Vitamins B3 and B6 are also key to adrenal function.

- VITAMIN C with bioflavonoids (500mg, twice daily) This vitamin is vital for healthy adrenal function. Producing cortisol uses huge amounts of vitamin C, so it's also crucial to replenish stocks. Bioflavonoids are potent immunity-boosting antioxidants. Take it as magnesium ascorbate, which is less acidic than the cheaper and more common ascorbic acid.

- VITAMIN E (300iu, daily) This vitamin is a fat-soluble antioxidant that plays an important part in keeping your adrenal function healthy.

- MAGNESIUM (300mg, daily) Known as nature's tranquillizer, this calming mineral helps balance blood-sugar levels. I suggest taking magnesium citrate, as it's easy to absorb.

- ZINC (15mg, daily) This mineral is essential for the production of adrenal and sex hormones. Take it as zinc citrate.

- GREEN TEA EXTRACT (50mg, daily) This contains an amino acid called theanine, which has a relaxing effect on the brain and body.

- OMEGA-3 FATTY ACIDS (1,000mg fish oil containing at least 700mg EPA and 500mg DHA, daily) Essential fats help boost your metabolism, balance your blood sugar, and reduce the inflammatory effects of too much cortisol in your system. (Use flax seed if you're vegetarian.)

HERBS

- RHODIOLA (*Rhodiola rosea*) This adaptogenic herb has a balancing effect on your body. Take 250mg in capsule form, daily.

- SIBERIAN GINSENG (*Eleutherococcus senticosus*) This adaptogenic herb, like other adaptogens, works according to your body's needs—boosting energy when needed and helping to beat stress and fatigue when you're under pressure. It also helps boost the function of the adrenal glands. If you're under extreme physical and emotional stress, take it for around three months. Take 250–300mg, in capsule form, twice daily.

- VALERIAN (*Valeriana officinalis*) This herb is superb for encouraging a restful night's sleep. Take 1 tsp. tincture in a little water before bedtime; or take one 300mg capsule, daily.

OTHER NATURAL TREATMENTS

Homeopathy Use a 30c potency of each of the following as relevant, but also consult a practitioner.
• Arg nit for irritability, anxiety, and constant crying
• Kali phos for nervousness and anxiety
• Phos ac for extreme exhaustion and loss of libido

Acupuncture The adrenals are linked to the kidney meridian, and an acupuncturist will probably treat points along that meridian to stimulate healing.

Osteopathy The nerves that connect to the spine also feed the adrenal glands. An osteopath may be able to strengthen your adrenal glands by releasing blockages that they can feel when examining you.

Aromatherapy Certain essential oils can help support and nourish the adrenal glands. Spruce is great for adrenal exhaustion; pine helps fatigue and nervous conditions; and citrus oils, such as bergamot, lemon, and lime, can boost energy without stressing the adrenal glands. Add one or a blend of several to a bath (use 5 drops of each), or create your own adrenal massage oil, by adding a total of 15 drops of one or several oils to 6 tsp. carrier oil, such as sweet almond. Use the blend to massage your back just above your kidneys.

SELF-HELP

Exercise Regular exercise is essential for easing stress, boosting mood and energy, and encouraging a good night's sleep. Don't go overboard, though, as too much exercise can have the opposite affect. Between 30 and 60 minutes a day is optimum.

Sleep If you suffer from adrenal exhaustion or overactivity, it's essential that you get between six and eight hours sleep a night, although you may need more.

Relaxation Because stress is the single biggest cause of adrenal problems, it's crucial that you find ways to deal with it. I highly recommend yoga (see opposite).

YOGA FOR ADRENAL HEALTH

The yoga Cobra pose gently stimulates your adrenal glands by massaging the area where the adrenals sit on top of your kidneys. Practice the pose daily on either a soft carpet or a yoga mat.

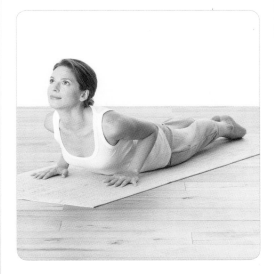

1 Lie face down, feet together, and your toes pointing behind you. Place your hands flat on the floor close to your body and beside your rib cage. Point your elbows upward.

2 Inhale and gently push upward from your hands, lifting your head and chest off the ground and tilting your head back. Feel your chest moving forward as well as upward to help prevent straining your lower back. Hold briefly and exhale as you lower to your starting position. Repeat four to six times.

YOUR BREASTS

Although often closely tied to a woman's sense of self-esteem, breasts are mounds of glandular, fatty, and fibrous tissue over the pectoralis muscles. They provide nourishment for a baby.

The tissue in your breasts consists of lobules, which are sphere-shaped sacs that produce milk, and mammary ducts, which are the canals that carry milk from the lobules to the nipples for breastfeeding. There are muscles in your nipple that allow them to become erect or aroused in response to sexual stimulation or breastfeeding, and muscle tissues around the lobules that help squeeze the breast milk into the ducts. Surrounding the nipple is a darker-pigmented circle of skin, the areola, which contains fluid-producing glands that keep the nipple lubricated.

Interestingly, women are the only female species in the animal kingdom to develop breasts long before they are needed to sustain a newborn. A baby girl is born with infantile milk ducts already in place. During puberty, when the ovaries begin to secrete estrogen, and usually alongside the appearance of pubic hair, the fatty tissues of the breasts begin to develop. Once ovulation starts, the breasts then swell as the milk ducts, glands, and nodules begin to mature. There's no set time it takes for breasts to reach their full size. Every woman is different.

YOUR CHANGING BREASTS

In the West, up to 70 percent of women will experience some kind of breast change (for example, tenderness, lumpiness, or pitting) during each menstrual cycle. Although these changes can be painful and uncomfortable, most cyclical breast problems are benign. However, because breasts have so much to do with our identity as women, it's not surprising that many women are increasingly concerned about the threat of breast cancer. It's for this reason that in this section I want to give you not only solutions to common, cyclical breast problems, but also all the tips I can on helping you to prevent breast cancer happening to you.

If you're prone to breast problems during your menstrual cycle, I want to make it absolutely clear that this does not mean you're at higher risk of developing breast cancer. Cyclical problems with your breasts tell you that your hormones are not in balance. If any pain or discomfort improves as soon as your period starts, the chances are there's no sinister cause. However, it is vital for all women to check their breasts regularly. Follow the step-by-step process set out in the box on page 77 to learn how.

As you already know, the two main female hormones circulating during your menstrual cycle are estrogen and progesterone. Your body uses the estrogen to turn your uterus into a nutritious cushion for the first bundle of cells that will become your baby, while progesterone inhibits your immune response to prevent your body from rejecting the embryo as a foreign body. Progesterone is also responsible for triggering your breasts to produce milk. Opinion varies as to whether it's high levels of estrogen, excess progesterone, or sensitivity to prolactin (the hormone secreted by the pituitary gland during breastfeeding) that is at the root of the problem of cyclical breast changes.

Over the following pages I shall look at the most common breast problems, whatever their cause, and explore natural ways to reduce their impact.

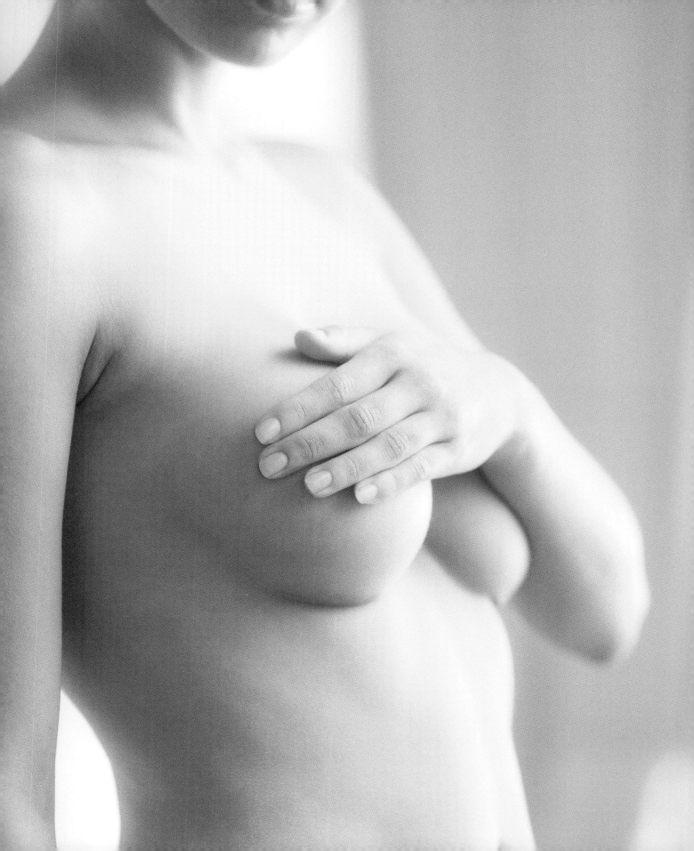

Breast problems

Over the course of your menstrual cycle, it's completely normal and natural that changes take place in your breast tissue. This is your body preparing for the possibility that you'll conceive.

Many breast problems are little more than an irritating interlude in your cycle. Sometimes, though, they cause excessive soreness, lumpiness, and pain; and sometimes they may not be related to your menstrual cycle at all. The following are some of the most common breast problems I'm asked to treat in my clinics. Although there's often a simple explanation for changes, check your breasts regularly for them.

FIBROCYSTIC BREAST DISEASE

This condition is the most common cause of lumpy, sore breasts in women aged between 30 and 50. It's completely benign, and its symptoms, which tend to be worse before your period, include swollen, tender breasts, and/or one or more lumps.

It's thought that fibrocystic breast changes are linked to the monthly hormonal roller coaster that your body goes through. Each month, as your body prepares for a possible pregnancy, your breasts ready themselves to produce milk. This response to hormonal triggers in your cycle may be responsible for the condition. You may be more likely to have fibrocystic breast disease if other women in your family have had it.

Diagnosing fibrocystic breast disease

Physical examination A doctor will usually diagnose fibrocystic breasts by feeling the lumpy areas in your breast(s), often close to your armpits. Unlike cancerous breast lumps, fibrocystic breast lumps tend to be mobile, often feel rounded, have smooth borders, and are rubbery or somewhat changeable in shape.

Mammogram If your doctor is unsure following a physical examination, he or she may recommend a mammogram. However, if you have entered menopause or are on HRT you're likely to have thicker than normal breast tissue, which often makes a mammogram difficult to interpret.

Ultrasound and biopsy Although an ultrasound breast scan can be expensive, it often provides a more reliable diagnosis of the state of your breast tissue than a mammogram. If after an ultrasound your doctor is still in any doubt as to whether or not the lumps are malignant, ask to be examined by a specialist. Although uncomfortable, a needle biopsy (in which tissue from the lump is extracted and examined in a lab) may be the most reliable diagnostic test.

CONVENTIONAL TREATMENTS FOR ALL BREAST PAIN

Medication For all types of breast pain and for breast lumps, the only non-surgical treatment your doctor can offer you is medication that tries to control your hormones or offer pain relief. For example, the drug bromocriptine works by lowering the levels of prolactin (the hormone that stimulates breast tissue and milk production), which will ease pain, while the contraceptive pill artificially alters the cycle of your hormones to give you better hormonal balance. The drugs danazol and tamoxifen are both anti-estrogens that suppress the menstrual cycle to relieve breast pain, while synthetic forms of gonadatrophin-releasing hormone

(GnRH) may be given as a nasal spray or injection to put the body into a temporary state of menopause, relieving pain. While all this seems good on the surface, hormone-suppression comes with side-effects. In the case of breast-pain medication, these range from nausea, dizziness, and mood swings to thrombosis, depression, and weight gain. Also, taking tamoxifen is associated with an increased risk of osteoporosis.

"Natural" progesterone cream One common "treatment" for fibrocystic and painful breasts is progesterone cream. Some women have rubbed the cream into their breasts at a given point in their cycle. The theory is that the fat cells in the breast tissue absorb the progesterone to equalize estrogen dominance and reduce pain. Fibrocysts usually disappear after applying the cream for two or three cycles. However, be aware that the word "natural" in this context does not mean "directly from nature," it means "the same as in nature"—only artificially produced. "Natural" progesterone cream is a man-made drug; it's not the same as, say, a plant or homeopathic remedy. Side-effects of using the cream include (weirdly) breast discomfort and enlargement. This makes sense if you think how many women say that these are also among the first signs of pregnancy, at a time when progesterone levels are high. Some studies suggest the cream may even give an increased risk of breast cancer.

Surgery Some doctors will suggest that the only way to eliminate cyclical breast pain is to cut out your body's major source of both estrogen and progesterone—that is, your ovaries. I strongly advise against this procedure, which would reduce the pain in your breasts, but it would also send you into menopause overnight. To compensate, your doctor would offer you estrogen-only HRT, but this in itself can cause breast pain, tenderness, and enlargement. I suggest, instead, that you adhere to the following recommendations so that you address the cause of your problem.

YOUR DIET
Before you take any medication, try my nutritional (and other natural) suggestions for three months to see

INVERTED NIPPLES

Inverted nipples are far more common than you might think— they occur in as many as one in five women. They happen because the nipple tissue is connected to a short milk duct and the muscle tone in the nipple can't overcome the inward pull. Although many women are concerned about inverted nipples, it's good to know that they will not stop you breastfeeding or having great sex.

When the nipples are "retracted" (meaning that occasionally they pull inward), rather than fully inverted, you can usually bring them outward by manipulating them with your fingers. For fully inverted nipples cosmetic surgery is one option, but it's important to bear in mind that sometimes breastfeeding itself can reverse the condition. If you plan to have a baby in the future, perhaps it might be worth waiting before you go into surgery. One UK cosmetic surgeon has invented a non-invasive device called the Avent Niplette (you can order it online throughout the world), which gently sucks the nipple outward into a plastic thimble-like cup. In many cases, the nipple remains permanently turned out and erect after only four weeks of use.

whether the natural approach eases your symptoms, without the need for medical intervention. If you show no signs of improvement, perhaps medication is the only way forward for you—however, I'm confident that using my approach you'll begin to see a change.

First and foremost, follow the recommendations in my hormone-balancing diet (see box, p.57). You'll need to be rigorous about this if you're going to make long-lasting changes to the balance of your hormones. In particular, adhere to the following nutritional advice:

Eliminate methylxanthines Substances found in coffee, tea, cola, chocolate, decaffeinated coffee, and certain medications, methylxanthines have been shown to cause breast discomfort. For this reason, it's important to eliminate them completely from your diet. Check labels when you buy.

Reduce saturated fat I recommend that you eat a low-saturated-fat diet because a high intake of saturated fat (found in red meat, cakes, pastries and so on) can increase estrogen levels in your body.

Eat phytoestrogens A good intake of phytoestrogens in your diet, especially from legumes such as chickpeas, lentils, soy, and so on, can have a balancing effect on your hormones. Breast problems tend to occur less frequently in cultures around the world where these foods are consumed on a regular basis.

Increase fiber Having a good intake of fiber can help with breast pain because it helps remove excess hormones from your body. If you're constipated or not passing a bowel movement regularly, then your body isn't eliminating waste products, toxins, and hormones efficiently. Soluble fiber, which is found in vegetables and whole grains such as oats and brown rice, has the most benefit in terms of breast pain because it contains the kind of fiber that binds to hormones. Make sure you're having at least one helping of whole grains and two servings of vegetables a day.

SUPPLEMENTS

■ B-COMPLEX (containing 25mg of each B-vitamin, daily) The B-vitamins in general are important for treating breast pain because they help your body to excrete excess hormones.

■ VITAMIN E (400–600iu, daily) Research shows that vitamin E can help ease breast pain. You can increase your intake of vitamin E from your food by including almonds, leafy green vegetables, oats, soy, and whole grains. Also add vitamin E in supplement form for three months while you're trying to increase your intake with your food. It's best to take it as d-alpha tocopherol, not dl-alpha tocopherol, which is a synthetic version.

■ EVENING PRIMROSE OIL (240–320mg, daily) The gamma linolenic acid (GLA) in evening primrose oil has a balancing effect on the good and bad prostaglandins in your body, reducing breast pain. If you have epilepsy check with your doctor before taking any capsules containing GLA.

■ PROBIOTICS (containing at least ten billion organisms per capsule; one capsule daily) Probiotics can help lower levels of the enzymes in your body that reabsorb old hormones. They also encourage regular bowel movements, which further reduce the chances of toxins being reabsorbed into your system.

HERBS

Herbal remedies can help balance your hormones and ensure that "old" estrogen is processed and excreted efficiently by your liver.

■ AGNUS CASTUS (*Vitex agnus castus*) This herb helps regulate prolactin levels, easing breast tenderness. Take 1 tsp. tincture in a little water or 200–300mg in capsule form, twice daily.

■ CLEAVERS (*Galium aparine*) Cleavers improves detoxification, helping to reduce swelling and bloating in your breasts. Take 1 tsp. tincture in a little water or 200–300mg in capsule form, twice daily.

■ GINKGO BILOBA (*Gingko biloba*) Ginkgo can help regulate your body's estrogen receptors. Take one 300mg capsule, daily.

Opposite: Cleavers (*Galium aparine*)

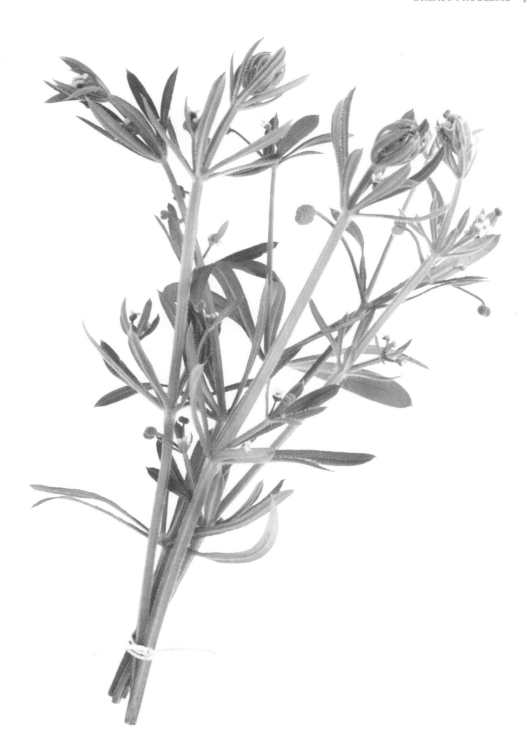

OTHER NATURAL TREATMENTS

Aromatherapy To ease discomfort, try a breast compress laced with essential oils. Add 3 drops each of ginger, German chamomile, and lavender oils to a bowl containing 1 cup warm water. Lay a folded gauze over the surface of the water for ten seconds, so that it soaks up the floating oil particles. Remove it and wring it out. Place the cloth over one bare breast for five to ten minutes. Repeat on the other breast, if necessary.

SELF-HELP

Exercise Regular exercise helps balance hormones. Aim for at least 30 minutes a day of any exercise that leaves you slightly breathless.

Check your breasts It's worth reiterating here how crucial it is that you check your breasts regularly (daily if you're concerned, otherwise once a month), using the technique described in the box, opposite.

GO BRALESS!

Some research has suggested that simply ditching the habit of wearing a bra can ease the discomfort of cyclical breast pain and even reduce fibrocysts, if you suffer from them. Some doctors believe that a bra can restrict the flow of lymph through your breast tissue (there are lymph glands just underneath each breast), allowing toxins to accumulate and cause pain. Although we've yet to discover a firm connection between breast problems and bra-wearing, try to avoid wearing underwire or tight-fitting bras. Opt instead for camisoles or tank-tops with built-in support, or at the very least use a wireless bra. Whenever you can (especially at nighttime), go braless altogether.

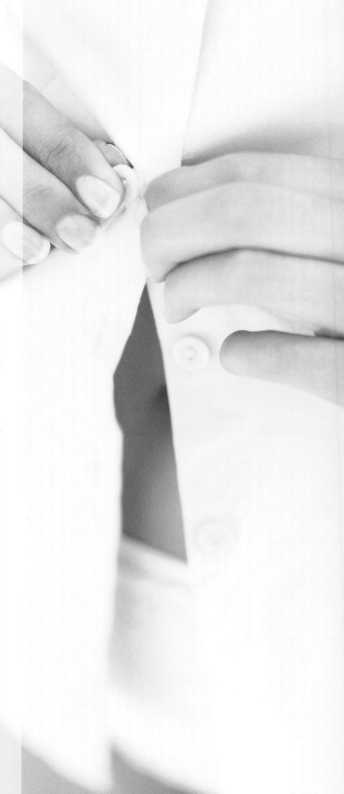

Preventing breast cancer

For many of the women I see, a fear of breast cancer is often almost as much to do with self-image as it is with illness. I want to turn this fear into a positive attitude towards checking your breasts regularly.

In the USA, the number of women with breast cancer is second only to the number of those with skin cancer. However, women everywhere are gaining awareness of how to arm themselves against this disease; just as the medical profession is improving its ability to fight it.

Checking your breasts could save your life—there's no more direct way to put it. Most breast lumps are picked up by women themselves rather than as a result of screening. Use the technique given in the box below at least once a month. If you notice any changes to your breasts, experience any continuous pain in them, or feel any lumps that aren't part of your normal cycle, see your doctor right away. Although serious problems are rare, it's important to rule them out. There have been concerns in recent years regarding the safety and effectiveness of mammograms, so discuss the option of an ultrasound with your doctor, or you can contact my clinic if you prefer (see p.320).

GET TO KNOW YOUR BREASTS

"Knowing" your breasts is essential if you're to spot when something changes. Examine them at least monthly, ideally seven to ten days after your period begins. This will allow the breast tissue to "settle" following any changes related to your hormonal cycle.

1 Stand topless in front of a mirror. Raise your arms. Look at your breasts. What's their position on your chest? How would you describe their shape? Where do your nipples point? Has one breast become larger or changed position (usually lower) since last month? Look for any redness, or ulcerated or scaly areas on the nipples or breasts and for any dimples. Is there any swelling under your armpit or around your collarbone? Is there discharge from your nipple?

2 Lie down on your back with your head on a pillow. Look at your right breast first. Raise your right arm, bend it at the elbow and put your forearm under your head. Using the tips of the fingers on your left hand, use a firm pressure to make small circles around the right breast and armpit. Can you feel any small lumps? Do any areas feel "thicker" or different to the rest of your breast tissue? Carefully feel over the whole right breast; then repeat on the left.

CAUSES

So far, we don't know for certain what causes breast cancer. However, there are certain risk factors that may put you at greater risk than others of developing the disease. Some of these risk factors we can do something about, and some we can't. It's important to keep everything in perspective to minimize the risks, but not to the detriment of living happily.

Being overweight, drinking too much alcohol, and lack of exercise are all risk factors that we have under our control, however age is also an important risk factor (breast cancer becomes more common after the age of 50). Heredity makes a different, too—if you have a family history of breast cancer, you may carry the BRCA genes, which are known to increase the risk of breast-cancer development. If you tell your doctor of your family history, you may be referred for genetic testing. Some women who know they have a BRCA gene have opted for an elective mastectomy, but this need not necessarily be your only option for prevention. Finally, there is overwhelming evidence that the female hormone estrogen plays a central role in causing breast cancer—women with excess estrogen appear to have a higher risk than women with normal levels.

YOUR DIET

Go Japanese Women in Japan have a much lower breast-cancer risk than women in the West: 39 cases of breast cancer per 100,000 Japanese women compared with 133 per 100,000 for Western women. Experts have suggested that the reason is dietary. Japanese women eat more phytoestrogens than Western women. One large study showed that a diet high in soy is associated with a 14 percent reduction in the risk of developing breast cancer. Phytoestrogens (see p.31) in soy seem to block the estrogen receptors in your breast tissue (in a similar way to the drug tamoxifen; see p.72), perhaps preventing the disease. They also stimulate the production of a protein called sex-hormone-binding globulin (SHBG), which controls how much estrogen circulates in your blood. Although phytoestrogens are found in their highest concentrations in soy products, other healthy sources include chickpeas, lentils, aduki beans, kidney beans, and other legumes. Japanese women also tend to eat more fish than Western women, especially oily fish. This boosts their intake of omega-3 fatty acids, which inhibit tumors.

Eat cruciferous vegetables Vegetables such as cabbage, Brussels sprouts, and cauliflower can help prevent estrogen overload because they contain a chemical called indole-3-carbinol that encourages the body to eliminate excess estrogen and prevents it from absorbing toxic estrogen. One study found that women eating one and a half cups of these vegetables daily decreased their breast-cancer risk by a quarter.

Eat fiber High-fiber foods encourage better elimination of waste products and toxins, including estrogens, from the body. Aim for 40g (1½oz.) fiber a day. Switching to a mainly vegetarian diet with an abundance of fruit and vegetables would give your fiber intake a fabulous boost. If you can, add in one or two handfuls of high-fiber flax seeds, which also contain lignans. These stimulate SHBG (see above) and inhibit the activity of aromatase, an enzyme that encourages the body to convert more male hormones to estrogen. (Some breast-cancer medications are aromatase inhibitors, which aim to stop the body converting testosterone to estrogen.)

SUPPLEMENTS

- FOLIC ACID (400µg, daily, perhaps in a multi-vitamin and mineral supplement) Studies show that people with a daily intake of 345µg or more folic acid (itself a B-vitamin) have a 38 percent lower risk of developing breast cancer than women with an intake of less than 195µg.

- PROBIOTICS (containing at least ten billion organisms per capsule; one capsule daily) One study has found that probiotics can help prevent the reabsorption of "old" estrogens from the colon, encouraging better elimination of these toxins from your body.

HERBS

■ BLACK COHOSH (*Cimicifuga racemosa*) This herb acts as a weak anti-estrogen, and research indicates that it may be able to slow the rate at which breast-cancer cells multiply. Take black cohosh either as a tincture (1 tsp. in a little water, two or three times daily) or in capsule form (250–350mg, daily).

SELF-HELP

Think twice about HRT Although hormone replacement therapy (HRT) was once considered a cure-all for a woman in menopause, we now know better. Research has concluded that this supposed "anti-aging" treatment can increase your risk of breast cancer. If you have a family history of breast cancer or are concerned about whether or not you're at risk, discuss this with your doctor before taking HRT and weigh up the risks. There are natural remedies available to eliminate the symptoms of menopause (see pp.252–5), without the need for HRT, so, in my opinion, the benefits don't make up for its dangers.

Avoid toxins All forms of cancer are the result of mutations in your DNA, so it's important to look at the environmental toxins you expose your body to and try to reduce this exposure. (See box, below.)

TOXINS AND POLLUTANTS

Toxicity surrounds us—it's in the air, the water, and the soil. I urge you to take responsibility for reducing the toxic load on your body by following a few simple lifestyle rules.

EAT CLEAN The most important thing you can do for cancer prevention is to eat organic food. Studies show that the breast tissue of women with breast cancer contains more pesticides than that of women with benign breast problems. If you do buy non-organic, wash it thoroughly and peel fruit and vegetables.

CHOOSE COSMETICS CAREFULLY Deodorants and antiperspirants contain preservatives called parabens, which have been found inside breast-cancer tumors and can have an estrogen-like effect on the body (and also aluminum, which has been linked to dementia). In addition, antiperspirants prevent the body from expelling toxins through sweat, so the toxins remain locked in your system. I advise you to avoid antiperspirants altogether and instead use a chemical-free or crystal deodorant that does not contain parabens and won't stop you from sweating, but will stop any body odor.

Whenever you use face creams, suntan lotions, body lotions, hair-removing agents, and so on, make sure you read the ingredient list and ask yourself if you could choose a more natural alternative. Many cosmetics, especially perfumes, contain xenoestrogens (see box, p.18) in the artificial "musks" that give them their scent. See page 320 for sources of natural cosmetics that won't cause you harm.

AVOID XENOESTROGENS EVERYWHERE In addition to all this, artificial estrogens may be found in baby bottles, plastic containers, water bottles, and tooth fillings, and in paints and plastics. Keep your exposure to anything contained in these items to a minimum.

Quit smoking—and alcohol Cigarettes and alcohol are your deadly enemies. Numerous studies show that any alcohol consumption can significantly increase your breast-cancer risk, and research suggests that women who smoke have up to a 60-percent higher risk of developing breast cancer than women who have never smoked. According to one study, even passive smoking for as little as one hour a day can triple your breast-cancer risk.

Watch your weight Being overweight can increase the production of estrogen from fat cells, which in turn increases the risk of breast cancer. However, it's not just what you weigh that impacts your likelihood of developing breast cancer, but also where you put on weight. If you're apple-shaped (you carry weight around your waist), you're at a higher risk than a woman who is pear-shaped (with weight around her hips). To check whether you could be at a higher risk, measure your waist and hips and divide the waist measurement by the hip. If the resulting figure is more than 0.8, you have too much fat sitting around the middle of your body. This may increase the levels of estrogen in your system and consequently increase your risk of developing breast cancer. You need then to take steps to reduce that fat around the middle by following a healthy diet (see pp.24–9) and exercising regularly (between three and five times a week), combining aerobic exercise with strengthening and toning.

Find time to relax Stress affects the way your body produces hormones and the effectiveness of your immune system, so it's not surprising that researchers have found links between stress and breast cancer. Give yourself 30 minutes to wind down each day.

Go out in the sun Manufactured by your body in response to sunlight, vitamin D has been shown to reduce the risk of breast cancer because it helps prevent abnormal cells from multiplying. One study in 2006 suggested that "vitamin D supplementation could reduce cancer incidence and mortality ... with few or no adverse effects." Try to get out in the sun for approximately 15 minutes a day without any sunscreen (check the skin cosmetics you use, as most contain in-built sun protection factors that would block the sunlight from getting through). Obviously, there are issues with skin cancer here, so keep your exposure to short bursts and, if you're worried, keep the sunscreen on, but also take vitamin D in supplement form (400–600iu daily of vitamin D3). You can also boost your levels of vitamin D by eating oily fish and egg yolks.

Get up and move Regular exercise is essential in the fight to prevent breast cancer. Studies show that all types of exercise have a positive effect, lowering estrogen levels, and can cut the risk of breast cancer significantly. One study suggested that women who exercise for more than four hours a week have a 58 percent lower risk of developing breast cancer; and those who exercise between one and three hours a week have a 30 percent lower risk. Aim for between 30 minutes and one hour of moderate exercise daily, and don't forget that housework and gardening count, too.

Breastfeed There are myriad reasons why breast is best for your baby—but we now know that breastfeeding is best for you, too. Preliminary research indicates that the hormones your body releases during breastfeeding cause a permanent, physical change in breast cells that can help protect them from the potentially cancer-inducing effects of estrogen.

Check your breasts I know I've already said it, but I can't stress enough how breast self-examination is the best method for detecting breast cancer in its earliest stages. The earlier you detect it, the greater the likelihood that you'll be able to prevent it from developing. Ninety percent of malignant lumps are found by women who have examined themselves. Please check—at least once every month—using the technique given in the box on page 77.

Opposite: Black cohosh (*Cimicifuga racemosa*; see Herbs, p.79)

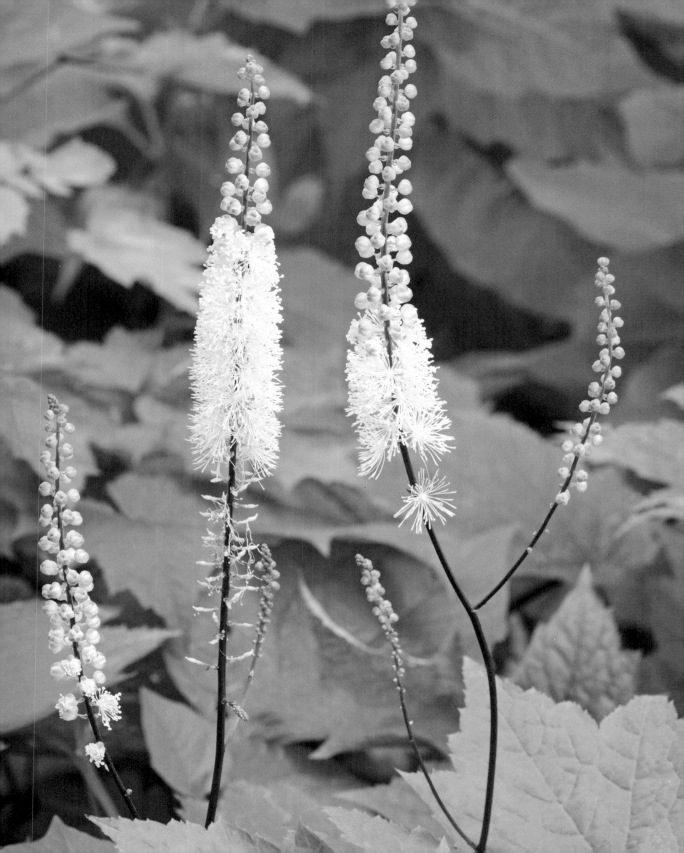

YOUR OVARIES

They may be only the size of almonds, but your ovaries are powerful organs that churn out estrogen, progesterone—the hormones that are instrumental in regulating your fertility—and also testosterone.

Through the action of estrogen, your ovaries could be said to play an important role in maintaining the health of your skin, heart, breasts, and bones, as well as regulating your metabolism and body temperature. Then there's the amazing miracle of ovulation. Every month your ovaries release a mature egg, and, if a healthy sperm meets it, the egg will become an embryo that will eventually become a baby.

However, despite their awesome power, your ovaries are not immune to dysfunction. Among the most common ovarian problems I see in my clinics are polycystic ovary syndrome (PCOS) and ovarian cysts. Fortunately, there are a number of natural treatments that can not only treat these problems successfully but also help prevent them from occurring in the first place.

In this section, I'm going to look in detail at the most common problems that are likely to affect your ovaries and the most effective ways to treat them. For now, it's worth noting the general guidelines that will help keep your ovaries in the peak of health for as long as possible. However, I do also want to stress that there are many ovarian problems that will need intervention or treatment by a medical doctor. Natural therapies, including nutrition and herbal medicine, can help hugely in the majority of cases, but it's vital that you obtain a correct diagnosis from your doctor and work with him or her to ensure the best, most effective treatment for you—perhaps including both conventional and natural approaches.

FLOWERING PLANTS have ovaries, too: the ripened fruit.

TAKING CARE OF YOUR OVARIES

Taking steps to balance your hormones will help ensure that your ovaries are working efficiently, keeping your fertility and overall health at optimum levels. Adopt the hormone-balancing diet (see box, p.57) and, in particular, be careful about the amount of sugar you eat. You need to try to keep your blood-sugar levels stable, so cut out refined carbohydrates and stimulants (such as caffeine) and opt for a low-GI diet.

Smoking is linked to problems with estrogen production from your ovaries, so if you haven't already, quit now. Balancing your weight (see pp.296–301) is also key. If you're overweight, your fat cells are likely to produce excess estrogen, and if you're underweight, you may not ovulate at all because your body goes into survival mode, thinking that it wouldn't be safe for you to have a baby during what it perceives is a time of famine. Stress can also inhibit ovulation, again because your body thinks there must be danger. Pay attention to your stress levels and try to make time to relax, even just for 20 minutes a day.

Finally, bear in mind that the Pill can sometimes play havoc with your hormonal balance, and also the action of your ovaries when you decide to stop taking it. If you take the Pill for contraceptive purposes and then decide you want to have a baby, give yourself at least three months after you stop taking it to get your body back into balance (use my pre-conception plan, see pp.168–73) before deliberately trying to conceive.

Polycystic ovary syndrome (PCOS)

Every month, follicles grow on a woman's ovaries. When the follicles don't develop properly they can form cysts on the ovaries' surfaces, which, when accompanied by hormonal imbalance, can lead to PCOS.

In a normal cycle, several follicles develop on the surfaces of your ovaries. In one of those follicles, a single egg matures more quickly than the eggs in the others, and is released into the Fallopian tube. All the remaining follicles then die away. If you have polycystic ovaries, you have a number of undeveloped follicles remaining on the surfaces of your ovaries, making the ovaries appear enlarged. In itself, this isn't necessarily a problem—many women have polycystic ovaries and have regular cycles and no problems getting pregnant. However, if you also have higher-than-normal levels of certain sex hormones, such as androgens ("male" hormones, including testosterone) and luteinizing hormone (LH), you have polycystic ovary *syndrome*, a condition that triggers symptoms such as irregular or absent periods, acne, excess hair, and weight gain.

CAUSES

The causes of PCOS continue to perplex even the experts who specialize in it. Although there's a strong genetic and hereditary link for the condition, many problems stem from the simple fact that the ovaries can't seem to produce hormones in the correct proportions. The pituitary gland then gets the message that the ovaries aren't working properly and releases more LH. Women with PCOS often have problems with blood-sugar swings, which cause the pancreas to release more insulin, which in turn targets the ovaries to produce more testosterone. The adrenal glands and liver are then affected, producing more male hormones in your system. All in all, you're in a vicious cycle.

DIAGNOSIS

If you suspect that you have PCOS, it's important you see your doctor as soon as possible, as early diagnosis can help prevent long-term complications of the condition, such as infertility and diabetes. If, after performing the following tests, your doctor confirms a diagnosis of PCOS, you may be referred to a specialist in endocrinology (hormones) or to a gynecologist.

Ultrasound Your doctor may decide to give you an ultrasound scan, which he or she will use to establish whether or not there are undeveloped follicles that remain on the surfaces of your ovaries.

Blood tests Your doctor will perform a blood test to check levels of follicle-stimulating hormone (FSH) and LH, androgens (male hormones), and SHBG (sex-hormone-binding globulin). High levels of LH and/or androgens, and/or low levels of SHGB can indicate a problem. Note that you don't have to have all these hormone imbalances to have PCOS, just one of them, plus the polycystic ovaries that showed on an ultrasound.

CONVENTIONAL TREATMENTS

There's no question that it's crucial to manage PCOS. Your doctor will probably offer you the following conventional treatments.

Hormone treatments As PCOS is essentially a problem with the balance of hormones in your body, it stands to reason that your doctor will offer you some

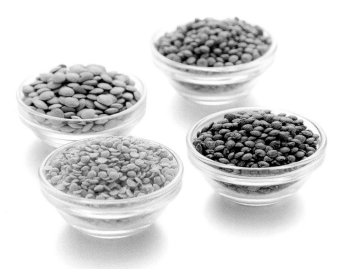

medication to regulate your body's hormone production. The standard treatment for women who aren't planning to have a baby is the anti-testosterone contraceptive pill. This drug can help eliminate some of the more "male" symptoms of PCOS, such as acne and excess hair, but it doesn't treat the cause.

If you're aiming to get pregnant, your doctor may offer you clomiphene citrate. Most women find that this stimulates ovulation, but it can also hamper your ability to carry your baby to term. Use clomiphene for a maximum of six months. If it's unsuccessful, your doctor may try medications such as gonadotrophins.

Insulin sensitizers The link between PCOS and insulin resistance means that some doctors prescribe type II diabetes medication to treat PCOS, too. You'll most likely be offered metformin. For some women, metformin doesn't work at all; while several studies show that it increases the efficacy of clomiphene (see above), so you may be prescribed both medications. A powerful drug, metformin causes stomach upsets in up to a fifth of the women who take it.

Surgery As a last resort, your doctor may advise a laparoscopic ovarian diathermy, also know as ovarian drilling. The procedure causes your levels of testoster-

one to fall in the hope that this will stimulate your ovary to release an egg. Although surgery works in the short term, it's likely the PCOS will return, which is why doctors use it only when all other treatments have failed.

YOUR DIET

There is overwhelming evidence to suggest that diet plays a significant role in the natural management of PCOS. Therefore, before you go on any medication for the condition, I strongly urge you to try the nutritional approach to managing it. Follow the nutritional recommendations below for six months (including taking the supplements). If, after this time, you see no signs of improvement (for example, if your hair growth hasn't slowed down, if your periods aren't more regular, and so on), go back to your doctor.

If you're overweight, it's crucial that you bring your weight down to the appropriate level for your height. Being overweight increases insulin levels dramatically and makes the symptoms of PCOS worse. Losing weight, on the other hand, results in lower insulin levels, which in turn reduce the testosterone levels that are interfering with ovulation. So follow the hormone-balancing diet (see box, p.57) and increase the amount of exercise you get. Aim to get your BMI in the right range for your age and height (see box, p.297).

Above: Lentils (see Phytoestrogens, opposite)

Adapting your eating habits so you keep your blood-sugar levels on an even keel throughout the day is an essential component of the natural approach to treating PCOS. If your adrenal glands are over-stimulated by ever-fluctuating sugar highs and lows, they produce too much adrenaline—the stress hormone—and also too much androgen (male hormone), preventing ovulation altogether. Although in the West we tend to base our day around "three square meals," this isn't the best way to eat if you suffer from PCOS. Try six smaller, well-balanced meals (ideally comprising low-GI foods) a day, instead.

Phytoestrogens Eating foods, such as soy, chickpeas, and lentils, that contain natural estrogens can be beneficial for women with PCOS because phytoestrogens help control levels of testosterone in the blood.

PREGNANCY AND PCOS

I believe that many women with PCOS can achieve pregnancy following the natural approach. However, never stop taking any prescribed medication without letting your doctor know first and asking for his or her support.

IF YOU'RE UNDER 35 Once you stop taking your medication, give your body six months using all the natural advice on these pages. Then stop taking the co-enzyme Q10 and the herbs and start trying for a baby.

IF YOU'RE OVER 35 Follow your doctor's advice about which medications to take. On top of this, take a reputable multi-vitamin and mineral supplement and follow all my nutritional advice. Do NOT take the herbs or co-enzyme Q10.

SUPPLEMENTS

The main aims of supplementation are to help your body regulate its insulin levels and by extension balance your blood sugar. The supplements below can also help you lose weight if you're overweight.

- B-COMPLEX (containing 25mg of each B-vitamin, daily) Deficiencies in B-vitamins can make symptoms of PCOS worse because all the B-vitamins, are essential for liver function (to excrete "old" hormones). One study found that B-vitamin supplementation boosted weight loss and improved ovulation in PCOS sufferers by 23 percent.

- CHROMIUM (200µg, daily) Low levels of chromium can trigger insulin resistance, a condition in which high levels of insulin circulate in the blood but are unable to control blood-sugar levels. Supplementing is a good way to keep your chromium levels at an optimum, but if you're diabetic and on medication, speak to your doctor before taking any chromium. If you need to lose weight, chromium has been shown to stem hunger and reduce food cravings.

- MAGNESIUM (300mg, daily, as magnesium citrate) Adequate magnesium intake is essential for controlling blood-sugar and insulin levels, fluctuations in which can worsen the symptoms of PCOS.

- ZINC (30mg daily, as zinc citrate) Zinc is not only vital for appetite control but also for insulin regulation and hormone balance.

- ALPHA LIPOIC ACID (100mg, daily) A powerful antioxidant, alpha lipoic acid releases energy by burning glucose, so your body has to release less insulin to deal with blood-glucose levels and has to store less fat. Over time this helps you lose weight. Alpha lipoic acid can also prevent high blood pressure, a long-term effect of PCOS. However, if you're diabetic and on medication, talk to your doctor before taking alpha-lipoic acid, so he or she can monitor its effects on your medication.

- CO-ENZYME Q10 (60–100mg, daily) This nutrient is important for normal carbohydrate metabolism, and so is vital for your body's energy output. It can also help lower levels of glucose and insulin in the blood, helping to stabilize blood sugar.

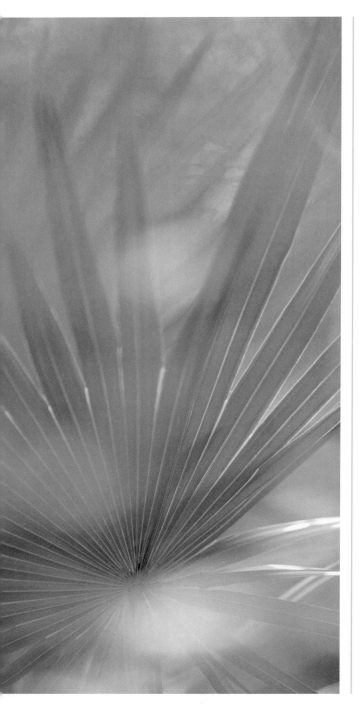

HERBS

The following herbs are from a great store of herbal hormone regulators I recommend for PCOS.

■ AGNUS CASTUS (*Vitex agnus castus*) By helping to normalize the function of your pituitary gland, agnus castus is often a good cycle regulator. Take 1 tsp. tincture in a little water, twice daily; or 200–300mg in capsule form, twice daily.

■ BLACK COHOSH (*Cimicifuga racemosa*) This herb helps suppress LH levels (see p.83). Although there have been some concerns about black cohosh causing liver damage, they appear unfounded. To be safe, avoid the Asian species and choose North American black cohosh. Take 1 tsp. tincture in a little water, two or three times daily; or 250–350mg in capsule form, twice daily.

■ DANDELION ROOT (*Taraxacum officinale*) and MILK THISTLE (*Silybum marianum*) These herbs may help PCOS because they cleanse the liver. Take 1 tsp. of either tincture in a little water, twice daily; or 200–400mg of either in capsule form, daily.

■ SAW PALMETTO (*Serenoa repens*) Saw palmetto can reduce high levels of androgens in your system. Take 1 tsp. tincture in a little water or 200–300mg in capsule form, twice daily.

OTHER NATURAL TREATMENTS

Homeopathy I have seen an excellent success rate in patients who have used homeopathy to treat PCOS. Your practitioner will probably prescribe you Sepia or Lachesis in 30c potencies (usually twice daily), although your precise prescription will depend upon an individual consultation with the homeopath.

Acupuncture Small studies show that acupuncture may regulate periods and even induce ovulation. However, it appears less effective for women with high levels of androgens or who are overweight.

Aromatherapy Use aromatherapy to balance your hormones. Add 5 drops each of myrrh, fennel, and

Above: Saw palmetto (*Serenoa repens*)

clary sage essential oils to 6 tsp. carrier oil, such as sweet almond, and massage the blend into your stomach. Alternatively, add 5 drops of each to your bath water and soak in it for 20 minutes or so each night. Add in 5 drops lavender essential oil to aid relaxation, too.

SELF-HELP

Reduce stress You need to keep your stress levels down in your efforts to reduce your symptoms of PCOS. Try to achieve at least ten minutes a day of deep breathing. Alternatively, if you find sitting still and tuning out difficult, you could try the walking meditation in the box, below.

Get up and go If you carry weight around your waist, rather than around your hips, you're said to be "apple-shaped." This makes you more prone to type II diabetes and PCOS (see p.84). As a result, an abdominal weight-loss program should be an essential component in your natural treatment plan. One of the best ways to reduce abdominal fat is to combine a healthy diet with regular exercise. Try to exercise for 30 minutes at least three times a week (five times a week is the ideal). Activities such as running, swimming, and hiking are good. Find something that increases your heart rate enough so that you can hold a conversation but are a little breathless.

WALKING MEDITATION FOR PCOS

Daily relaxation is a key component in managing the effects of PCOS. I've chosen a walking meditation because I hope you'll be able to slot it into your lifestyle easily and so make relaxation part of every day. Ideally, practice the following with bare feet and try to make sure you practice in a place where you'll be undisturbed. If you can, stay mindful of every step as you take it.

1 Stand up straight and breathe deeply. Allow your arms to hang loosely by your sides. Close your eyes for a moment and feel your weight running down through you into your legs and into the floor. Feel the floor beneath your feet.

2 Open your eyes and gently focus in front of you. Make sure you don't strain or stare, simply allow your eyes to rest upon a point ahead. Pick up one foot to take your first step, focusing on the sensations that run through you, both in the leg you're using and the one on the ground. Feel the motion resonate through your whole body.

3 As you step the foot forward and down, focus on the sensations that this brings. Try to really experience the sensation as the foot makes contact again with the ground. Put your foot down purposefully: heel, ball, and toe.

4 Now move the other foot with the same level of mindfulness. If your mind wanders from the feeling of walking, refocus it on the minute sensations in your foot and work outward from there. Try not to look around; keep your gaze in front of you. Continue walking mindfully like this for as long as you feel absorbed by it.

Ovarian cysts

Not to be confused with the unruptured follicles that occur in polycystic ovary syndrome (PCOS), ovarian cysts are fluid-filled sacs that form in or on your ovaries and may be benign or malignant.

For many women, ovarian cysts are simply a by-product of their monthly cycle—and indeed doctors believe that such cysts are common. Often, the cysts are small, so show no symptoms and present no problems. They can even disappear of their own accord over time. You may never know that you had them, or you may discover them only when you have a scan for something else. Occasionally, however, the cysts are large and can rupture. This may cause abdominal pain and bloating, or you may experience spots of blood between your periods. Very occasionally, the cysts may be cancerous. Although rare, the possibility makes it vital that you visit your doctor if you experience any symptoms that concern you.

Natural medicine can provide wonderful, long-lasting relief from ovarian cysts, primarily by giving you the tools with which to balance your hormones. However, as ovarian cysts can be cancerous, it's important that you follow any natural healthcare program in conjunction with advice from your medical doctor.

TYPES OF OVARIAN CYST

There are two categories of ovarian cyst. They are functional cysts and abnormal cysts.

Functional cysts

As the name implies, functional cysts are caused by the abnormal functioning of the ovaries and are the most common kind of ovarian cyst. Cysts may form at any time in your cycle but are given different names according to when in the cycle your ovaries malfunction to cause them. As the first half of your cycle is called the follicular phase, cysts occurring at this stage are called follicular cysts. The second half is called the luteal phase and so may produce luteal cysts (sometimes called corpus luteum cysts).

The follicular phase is characterized by the gradual maturation of follicles on your ovary, one of which will usually release an egg. If the follicles fail to release an egg, and instead keep growing, filling up with fluid, you'll develop follicular cysts. If an egg is released, you enter the luteal phase. A luteal cyst forms when, instead of withering away, the follicular sac that once held the egg, seals up again and becomes engorged with blood and fluid. Sometimes a luteal cyst can twist the ovary and cause pain. If the cyst ruptures, you'll experience a sharp pain and have internal bleeding. You may need emergency surgery.

Abnormal cysts

These kinds of cyst come in three types: cystadenoma cysts (which develop from cells on the outer surface of the ovaries), endometrial cysts, and dermoid cysts. Dermoid cysts are classed as tumors because they are solid structures, filled with pieces of teeth, skin, hair and bone, rather than being filled with fluid. It's thought that dermoid cysts occur because an unfertilized egg starts to produce various body tissues.

A SIMPLE ultrasound scan can detect ovarian cysts.

Although they're caused by abnormal cell growth, abnormal cysts are not necessarily cancerous and in some cases they will not cause you any problems at all. However, if abnormal cysts rupture, or if the stem on which they have grown twists, you may be forced to have emergency surgery to remove the cyst. The symptoms of a burst cyst are pain in the lower abdomen, bleeding, or abdominal infection. A twisted cyst stem will cause severe pain and sometimes vomiting.

CAUSES

Research has yet to uncover why women develop abnormal ovarian cysts, but there are several risk factors we know about when it comes to the functional kind. Cysts are a natural by-product of ovulation every month, and every woman has the potential to get them. If you delay childbearing, you have more periods and so there is more chance that your ovaries will develop functional cysts. Pregnancy, breastfeeding, and even being on the Pill mean that your body has a "rest" from ovulation, which reduces your likelihood of functional cysts occurring. You're also more at risk if you're a smoker.

DIAGNOSIS

Pelvic examination The first thing your doctor will do to diagnose whether or not you have ovarian cysts will be to give you a combined internal and external pelvic examination. To do this, he or she will insert two fingers into your vagina and use the other hand to press on the outside of your lower abdomen. In this way, he or she can feel whether or not your ovaries and uterus are the right size and free of cysts or fibroids.

Ultrasound scan If, as a result of the pelvic examination, your doctor suspects you have ovarian cysts, he or she will refer you to a gynecologist for a pelvic ultrasound scan. By passing an ultrasound device over your abdomen or inserting it into your vagina, your doctor can find out where your cysts are, how many you have, and whether they're filled with fluid or more solid matter (and so more likely to be cancerous).

CONVENTIONAL TREATMENTS

As functional cysts are more likely than not to disappear of their own accord, your doctor will probably at first ask you to come back for a follow-up scan in a few months. This could show that your body has reabsorbed your cysts and they have gone. However, if the

OVARIAN CANCER: SYMPTOMS

One in 67 women in the USA suffers from ovarian cancer, making it the fifth most common cancer among women. Being aware of early warning signs can help early detection and improve your chances of a full recovery. If you experience any of the following symptoms, talk to your doctor immediately:

• General abdominal or pelvic discomfort and/or pain (gas, indigestion, nausea, pressure, swelling, bloating, cramps)
• Constant diarrhea and/or constipation
• Urinary frequency or urgency
• Loss of appetite
• Unexplained weight loss or weight gain
• Pain during intercourse
• Irregular periods or abnormal bleeding from your vagina
• Overwhelming fatigue
• Lower back pain

Be aware that symptoms of ovarian cancer can be similar to those of digestive disorders. However, with a digestive disorder your symptoms will come and go, whereas with ovarian cancer they will be unrelenting, worsening over time.

cysts persist, your doctor will probably suggest treatment that suppresses ovulation. If your cysts are abnormal, he or she will probably suggest surgery.

The contraceptive pill Cysts form as a result of your body's natural process of ovulation. If you can prevent ovulation, such as by taking the Pill, your body won't form cysts. However, bear in mind that the temporary cessation of your cycle in this way won't fix the root of the problem.

Surgery Abnormal cysts may develop into ovarian cancer (see box, p.89), so your doctor will probably advise a laparoscopy to remove them. A laparoscopy is performed in the hospital under general anaesthetic. The cyst isn't cut away, but instead a doctor collapses it by suctioning out from it any fluid or solid mass. Find a gynecologist whose aim is to remove your cyst but not your ovary. If your cyst is very large, the partial or total removal of your ovary may be unavoidable. Unfortunately, the chances are that no one will know until the surgery is taking place. For this reason, make your wish to save your ovary (if at all possible) clear to your surgeon before surgery begins.

YOUR DIET

Functional cysts are the result of hormonal imbalance, so it's crucial that if you suffer from them, you follow the hormone-balancing diet (see box, p.57). The diet also helps boost your body's natural processes of detoxification, which will in turn encourage your body to control abnormal cell growth. This means that the diet is also essential if you have abnormal cysts.

In addition, make a real effort to boost your intake of antioxidants, which help clear free radicals (see p.28) from your body. Free radicals are unstable atoms that can cause abnormal cell growth, which in turn can lead to cell mutation and cancer. Antioxidant-rich foods include leafy green vegetables and all foods that contain lots of vitamin C, such as citrus fruits (oranges, grapefruit, and so on), kiwi fruit, and green beans.

SUPPLEMENTS

■ B-COMPLEX (containing 25mg of each B-vitamin, daily) The B-vitamins help detoxify any "old" or excess estrogen in your body, and this, in turn, improves overall hormone balance.

■ VITAMIN C with bioflavonoids (1,000mg, daily, as magnesium ascorbate) This crucial antioxidant helps fight free-radical damage and is vital for boosting your immunity.

■ ZINC (15mg, daily) Your body needs zinc to ensure the normal development of eggs within your ovaries, and it also helps protect your body against damage by free radicals.

HERBS

■ ECHINACEA (*Echinacea purpurea*) This well-known immunity-booster helps improve the number of white blood cells (which are the cells that fight foreign invaders or other abnormal cells) in your body. Echinacea is more effective when you take the herb non-continually—that is, with breaks. So, take it for ten days, stop taking it for three days, and then take it again for another ten days. When taking it, take 1 tsp. tincture in a little water, two or three times daily; or take 300–400mg in capsule form, twice daily.

■ FALSE UNICORN ROOT (*Chaemaelirium luteum*) This adaptogenic herb helps regulate your body's hormones and the cycle of changes that take place in your ovaries. Take 1 tsp. tincture in a little water, twice daily; or take 600–900mg in capsule form, daily.

■ GARLIC (*Allium sativum*) This common cooking herb has a protective effect on the body's cells. A particularly good garlic supplement is "aged garlic." Take 1,000mg, daily. Alternatively, you could aim to eat two to five cloves of raw or cooked garlic a week.

■ MILK THISTLE (*Silymarin marianum*) This well-known liver tonic can boost the body's ability to detoxify. Milk thistle encourages the body to excrete excess hormones and destroy abnormal cells. Take 1 tsp. tincture in a little water, twice daily; or take 200–400mg in capsule form, daily.

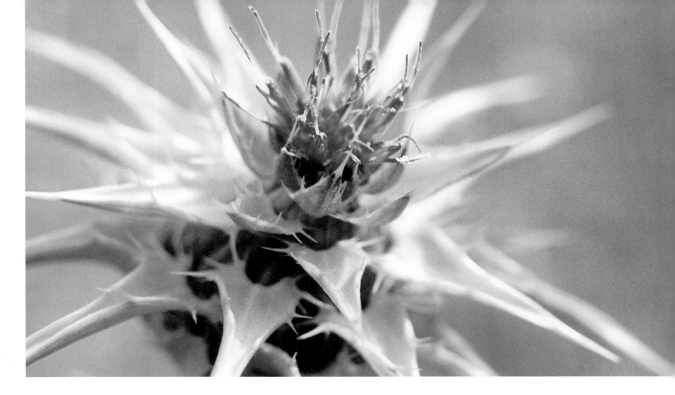

Above: Milk thistle (*Silymarin marianum*)

OTHER NATURAL TREATMENTS

Acupuncture An acupuncturist will treat your body for hormone imbalance (working on your endocrine and reproductive systems) and try to regulate or induce ovulation, as required. If you have specific symptoms of ovarian cysts, such as bloating, the acupuncturist will aim to treat those, too. In my experience, acupuncture has had varying degrees of success for treating functional cysts, and I think it's certainly worth trying if you've had success with acupuncture in the past.

Aromatherapy If you have to have surgery, to speed healing and reduce any scarring, try a blend of lavender, sage, and rosemary essential oils, diluted in a carrier oil such as sweet almond (use a dilution of 15 drops of essential oil per 6 tsp. of carrier oil), applied to the site of the wound once a day for two weeks.

SELF-HELP

If you have suffered from cysts in the past, focus your treatment on prevention so the cysts don't come back.

As well as the nutritional and supplementation advice, try the following recommendations.

Don't use talcum powder This applies specifically to on or around your genitals. Anything you put on your genitals can make its way into your vagina, uterus, Fallopian tubes, and ovaries. Some experts believe talcum powder can increase your risk of developing ovarian cancer.

Quit smoking Research shows that women who smoke are one and a half times more likely to suffer from ovarian cysts than non-smokers. There's no other way to put it—quit if you want to protect your fertility and your overall health.

Avoid alcohol All toxins are bad for your hormone levels, and alcohol is a toxin. Keep your intake low—this means, not more than one glass of wine (or equivalent) a day. If you can abstain from alcohol altogether, so much the better.

YOUR UTERUS

The uterus's impact on "womanhood" is perhaps greater than that of any other organ. From your first period to pregnancy and menopause, life constantly reminds you of this most significant part of yourself.

As you already know, your uterus is an incredibly dynamic organ that can expand dramatically to host a full-term pregnancy and then shrink back to just the size of a pear (see pp.14–15). It's the heart of new life.

Every month, over the course of your menstrual cycle, the two innermost layers of your uterus go through several changes. In the weeks leading up to your period, as levels of estrogen rise in your blood (thanks to your ovaries), the lining of your uterus (the endometrium) and the layer of uterine muscle (the myometrium) begin to thicken and grow. They are thickest and engorged with blood vessels to nourish and sustain a fetus immediately after ovulation.

If fertilization does not occur, the levels of estrogen and progesterone in your blood decrease, which causes the uterus to shed its lining of blood and tissue through the cervix and vagina during menstruation.

Unfortunately, like all sophisticated equipment, your uterus may malfunction. Among the problems you could face are benign growths, called fibroids, which can cause pain and bleeding; endometriosis, a condition in which the tissue that forms the lining of the uterus grows outside it; bleeding problems; and prolapse, in which the uterus dips down from its normal position causing pain and discomfort. The conventional, most dramatic method for treating serious problems with the uterus is a hysterectomy (see pp.128–31), surgery to remove the uterus. However, I feel very strongly that in many cases surgery is entirely avoidable and you can treat problems with your uterus perfectly effectively with the natural approach.

TAKING CARE OF YOUR UTERUS

Like all organs in your body, your uterus needs optimum nutrition and hormone balance to function efficiently and have healthy cells. Even when you don't have a specific problem to treat, to this end you should follow the hormone-balancing diet (see box, p.57) and take herbal remedies such as raspberry leaf (*Rubus idaeus*) and pennyroyal (*Mentha pulegium*), both of which help your uterus. You can also take herbs and supplements that have beneficial effects on your hormone levels. Agnus castus (*Vitex agnus castus*), milk thistle (*Silybum marianum*), and dandelion (*Taraxacum officinale*), as well as the B-vitamins and omega-3 fatty acids are all great for hormonal balance (and come up time and again throughout this section).

Cut down on your caffeine intake and try to steer clear of mucus-producing foods, such as dairy products and red meats, as they contribute to tissue congestion and inhibit your uterus's ability to cleanse itself. Alcohol also negatively affects the uterus by contributing to inflammatory problems and interfering with your liver's ability to remove estrogen.

Finally, I urge you to get to know your body and watch for the signals it sends you. It goes almost without saying that your uterus is a fundamental piece of the puzzle when it comes to your menstrual cycle and your fertility. Learn what is "normal" for you and, if you need to, keep a written diary of your cycle, level of bleeding, and so on. If you show any signs of unusual bleeding or experience any unusual menstrual-like pain, let your doctor know about it right away.

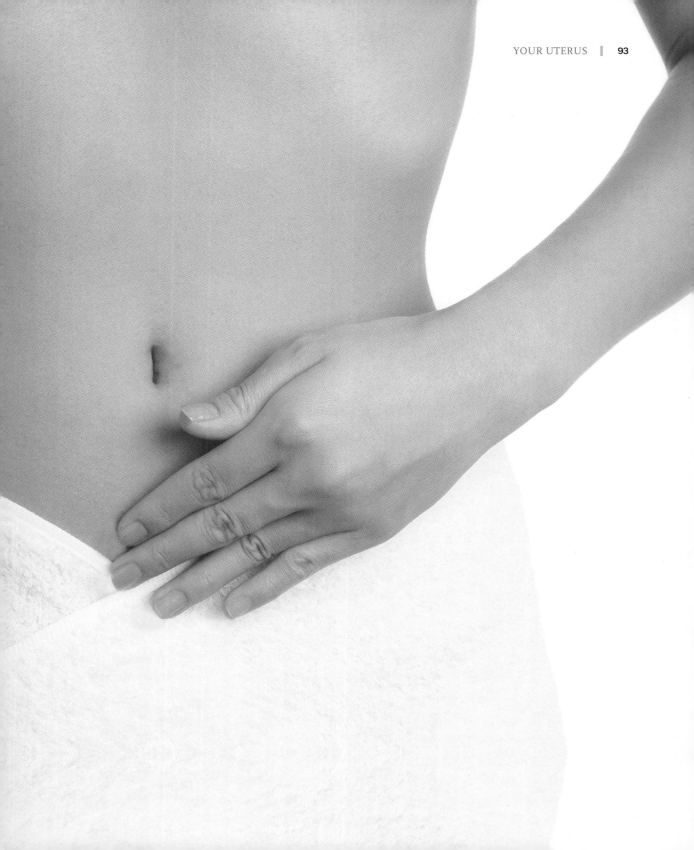

Regulating your cycle

Your menstrual cycle is a reflection of your overall well-being. Regular periods indicate your uterus is healthy, your hormones are balanced, and your body is getting the food, exercise, and sleep it needs.

I think making sure your cycles are regular is step one towards ensuring you're in general good health. To do this, you need to understand what "regular" means.

WHAT IS REGULAR?

It's a common misconception that a menstrual cycle should last for 28 days. Regular cycles can vary from 23 to 35 days, and they're considered regular if your periods occur over roughly the same number of days each cycle. Ovulation occurs about 14 to 16 days before menstruation, not 14 days after menstruation starts. The second half of the cycle—from ovulation to menstruation—is typically the same length, but the first part may vary from cycle to cycle. So if your periods always appear, for example, around day 24, they would be classed as normal. Irregular periods, on the other hand, can be difficult to predict. There may be long gaps between them, or they may come too frequently; or you may have gaps of no periods at all, followed by continuous bleeding for a few weeks as well as spotting in between periods.

I want to reassure you that minor or occasional cycle irregularities are common for most women because dieting, travel, stress, exercise, and seasonal changes can all have an effect on your period. It's perfectly normal to have erratic cycles on the run-up to menopause, too. However, if you aren't approaching menopause and experience irregular menstrual patterns for more than three cycles in a row, follow all the advice in this section to try to restore some balance—and please visit your doctor. He or she will be able to rule out any medical cause, such as polycystic ovary syndrome, a build-up of your uterine lining, fibroids, or an infection. In rare cases, irregular periods can be a symptom of uterine or cervical cancer, and they may also be caused by certain medications, such as corticosteroids. Let your doctor investigate what's going on.

YOUR DIET

The first stop for anyone experiencing irregular periods has to be the hormone-balancing diet (see box, p.57). In particular, stock up on the phytoestrogens (see p.31), which help control levels of excess estrogen in your blood, and on fiber, which optimizes the transportation of waste products (including "old" estrogens) out of your body. Reduce your intake of saturated fat, which can raise levels of estrogen in your body.

If there can be a "star" food for regulating your hormones and your cycle, I think it's flax seeds, which contain good phytoestrogens, as well as omega-3 and omega-6 essential fatty acids. Use ground, organic flax seeds and sprinkle them over your food. I like to eat them added to my morning oatmeal.

While being the right weight for your height is certainly good for your well-being, avoid crash dieting or fad diets because losing weight rapidly may cause erratic periods or stop them completely. If you're overweight, following the hormone-balancing diet should restore your natural weight gently and without a shock to your system. If obesity has caused your periods to stop, losing weight slowly can trigger ovulation. As with everything in life, balance is the key.

SUPPLEMENTS

- B-COMPLEX (containing 25mg of each B-vitamin, daily) The B-vitamins can boost your body's ability to cope with stress and are important for thyroid and adrenal function, which can affect your menstrual cycle.

- MAGNESIUM (300mg, daily) This calming mineral helps your body cope better with the effects of stress.

- ANTIOXIDANTS (see below for dosages) These nutrients protect your cells from free radicals, and they are extremely important if endometrial hyperplasia (excess uterine lining; see box, p.125) has caused your irregular periods. Vitamins A, C, and E and the minerals zinc and selenium are all antioxidants. Find an antioxidant supplement that contains, or take separately, the following: vitamin A (2,500iu, daily), vitamin C (500mg, twice daily, as magnesium ascorbate), vitamin E (400iu, daily), selenium (100µg, daily), and zinc (15–25mg, daily).

- OMEGA-3 FATTY ACIDS (1,000mg fish-oil containing 500mg DHA, daily) DHA has been shown to lower levels of estrogen in the body. (Use flax seed oil if you're vegetarian.)

HERBS
For your hormones

- AGNUS CASTUS (*Vitex agnus castus*) This herb works on the action of your pituitary gland to restore hormonal balance. Take 1 tsp. tincture in a little water, or 200–300mg in capsule form, twice daily.

- FALSE UNICORN ROOT (*Chamaelirium luteum*) This herb helps normalize ovarian function. Take 1 tsp. tincture in a little water, twice daily; or 600–900mg in capsule form, daily.

For stress

If your irregular periods are stress-related, take the hormone-regulating herbs (above), as well as:

- SIBERIAN GINSENG (*Eleutherococcus senticosus*) This herb is an adrenal tonic. Take 1 tsp. tincture in a little water twice daily; or a 250–300mg capsule daily.

- VALERIAN (*Valeriana officinalis*) and SKULLCAP (*Scutellaria lateriflora*) Take 1 tsp. each tincture in a little water twice daily; or a 300mg capsule of each daily.

SELF-HELP

Exercise Regular, moderate exercise is great for hormone balance as well as for your heart and weight loss. However, don't do too much too vigorously because extreme exercise can cause your periods to become irregular or to stop altogether. Aim for between 30 and 60 minutes daily of moderate exercise, such as walking, cycling, swimming, or even gardening.

Cut out alcohol Try to eliminate alcohol from your lifestyle completely as it severely upsets the function of your liver, meaning that you can develop estrogen excess, which in turn can unsettle the good hormones in your body and encourage the growth of fibroids.

Limit stress When you're under physical or emotional stress your body releases hormones that interfere with ovulation. This is nature's way of saving you from pregnancy when you would find it hard to cope. If you're under severe stress, perhaps through bereavement or divorce, your periods may stop altogether. Go to your doctor—if there's no physical cause for your menstrual irregularities, take it as a clear warning sign that you need to take time out to relax. Examine your life carefully—what's causing the stress? What steps can you take to overcome it? If it's a job situation, perhaps you need to rethink your work–life balance; if it's a bereavement or divorce, consider going to a counselor, or seeking the support of a good friend to talk things through with.

Make a point of taking time out every day, even if it's just for ten minutes, to spend time in quiet contemplation. If walking or swimming relax you, all the better, because the gentle nature of these activities will release endorphins in your system to lift mood, too. You could also treat yourself to a weekly massage or use essential oils in your bath (lavender is a great relaxer). Find what works best for you. Finally, remember to take those stress-busting supplements and herbs (see p.310). You should find that as your stress ebbs away, so your periods become more regular.

Premenstrual syndrome (PMS)

You feel bloated and achy, and your breasts are tender. You're tired and keep craving sweet food. Even worse, you feel like you'll lose your temper if anyone upsets you. All these are classic symptoms of PMS.

If symptoms of PMS affect you, you're not alone—nine out of ten women of childbearing age have them. Your symptoms may be so bad that they affect your home life and work, and may even to lead to depression.

SYMPTOMS

The term premenstrual syndrome (sometimes referred to as premenstrual tension) has come to mean many different things: A staggering 150 symptoms are now believed to form part of the condition. These symptoms tend to fall into one of two categories: emotional or physical. Among the most common emotional symptoms are dramatic shifts in mood, irritability, worry, tension, fatigue, tearfulness, and depression. Physical symptoms usually include bloating and water retention, sore or tender breasts that may feel swollen or lumpy, spotty skin (or even acne), weight gain, headaches or migraines, cravings for sweet foods, constipation, and feelings of lightheadedness.

PMS affects every woman in a different way—and although we've talked about the negative symptoms, sometimes the effects aren't all bad. Some women find that in the run up to their period they experience a burst of creativity or productivity. And one of my patients told me she didn't want to get rid of her PMS symptoms because that's when she took everything back to the stores to complain!

CAUSES

No one knows for sure what causes PMS, although lowered levels of progesterone in relation to estrogen, as part of your normal, monthly hormonal fluctuations, are suggested by some experts to cause some of the symptoms, such as mood swings. High levels of stress and a poor diet also seem to have an effect.

It's these latter triggers that I think provide the key to dealing with PMS because these will upset your hormone balance. If this is the case, correcting the lifestyle triggers should produce a vast improvement in your body's response to your menstrual cycle, reducing the symptoms of PMS.

DIAGNOSIS

Although it's easy to focus on lists of symptoms, it's important to look at the full picture. A diagnosis of PMS relies not just upon which of the 150 or so symptoms you have, but the point in your cycle when you have them. If your symptoms occur frequently—say, for at least two out of three menstrual cycles—and they always occur in the second half of your cycle (the luteal phase, after ovulation), and if you're symptom-free for one or two weeks after your period starts, then a diagnosis of PMS is likely.

CONVENTIONAL TREATMENTS

The following are the most common medications prescribed to women who suffer from PMS.

Ovulation suppressors The contraceptive pill, danazol (a weak male hormone), and GnRH analogues all have the effect of suppressing ovulation by various hormonal actions on the body, and you may be

WHO GETS PMS?

While the causes of PMS still evade us, there are several circumstances that we know seem to predispose women to the condition. So, you're more likely to suffer from PMS if you're between the ages of 30 and 50, or if you've had more than one child, have given birth recently, had a termination or miscarriage, or have had several pregnancies in quick succession. PMS also appears to run in families, so if your mother suffered from the condition, you're more likely to suffer from it, too.

prescribed any one of these. However, they all also have unwelcome side-effects, including some of the symptoms of PMS itself, such as mood swings, and menopausal-like symptoms, such as hot flashes. Your doctor may suggest you wear estrogen patches, which some women find offer relief from symptoms. However, I urge you to bear in mind that these are basically hormone replacement therapy (HRT), which carries with it some serious side-effects (see pp.249–51).

Progesterone supplements Some experts believe that PMS may result from low levels of progesterone in the second half of your cycle, so your doctor may prescribe a synthetic form (known as progestin or progestogen) of this hormone. It'll raise your progesterone levels to reduce your symptoms. In the USA, women are able to buy (literally over the counter) what's known as "bioidentical" progesterone—that is, progesterone that is chemically identical to the progesterone produced in your ovaries. It's usually available as a cream or a pessary. (In the UK, bioidentical progesterone

IT CAN TAKE UP to five years to get a diagnosis of PMS.

has to be prescribed by a doctor.) However, to make things really clear, although bioidentical hormones match the chemical structure of the natural versions, they're still powerful hormonal drugs. Taking a synthetic hormone is not the same as using a wholly natural herb to balance your hormones.

Specific symptom relief If you suffer from PMS-related breast pain, your doctor may prescribe the drug bromocriptine. Its side-effects include nausea, vomiting, and headaches, and I personally think its effects are too strong to justify its prescription for PMS symptoms alone. For help with bloating, your doctor may give you diuretics, which help your body to flush away fluids—and vital nutrients, too.

Surgery In my opinion, surgery is the most drastic option your doctor could recommend to treat PMS. The logic is that if you don't have a menstrual cycle, you can't have PMS. In order to prevent the cycle, a doctor can suggest removing your ovaries. However, doing so sends you into immediate menopause, which means you'd then have to take estrogen-only HRT to protect your bones (see p.251). Please make sure you've considered all the options—including the natural approach—before you consider this serious surgery.

Because the causes of PMS elude us, conventional medicine tends to relieve only its symptoms—if you take medication for PMS and then stop, your symptoms will return. For this reason alone, I urge you to try my natural methods first. With nutrition, herbal, and lifestyle approaches, you can treat not only the symptoms but also the causes (even the ones we don't know about yet!), for long-lasting relief. Many of my patients have eliminated their PMS symptoms completely using my natural approach. You should allow three months to see the full effects, but you should start to see an improvement after even one cycle.

YOUR DIET

If you want to eliminate PMS, the most important thing you can do is to follow the hormone-balancing diet (see box, p.57), and, in particular, take steps to balance your blood sugar. This means cutting out refined sugar and refined carbohydrates, eliminating alcohol, and eating six small meals a day (including three healthy snacks, such as a handful of nuts), always with a little protein, to keep your energy levels stable. Balancing your blood sugar reduces the strain on your adrenal glands, which, when overloaded, can upset the balance of progesterone in the latter part of your cycle.

Foods to treat PMS symptoms

The hormone-balancing diet will increase your intake of unrefined whole carbohydrates (brown rice, oats, and so on), which will help balance your blood sugar and encourage your body's production of serotonin, a natural feel-good hormone that can make you feel brighter and happier (improving dark moods) and also reduce your cravings for certain foods.

To combat water retention or bloating, limit your intake of salt and fatty foods and drink plenty of pure water, or juice or herbal tea. If you don't drink enough, your body thinks there is a drought and tries to retain any water you have, storing it in your tissues and contributing to water retention. Aim for six to eight cups of healthy fluids a day. This means that sugary, sweet drinks don't count. Nor do drinks containing caffeine (including black and green tea), which are diuretic and will worsen the PMS symptoms of breast tenderness and pain if you suffer from them.

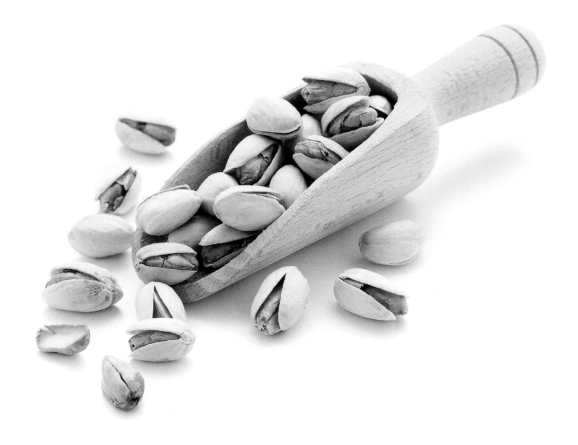

SUPPLEMENTS

Providing your body with the right levels of nutrients can help relieve many of the most debilitating symptoms of PMS. Take good-quality versions (see p.320) of the following.

- VITAMIN B6 (50mg, daily) Many studies indicate that vitamin B6 shows promise in the treatment of PMS-related symptoms, but a combination of magnesium (see right) and B6 together is even more effective. (In fact, a good daily multi-vitamin and mineral supplement should provide both these vital nutrients.) Make sure you take B6 as pyridoxal-5-phosphate (P-5-P) rather than pyridoxine (the cheaper form, found in many supplements). P-5-P is the active form of vitamin B6, saving your body the job of converting the inactive form (pyridoxine).

- VITAMIN E (400iu, daily) Vitamin E will help treat breast problems, mood swings, and irritability. Take the vitamin as d-alpha tocopherol.

- MAGNESIUM (200mg, daily) This vital nutrient is often deficient in women who suffer from PMS. Magnesium is a calming nutrient, having a relaxing effect on the nervous system, including easing menstrual headaches and migraines. Take magnesium as magnesium citrate, or amino acid chelate.

- ZINC (25mg, daily) This important mineral plays a major part in balancing your sex hormones and women with PMS are often deficient in it.

- EVENING PRIMROSE OIL (150mg GLA, daily) Evening primrose oil is a source of gamma linolenic acid (GLA), an essential fat that according to some studies is effective in reducing PMS-related breast tenderness—although other research has shown no effect at all. The most positive results happened when women were also taking a multi. I've noticed that women need to take evening primrose oil for three months before they see any effects.

HERBS

The following herbs help balance hormones and ease symptoms of PMS. You should be able to get good combined herbal supplements that include agnus castus, black cohosh, and skull-cap (as well as perhaps milk thistle) from your local natural pharmacy, or order one online (see p.320 for sources). Alternatively, take them individually in the dosages below.

- AGNUS CASTUS (*Vitex agnus castus*) This hormonal wonder-herb helps stimulate and normalize the function of your pituitary gland. One study in the *British Medical Journal* stated that agnus castus is an "effective and well-tolerated treatment" for PMS, specifically. Furthermore, in studies comparing the anti-depressant effects of agnus castus against those of conventional medication in cases of PMS, the results were almost the same. Take 1 tsp. tincture in a little water, or 200–300mg in capsule form, twice daily.

- BLACK COHOSH (*Cimicifuga racemosa*) With its calming effect on the nervous system and balancing effect on the hormones, black cohosh may be helpful if you suffer from anxiety, tension, depression, and premenstrual headaches. Take 1 tsp. tincture in a little water, twice daily; or 250–350mg in capsule form, daily.

- DANDELION (*Taraxacum officinale*) A liver tonic and natural diuretic, dandelion helps flush out excess fluid to relieve bloating but doesn't flush out nutrients at the same time. Take 1 tsp. tincture in a little water,

twice daily; or 200–400mg in capsule form, daily.

- DONG QUAI (*Angelica sinensis*) This herb can help promote normal hormone balance and prevent muscle spasm, so reducing abdominal cramping. Take 1 tsp. tincture in a little water, or 300mg in capsule form, twice daily.

- SKULLCAP (*Scutellaria lateriflora*) Another herb good for the nervous system (so helpful for symptoms of anxiety) is skullcap. Take 1 tsp. tincture in a little water, twice daily; or 300–600mg in capsule form, daily.

OTHER NATURAL TREATMENTS

Homeopathy The following homeopathic remedies have a good track record for treating the symptoms of PMS. Take them 24 hours before your symptoms usually begin. Use a 30c dilution every 12 hours for up to three days, unless your homeopath advises otherwise (a constitutional-based treatment is always best).
• Causticum when you get pains in your lower abdomen and feel the need to urinate frequently
• Lachesis for tender breasts
• Nat mur for breast pain, depression, and bloating
• Sepia when you feel tearful and crave comfort food.

Acupuncture and osteopathy Both these natural therapies have been shown to be effective at treating the symptoms of PMS. You'll need to see a specialist practitioner in each for individual treatments.

Aromatherapy Essential oils can help with problems such as hormonal imbalance, impaired liver function, stress, and poor sleep. Use the oils most relevant to your symptoms from the list below. Add five drops of each oil, up to three at a time, to your bath water, or add 15 drops of oil per 6 tsp. of sweet almond oil to use in a massage (over the abdomen is best for PMS).
• Clary sage to lift mood and balance your hormones
• Fennel and rosemary for water retention
• Jasmine to ease depression, tension, and anxiety
• Juniper to ease bloating and detoxify the liver (so balancing your hormones)
• Grapefruit to ease constipation and headaches
• Geranium to cool and regulate your system, easing depression and anxiety
• Bergamot and Roman or German chamomile to reduce depression and ease irritability
• Lavender to reduce tension, balance the whole body system, and improve sleep, if your sleep is affected.

Reflexology Various studies prove the effectiveness of reflexology in the treatment of PMS, and many women report feeling calmer and finding it easier to stay in control when they're having reflexology treatments. At home, try the reflexology exercise opposite.

SELF-HELP

Keep a journal If your problems occur always in the second half of your cycle, you almost certainly have PMS, but it may also be useful to keep a symptom journal to rule out any other possible causes. It's important to get to know your body. If you encounter any unusual or erratic variations, tell your doctor.

Take care of your liver Follow my recommendations for improving liver function (see box, p.43), so your liver can efficiently eliminate "old" hormones during each cycle. This is particularly important if you suffer from premenstrual or menstrual migraines and/or premenstrual headaches.

Stay active Exercise is particularly beneficial for women who suffer from premenstrual stress, anxiety, and depression because exercise releases brain chemicals called endorphins. These help us to feel happier, more alert, and calmer. Try to exercise for at least 30 minutes a day. Anything that raises your heart rate a little is worthwhile.

Beat stress During times of stress, your adrenal glands release the hormone adrenaline, and this prepares your body to fight or flee from danger. When this happens during the luteal phase (latter half) of your cycle, the adrenaline inhibits the body's ability to use progesterone, leading to hormonal imbalance. I advise my patients to make time for dedicated relaxation at least twice weekly. See p.311 for ideas on how.

Come off the Pill If your symptoms get worse when you're on the Pill, make an appointment with your doctor to discuss another form of contraception. In your case the medication is causing your PMS, not your natural cycle. (Never take herbs if you're on the Pill unless you're supervised by a qualified herbal practitioner.)

REFLEXOLOGY FOR PMS

In one study, women with PMS were given either "real" reflexology (pressure applied to the reflex points) or a "placebo" foot massage, which avoided the reflex points. The women getting the "real" reflexology showed improvement far quicker than the placebo group. Practice the following exercise every day in the week running up to your period.

1 Sit comfortably so that you can reach your feet easily. Take off your shoes and socks or tights. Relax both your feet by wiggling your toes and consciously letting tension ebb out of them. Rub the centers of your feet beneath the balls, using the heel of your hand.

2 Find the pancreas reflexes (these help control blood sugar), which lie on the inside edge of the sole of your right foot and about half way down the center of your left foot (see below). Use the side of your thumb to rub the area.

3 Still using your thumb, rub the kidney reflexes, which lie about halfway down each sole in the center of your feet. This will help relieve water retention (bloating).

4 Working on the adrenal points helps with mineral balance, renews energy, and releases a natural form of cortisone, which can help reduce swelling (good if you get painful breasts or cramping). Using the top of your thumb, apply pressure to the point on the inside soles of both feet, just above the halfway point, about ½in. in from the edge of the foot.

5 Finally, to ease headaches and irritability, massage your two big toes, pulling each of them gently to extend them outward.

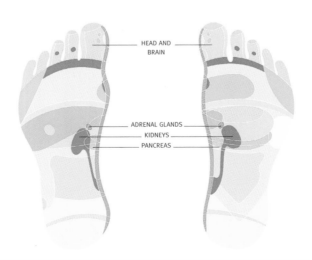

HEAD AND
BRAIN

ADRENAL GLANDS
KIDNEYS
PANCREAS

Period pain

Known medically as dysmenorrhea, period pain is caused by substances called prostaglandins. Many prostaglandins are healthy, but some are unhealthy and can increase your sensitivity to pain.

Around ten percent of the women who suffer from period pain (and about half of us do) describe their pain as severe, starting anything from one hour to a day before a period begins and typically lasting for around 24 hours.

In all types of period pain, from the mild to the severe, cells in your uterine lining release unhealthy (or "bad") prostaglandins when the uterine lining begins to shed during your period. This release stimulates your uterus to contract. If you have high levels of "bad" prostaglandins, these natural muscular contractions will become painful.

A woman typically gets period pain only when she is ovulating normally, so the good news is that cramping is usually a sign that there's nothing wrong with your cycle. In some instances, though, your period pain may be as a result of another condition, in which case it is known medically as secondary dysmenorrhea. The conditions that can cause cramping tend to be more serious than simple period pain itself and include fibroids (see pp.114–15) and endometriosis (see pp.118–19). As a result, if you suffer from period pain, particularly if your period pain is severe and it is accompanied by heavy or prolonged bleeding, it's important to visit your doctor to have these other conditions ruled out.

CONVENTIONAL TREATMENTS

Most conventional medical help for dealing with period pain is fairly limited because it treats the symptoms (the pain), but not the cause (the "bad" prostaglandins). If you don't take your medication, your symptoms will return.

Painkillers The most likely treatment your doctor will offer you is a painkiller, such as ibuprofen. Be aware, however, that taking painkillers can cause stomach upset and nausea.

The contraceptive pill Because the Pill leaves you with no real period, you experience no pain. However, headaches and breast tenderness may occur.

YOUR DIET

What you eat can decrease or increase the levels of "bad" prostaglandins in your system. The hormone-balancing diet in the box on page 57 should become your staple diet. In particular, cut down on caffeine (in coffee, tea, and chocolate) and saturated fat (mainly in dairy and animal products) because they encourage the body to produce bad prostaglandins. Also, increase the amount of essential fats in your diet, from foods such as oily fish, as well as nuts and seeds. You body needs essential fats to produce good prostaglandins to counteract the bad.

Although it's unclear why, heavy or spicy meals can sometimes contribute to period pain. In the week running up to your period, keep your diet light and spice-free to see if this helps relieve the cramping.

UP TO 50 PERCENT of all women suffer from pain during their period.

SUPPLEMENTS

I strongly recommend you take a good-quality multi-vitamin and mineral every day (see p.320). The dosages below are total daily dosages, including anything in your multi. So, if the multi contains 100mg magnesium, you need to add in a separate supplement containing only 200mg magnesium per day—the same principle applies for all the other vitamins and minerals.

■ B-COMPLEX (containing 25mg of each B-vitamin, daily) Your body needs vitamin B6 to produce good prostaglandins and studies show that vitamin B6, B1, and B12 significantly reduce the intensity of period pain.

■ VITAMIN C with bioflavonoids (1,000mg, twice daily, as magnesium ascorbate) Vitamin C is an antioxidant that may ease period pain in the same way as vitamin E (see below).

■ VITAMIN E (400iu, daily) This vitamin has antioxidant properties that can help control the levels of bad prostaglandins in your system, which is why studies show that women who take vitamin E have reduced painful periods. Take it as d-alpha tocopherol.

■ MAGNESIUM (300mg, daily) This mineral acts as a muscle relaxant. Take it as magnesium citrate.

■ ZINC (15mg, daily) Your body uses zinc (as well as magnesium and vitamin B6) to convert omega-3 and -6 essential fatty acids into beneficial prostaglandins.

■ BROMELAIN (500mg, three times daily between meals, making 1,500mg per day) This enzyme (found naturally in pineapples) has anti-inflammatory properties, helping to ease pain. It also acts as a muscle relaxant.

■ OMEGA-3 FATTY ACIDS (1,000mg fish oil containing at least 700mg EPA and 500mg DHA, daily) Omega-3 oils (or essential fatty acids) are vital nutrients that provide the raw materials for the production of good prostaglandins, which is why you should both increase them in your diet (see opposite) and take a supplement.

HERBS
For uterine function

The following two herbs in particular have a wonderful ability to normalize the functioning of your uterus in the long term. Take them throughout the month and then stop when the pain starts (you can continue black cohosh for pain relief, too; see below). Start them again when your period is over.

■ BLACK COHOSH (*Cimicifuga racemosa*) Black cohosh has a relaxant effect on the uterus. Take 1 tsp. tincture in a little water, two or three times daily; or 250–300mg in capsule form, daily. You can also take this herb as short-term pain relief.

■ DONG QUAI (*Angelica sinensis*) This herb improves the circulation to your uterus and acts as a natural painkiller. It can also regulate your body's production of bad prostaglandins. Take 1 tsp. tincture in a little water, or 300mg in capsule form, twice daily.

For pain relief

For short-term relief, take the following herbs as soon as the pain begins and stop when it subsides.

■ BLACK HAW (*Viburnum prunifolium*) and CRAMPBARK (*Viburnum opulus*) Both these herbs help relax the muscles of the uterus. Take both as tinctures (1 tsp. of each in a little water, twice daily) or in capsule form (600mg of both, daily). Alternatively, you could make a crampbark decoction. Boil a small piece of the bark in a cup of water for ten minutes. Strain the liquid into a cup and allow to cool before drinking. You can take one cup of decoction up to five times daily to relieve cramping.

■ SKULLCAP (*Scutellaria laterifolia*) This herb helps relieve muscle spasms in the uterus. Take 1 tsp. tincture in a little water, twice daily; or 600mg in capsule form, daily.

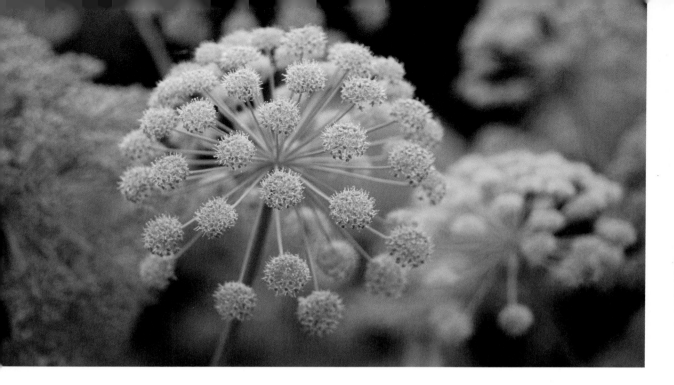

Above: Dong quai (*Angelica Sinensis*; see Herbs, p.103)

OTHER NATURAL TREATMENTS

Homeopathy A homeopath will usually prescribe the following for period pain, as well as others suited to your constitutional type. Take a 30c potency as relevant, twice daily for up to three days during your period.
• Belladonna for throbbing, harsh menstrual pain accompanied by a particularly heavy period
• Chamomilla to treat deep, dragging period pain.

Acupuncture Some small studies in the USA have revealed that acupuncture can reduce the need for medication to relieve period pain, sometimes totally. An acupuncturist will first investigate the spleen and liver meridians, where blocked *qi* causes period pain.

Aromatherapy The essential oils of rose, marjoram, and rosemary encourage the body to relax, helping you cope better with period pain. Use up to 5 drops of each of these oils diluted in 6 tsp. sweet almond oil for an abdominal massage (see box, opposite). Another good combination for massage is 5 drops each of clary sage (don't use this if you've drunk any alcohol in the preceeding 12 hours), geranium, and cypress essential oils in 6 tsp. sweet almond oil. For a gentler effect, add a few drops of any of these oils to a bath.

SELF-HELP

Move it Regular exercise can help keep cramps to a minimum because it releases endorphins, which are natural painkillers. Aim to exercise for at least 30 minutes a day—walking or swimming are gentle and won't place a strain on your uterus. Alternatively, try pelvic rocking, which helps relieve the pressure on the blood vessels in the area around the uterus and also helps strengthen the abdominal muscles and those of the lower back. Try it two or three times a day during a painful period. Position yourself on your hands and knees with your hands directly under your shoulders and your knees directly under your hips. Take a deep breath and then while exhaling slowly, pull in your abdomen, tighten your buttocks and pull up your pelvic floor muscles. This lifts up the spine to form a "C" shape. Release, and return to the start position with your spine flat. Repeat the lift at least ten times.

SOOTHING ABDOMINAL MASSAGE

This abdominal massage will help soothe away cramping period pains. You can practice it sitting, standing, or lying down. If you want to lie down, place a pillow under your knees to avoid back strain. Most importantly of all, make sure you're comfortable.

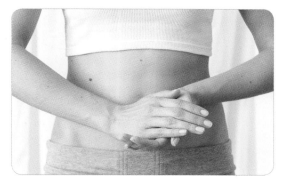

1 Put a little of your chosen massage blend (see opposite) into the palm of one hand and rub your hands together to warm the oil.

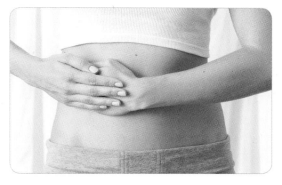

2 Place one hand on top of the other, palms down, above your belly button. Move your hands together in a clockwise (towards your left and downward) direction around your middle. Apply gentle pressure. Make 20 circles.

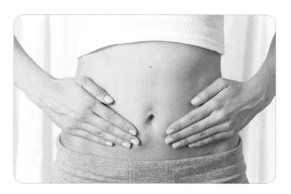

3 Put one hand below your rib cage on either side of your torso, fingers pointing to the middle. Massage by sweeping your hands down towards your pelvis. Make five sweeps altogether.

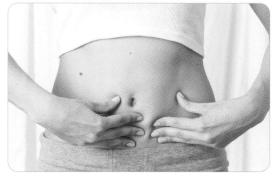

4 Using the fingers and thumbs of both your hands, knead your abdomen in a clockwise direction around your belly button. Make three complete revolutions altogether.

Lack of periods

If you're pregnant, breastfeeding, or approaching menopause, it's perfectly normal for your periods to stop. But if they stop at any other time, you have a condition called amenorrhoea—lack of periods.

There are two kinds of amenorrhoea, primary and secondary. Primary amenorrhea occurs when a girl's periods don't start before she reaches the age of 12. Its main cause is low body fat. A young girl's body must contain at least 17 percent fat before menstruation will begin because fat provides the factory that makes estrogen for each menstrual cycle. Secondary amenorrhoea, on the other hand, is when a girl's periods start normally, but then stop for a number of months. This section is about this second kind of amenorrhea, and it's all to do with hormonal balance.

CAUSES OF SECONDARY AMENORRHEA

Many of the reasons why periods suddenly stop are not serious, but if you have had no periods for three months or more, as a precaution, please see your doctor. Periods may stop because of pregnancy, and under- or overactive thyroid (see pp.58 and 62), polycystic ovary syndrome (PCOS; see pp.83–7), high levels of prolactin (the hormone normally produced during breastfeeding, but also during times of stress), and premature menopause, among other reasons.

Of the more treatable reasons for secondary amenorrhea, weight (being under- or overweight) is probably the most common. If you're underweight, or lose 15 percent of your body weight quickly, your body begins to assume that famine is around the corner. The result of this is that it shuts down systems that are not essential for your immediate survival—among them your reproductive organs. This also prevents a pregnancy when, as far as your body is concerned, there is not enough food to sustain both you and a baby.

Being overweight can also stop your periods because the more body fat you have, the more estrogen you produce. While some fat is essential for ovulation, excessive levels can inhibit it.

In short, then, it's essential for a normal menstrual cycle that your weight is at its optimum. The best way to assess whether or not you are over- or underweight is to check your Body Mass Index (BMI), a measure that represents the ratio of your height to your weight (see box, p.297). If you're underweight, take steps to gain weight by increasing your intake of healthy calories, especially of complex carbohydrates; if you're overweight, it's time to consider a sensible weight-loss program (see pp.299–301).

Other reasons your periods might stop include over-exercising (which can make your body fat too low) and stress. Studies conclude that emotional trauma, or any kind of pressure that places extra demands on your system, causes your body to release stress hormones. These interfere with the hormones your body needs to stimulate your ovaries to produce and release eggs.

If you're on the Pill and come off it, you may experience amenorrhoea (in this case, your periods aren't starting up again). This can mean that being on the Pill has masked another problem, such as PCOS or a thyroid condition. Your doctor will perform an ultrasound to check your ovaries and blood tests to check your hormone levels. If everything is normal, you probably have a "hangover" hormone imbalance from taking the Pill.

Follow the advice below on how to make changes to your diet and lifestyle that will help redress the balance and kick-start your ovaries.

CONVENTIONAL TREATMENTS

Modern medicine can treat only some of the specific causes of amenorrhea—the rest will be down to you. If your doctor can't find a physiological cause for the problem, you'll need to make your own diet and life-style changes to restore balance in your body and hope-fully restart your periods. So you can treat yourself in the most appropriate way possible, press your doctor to do all he or she can to find a cause for your amenor-rhoea. Make sure he or she tests for all the causes I've given above and even ask for a referral to a gynecologist if you need one. The following are the most common drug treatments you'll be offered, depending on your specific diagnosis.

Bromocriptine Your doctor will probably prescribe you bromocriptine if your amenorrhoea is caused by high levels of prolactin (hyperprolactinemia). Side-effects include nausea, headaches, and dizziness.

Hormone replacement therapy (HRT) If a blood test reveals you have high levels of follicle-stimulating hormone (FSH), your lack of periods may be the result of an early (premature) menopause. Not only does an early menopause mean that you won't be able to con-ceive naturally (if you wanted to), you'll also be suscep-tible to the health issues associated with menopause (see pp.246–8). Your doctor will advise you to take HRT to boost your levels of hormones essential to the health of your bones and your general well-being.

YOUR DIET

Your body needs to be well nourished in order to sup-port a regular menstrual cycle—and this doesn't mean necessarily being thinner or fatter, but being healthy. Begin by following my hormone-balancing diet (see box, p.57), which will help you manage your weight without the need for dieting. It's especially important to keep your blood-sugar levels and your hormones in balance by cutting down on caffeine, sugar, and refined food. Try to eat little and often (even as often as every three hours) and include a wide variety of healthy, pref-erably organic, whole grains, fruits, vegetables, leg-umes, nuts, seeds, and oily fish in your diet.

SUPPLEMENTS

Because your body needs to be in good health in order for your periods to return, as well as following the hor-mone-balancing diet, take a quality multi-vitamin and mineral every day (see p.320). Pay particular attention to the following supplements. The dosages given are total daily dosages, so take into account anything in your multi-vitamin and mineral supplement, when deciding which nutrients you need to boost.

■ B-COMPLEX (containing 400µg folic acid and 25mg of each other B-vitamin, daily) Any help you can give your body to produce and release an egg at ovulation can help restore your periods. Your body needs B-vitamins, especially folic acid, for your cells to divide and create, including making a new egg each month. Restoring your levels of B-vitamins is especially important if you've just come off the contraceptive pill.

■ MAGNESIUM (300mg, daily) If stress may be causing or worsening your amenorrhoea, magnesium will help calm you.

■ ZINC (15mg, daily) Zinc helps ensure your body has a healthy balance of estrogen and progesterone, the hormones essential for normal egg development and a healthy menstrual cycle. Zinc is an especially important supplement if your amenorrhoea occurs after coming off the Pill (which can cause zinc deficiency). Take the supplement as zinc citrate.

■ OMEGA-3 FATTY ACIDS (1,000mg fish oil, daily, containing at least 700mg EPA and 500mg DHA). Most of the women I see with amenorrhoea are deficient in essential fats. A supplement boosts your body's supply to help kick-start menstruation.

HERBS

The herbs below will help your body restore hormone balance and reduce the impact of stress, with the ultimate aim of restoring your periods.

■ AGNUS CASTUS (*Vitex agnus castus*) High levels of the hormone prolactin and imbalances in levels of follicle-stimulating hormone (FSH) and luteinizing hormone (LH) can all inhibit ovulation and your menstrual cycle. Agnus castus helps regulate the action of your pituitary gland, which stimulates the release of all these hormones, to bring your body back into balance. Take 1 tsp. tincture in a little water, or 200–300mg in capsule form, twice daily. It can take up to six months for the herb to take effect in your body, so you'll need to be patient. However, keep taking it until your periods are regular again. Then, once you've restored a regular cycle, gradually reduce your daily dosage of agnus castus, so that after a couple of months of winding down, your menstrual cycle continues without the trigger of the herb.

■ BLACK COHOSH (*Cimicifuga racemosa*) Traditional herbalists use this herb for its hormone-balancing effects and its ability to kick-start periods. Take 1 tsp. tincture in a little water, twice daily; or 250–350mg in capsule form, daily—until you have re-established a regular menstrual cycle.

■ FALSE UNICORN ROOT (*Chamaelirium luteum*) This herb can help normalize and even improve ovarian function, including the levels of hormones they produce. Take 1 tsp. tincture in a little water, or 600–900mg in capsule form, daily—until you have re-established a regular menstrual cycle.

■ SIBERIAN GINSENG (*Eleutherococcus senticosus*) Use this herb if you think your amenorrhoea is caused by stress. An adaptogenic herb, Siberian ginseng can support your body, reducing the impact of stress and boosting your energy levels as required. Take 1 tsp. tincture in a little water, or 250–300mg in capsule form, twice daily. Be prepared to take Siberian ginseng for approximately three months before you begin to see its effects.

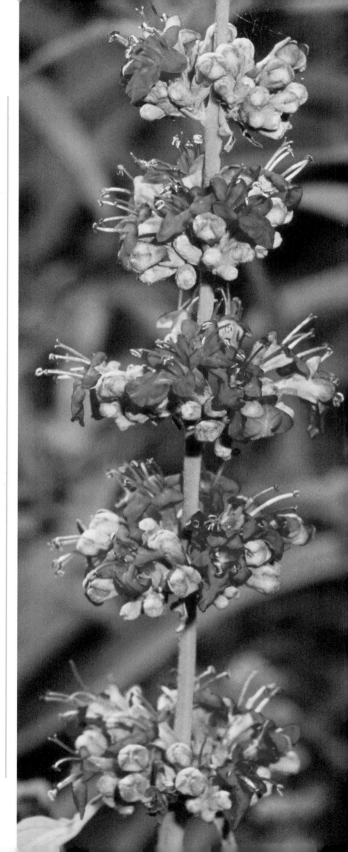

Right: Agnus castus (*Vitex agnus castus*)

OTHER NATURAL TREATMENTS

Homeopathy A homeopath is likely to prescribe the following remedies to help re-start your periods. If you're self-prescribing, take those that are relevant in a 30c potency, twice a day, for up to three days. However, also make an appointment with a homeopathic practitioner, who can advise you further according to your own particular symptoms and constitution.

• Aconite for when your periods stop suddenly, perhaps after a sudden trauma or shock, such as a serious accident or a bereavement

• Nat mur can help restore menstruation if you think its absence might have been caused by feelings of deep sadness or even depression.

• Pulsatilla is useful if your periods have stopped perhaps as a result of exhaustion or anemia (lack of iron in the blood)

• Sepia is particularly useful if your periods have not started again after a pregnancy or after you've stopped taking the contraceptive pill

Acupuncture When you consult an acupuncturist with secondary amenorrhoea, he or she will want to establish whether your problem is caused by stagnant *qi* energy and blood in your system, or a deficiency of *qi* and blood. To do this, the practitioner looks at your overall health and asks you questions (about such things as your sleep patterns and stress levels) to try to establish any other possible signs and symptoms. He or she will examine the health of your tongue and the strength and rhythm of your pulse. Once the acupuncturist has established the apparent cause of your absent periods, he or she will treat the appropriate, corresponding acupuncture points to rebalance both *qi* and blood-flow through your body.

Aromatherapy A regular aromatherapy massage can help re-start your periods by stimulating the pelvic organs and helping you to relax. Visit a local practitioner or try a self-massage. For self-massage use the technique on page 105, using an aromatherapy blend of

QUICK ABDOMINAL MASSAGE

Blend 15 drops of lavender oil into 6 tsp. of sweet almond oil. Rub the oil into your hands and, starting at the lower right side of your abdomen, place your fingers flat and make small circular movements over the area. Press your abdomen as deeply as you comfortably can. Using slow, circular movements massage up the right of the abdomen, across the center just above your navel and down the left side. Make several large circuits of your abdomen in this way and finish by rubbing your abdomen with the palms of your hands in the same clockwise direction, using smooth, gliding strokes.

15 drops rose essential oil diluted in 6 tsp. sweet almond oil; or try the quick abdominal massage above. Aim to practice the self-massage every day, if you can.

Reflexology A reflexologist will aim to restore balance to your system, and so your periods, too, by massaging the reflex points for the pituitary, thyroid, and adrenal glands, as well as those related to the kidneys and reproductive system.

SELF-HELP

Relax and sleep Stress and poor-quality sleep can trigger hormonal imbalances that in turn can lead to amenorrhoea. Include some relaxation time in your daily routine, even if it's just half an hour a day. Practice a daily meditation—any of the meditations or visualizations in this book can provide a starting point. Or try a dedicated relaxation exercise, such as tensing and releasing all the muscle groups in your body, in turn, to create a sense that you're "letting go" of your tension. Feel tension ebb away as you release each muscle.

Heavy periods

Is there ever such a thing as a "typical" bleed for an "average" woman? Probably not. But there's no question that for some women a monthly bleed is both longer and heavier than is healthy.

For the purposes of diagnosing problems with menstrual bleeding, we assume that typically you lose around 1¼oz., or just under 3 tbsp., of blood in each period. Of course, it's not practical to measure blood loss in this way at home, so I think the best way to decide whether or not your periods are unusually heavy is to consider how often you have to change your sanitary protection. If you have to change your tampon or pad every hour, the chances are you're suffering from menorrhagia, or heavy periods.

CAUSES
Heavy bleeding can be a symptom of a gynecological disorder, such as any of the following:

• Polyps in the uterus
• Underactive thyroid (see p.58–61)
• Fibroids (see pp.114–17)
• Endometriosis (see pp.118–124)
• Uterine cancer (see p.125)
• Pelvic inflammatory disease (PID; see box, p.140)

Although this list suggests that suffering from menorrhagia is a symptom of a more serious gynecological problem, for many women there is no particular cause for heavy bleeding at all. This is known as dysfunctional bleeding, and, happily, it means there's nothing seriously wrong with you. Perhaps your body is producing a particularly thick uterine lining, itself caused by an imbalance between estrogen and progesterone in your system. (Bear in mind, though, that hormonal imbalance can indicate you didn't ovulate in this cycle, which would create an estrogen dominance. You should ask your doctor to investigate this, if necessary.) If your blood doesn't clot efficiently in your uterus, but otherwise you're healthy, you may still experience heavy monthly bleeds. Stress can also lead to more heavy bleeding and, ironically, so can anemia (lack of iron in the blood), and then your extra blood loss makes you more anemic—in a vicious cycle. Finally, if you use a intrauterine device (IUD), you may experience heavier bleeds. However, if you have a levonorgestrel (LNg) IUD, also known as Mirena (see opposite), which contains progestin, you'll find this can control heavy bleeding because it thins the lining of the uterus.

DIAGNOSIS
Heavy periods are usually a harmless by-product of your body's uniqueness, but it's always important that you have a check up with your doctor to rule out anything more serious, including uterine cancer. If you're told that there's nothing seriously wrong, use the natural approach (my diet, supplement, herb, and lifestyle advice) to help control your bleeding. The following are the diagnostic tests your doctor is likely to request.

Ultrasound scan In this procedure, a gel is put on your abdomen and a sonar device moved over the area to create an image of your uterus on a screen (sometimes the scan is taken from inside your vagina). This procedure helps establish whether or not a condition such as fibroids is the cause of your heavy bleeding.

Hysteroscopy In this test, a microscopic camera is inserted through your cervix to view the inside of your uterus. Your doctor can see whether any abnormalities, such as polyps, could be causing your heavy bleeding.

Blood tests These will establish whether or not hormonal imbalances are at the root of your menorrhagia. Ask your doctor to test you for anemia, too. Heavy bleeding means you're losing a lot of iron, and this can make you feel tired and lethargic.

Swab testing If your doctor thinks an infection (such as pelvic inflammatory disease) might be causing your bleeding, he or she will order a swab to be taken from your vagina to confirm or refute the diagnosis.

CONVENTIONAL TREATMENTS

Make sure your doctor establishes the cause of your heavy bleeding (even if it's to decide there's no medical reason) before you take any medication. Taking medication to control clotting, for example, may hide the fact you have large fibroids. If the bleeding is a symptom of another problem, usually treating the other problem will reduce blood loss. The following apply especially to dysfunctional bleeding.

Tranexamic acid Of all the medications a doctor may prescribe for heavy bleeding, this appears to be most effective. It works by improving blood clotting in your uterus. However, it can have some unpleasant side-effects, including nausea and stomach upsets.

The contraceptive pill The Pill controls heavy bleeding by (in effect) taking the responsibility for a menstrual cycle out of your body's hands. The period you experience during the week's break between Pill cycles is really only a symptom of your body's withdrawal from the Pill's hormones; it isn't a real period. Although this fixes the problem of menorrhagia, taking the Pill has some unpleasant side-effects: nausea,

loss of libido, depression, breast pain, and blood clots, among them.

Progestins If your doctor suspects you have a problem with progesterone production (so you have an estrogen dominance in your system), he or she may prescribe progestins, which are synthetic progesterone. They will help your bleeding return to normal, but side-effects include nausea, acne, breast tenderness, bloating, and mood changes.

Mefenamic acid This drug, shown to reduce blood loss significantly, falls under the category of non-steroidal anti-inflammatory steroids (NSAIDs), which reduce the levels of "bad" prostaglandins in the blood. Fewer "bad" prostaglandins mean less inflammation in the uterus and better blood-clotting, both of which will reduce blood-flow. Your doctor will probably prescribe the drug for you to take only while you're bleeding. Although it's effective, its side-effects include fatigue, rashes, and stomach upsets.

Danazol A modified, synthetic version of the male hormone testosterone, danazol alters your hormone balance so that you don't ovulate. This, in turn, prevents a build-up of your uterine lining, so you have less to shed during your period. Its side-effects can include irritability, headaches, acne, weight gain, hoarseness, smaller breasts, and facial hair.

Gonadotrophin-releasing hormone (GnRH) analogues These synthetic hormones put your body in a state of temporary menopause, preventing periods altogether. Side-effects include hot flashes, headaches, mood swings, vaginal dryness, and insomnia.

Levonorgestrel IUD (Mirena) This intrauterine device contains the synthetic hormone progestin, which it releases directly into the uterus lining, stopping it from building up and so regulating bleeding. Over time, it can prevent bleeding altogether, but it doesn't mean you're in menopause: you can still ovulate, but, because the IUD prevents your uterine lining from growing, you don't have any blood to shed.

Surgery There are three kinds of surgery your doctor may suggest if it turns out that medication can't control your menstrual flow. The first, and least intensive, is a D&C (dilation and curettage). Your gynecologist opens your cervix (the "dilation" part) so that he or she can scrape away or suck out a layer of tissue from your uterus. Although the procedure is effective in the short term, eventually your uterine lining will build up again, so you may need repeat D&Cs. The second type of surgery is endometrial ablation or endometrial resection, in which your uterine lining is permanently destroyed using a laser or a wire respectively. Although this surgery is effective, it will almost certainly reduce your fertility. Hysterectomy (see pp.128–31), a major operation, is the final and most dramatic kind of surgery for menorrhagia. I strongly urge you to avoid it if you can.

YOUR DIET

Because hormonal imbalance is a common cause of heavy bleeding, follow the hormone-balancing diet (see box, p.57). In particular, avoid coffee and alcohol, which increase menstrual flow. Do eat plenty of phytoestrogens (see p.31) and essential fatty acids (see p.26). Both these nutrients increase the levels of beneficial prostaglandins in your system to reduce blood flow.

The other part of the diet you should be especially aware of is reducing your intake of saturated fat, such as that found in meat and dairy products. Foods rich in saturated fat also contain arachidonic acid (AA), which is found in high levels in women who suffer from heavy periods. AA triggers the production of PGE2, a "bad" prostaglandin that leads to "thickening" of the blood and increased blood flow.

Finally, avoid drinking black tea and carbonated, caffeinated drinks with your meals because they block the uptake of iron from your food. Iron is essential for regulating blood flow (see right).

SUPPLEMENTS

Take a good-quality multi-vitamin and mineral supplement (see p.320) every day and increase your intake of the following. Take into account what's already in your multi when topping up to the following amounts.

■ VITAMIN A (10,000iu, daily) Studies show that women who have heavy periods may have a deficiency in vitamin A. Take it as beta-carotene, not retinol.

■ B-COMPLEX (containing 25mg of each B-vitamin, daily) The B-vitamins are crucial for your body's production of beneficial prostaglandins.

■ VITAMIN C with bioflavonoids (500mg, twice daily) Vitamin C helps strengthen your blood capillaries, so helping to stem blood loss. Take vitamin C as magnesium ascorbate.

■ VITAMIN E (400iu, daily) Vitamin E has been shown to reduce blood loss, but it isn't clear how. It's possible that the vitamin helps improve blood clotting or helps regulate the hormones, especially estrogen.

■ IRON (14mg, daily) In order to stem blood flow, your blood vessels need to contract. Iron helps this process. If tests reveal you have an iron deficiency, take iron as amino acid chelate or citrate along with your vitamin-C supplement, on an empty stomach.

■ ZINC (15mg, daily) If your menorrhagia is caused by excess estrogen in your system, zinc will help improve your overall hormone balance.

HERBS

If you can't control your bleeding naturally, you may need to use medication. However, you can try to reduce the amount of medication you take by also taking herbs (although avoid herbs if you're taking artificial hormones). After a few cycles, as the herbs begin to do their work, you may find that they start to control your flow. You'll know they're working if, little by little, you lower your medication dosage until you're able to take the herbs alone—and have "normal" cycles. Eventually, your need for herbs should disappear completely, too.

■ DONG QUAI (*Angelica sinensis*) and LADIES' MANTLE (*Alchemilla vulgaris*) Use dong quai and ladies' mantle in the long term to improve uterine function, help stop excessive blood flow and balance your hormones. Dong quai helps reduce the amount of "bad" prostaglandins in your system, so improving your blood-clotting ability. Ladies' mantle can boost circulation to your uterus, improving its general health. Take 1 tsp. of the combined tinctures (equal parts) in a little water, two or three times daily; or take 300mg of both herbs in capsule form, twice daily. Use throughout the month, including during your period.

■ ASTRINGENT HERBS These herbs help constrict your blood vessels and so control the flow of blood. Take 1 tsp. of the combined tinctures (equal parts) in a little water, two or three times daily; or take 200–300mg of each herb in capsule form daily.

• Cranesbill (*Geranium maculatum*)

• Goldenseal (*Hydrastis canadensis*)

• Shepherd's purse (*Capsella bursa pastoris*)

• Yarrow (*Achillea millefolium*)

OTHER NATURAL TREATMENTS

Homeopathy The remedies commonly prescribed for heavy periods are Lachesis and Sanguinaria. Take them in a 30c potency, twice a day, for up to three days. Also make an appointment to see a practitioner, who can advise you according to your symptoms.

Acupuncture An acupuncturist will help control your blood flow by regulating how much blood passes through your uterus, and optimizing your liver function (to ensure "old" hormones are flushed out).

SELF-HELP

Stay fit If you suffer from heavy periods, the most useful thing you can do for your health is exercise. In addition to helping balance your hormones (and ease any period pain), exercise improves your circulation throughout your body, including through your uterus. If blood isn't allowed to build up in your uterus, your periods should become lighter.

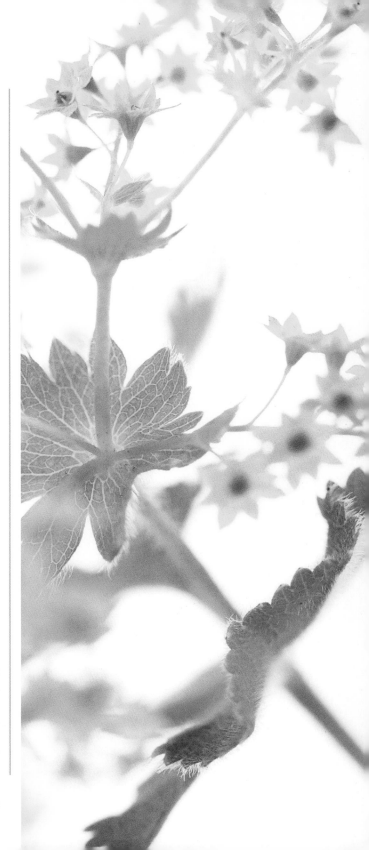

Right: Ladies' mantle (*Alchemilla vulgaris*)

Fibroids

Non-cancerous growths located in the uterus, fibroids may affect up to 20 percent of women. They sometimes run in families and are most common in women between the age of 30 and menopause.

A fibroid itself is like a pale-colored rubber ball. Although it may not be perfectly round, it is a tough bundle of cells that forms a hard mass. It begins as a single uterus cell that then divides abnormally.

SYMPTOMS

Large or small, within the uterine wall muscle, or on top of it, fibroids are remarkably common—and can go unnoticed. A large fibroid (perhaps even as big as a seven-month-old fetus) can cause long, heavy periods and/or bleeding between your periods. This is because fibroids increase the surface area of your uterine lining, giving you more lining to shed. You may also experience pain in your lower back or pelvis, often during your period or during intercourse. Or, you may have no symptoms at all. I have had many women come to me because they are having difficulty getting pregnant, to discover only then that fibroids are the cause. Fibroids can affect fertility as they enlarge and distort the uterus, making it harder for a fertilized egg to implant.

CAUSES

There is no known cause for fibroids, although we do know that excess estrogen makes them larger. This is why if you're overweight, you're more prone to fibroids because fat cells manufacture estrogen.

DIAGNOSIS

If you suffer from heavy bleeding, along with any of the other symptoms mentioned earlier, and have a swollen abdomen, and suffer from constipation or the need to urinate frequently, or if you're having trouble conceiving, visit your doctor to investigate fibroids.

He or she will give you a pelvic examination, and (if fibroids appear to be present) you'll probably be sent for an abdominal or vaginal ultrasound scan to establish the size and location of the growths.

CONVENTIONAL TREATMENTS

In many cases, fibroids require little or no treatment at all. However, if they are large and causing you unwanted symptoms, such as menorrhagia or constipation, or if they're pressing on your bladder or affecting your fertility, your doctor may recommend treatment.

I urge you to see a gynecologist before you begin any medication, to make sure you're offered the most appropriate treatment for your problem.

Gonadotrophin-releasing hormone (GnRH) analogues These drugs interrupt your normal hormonal cycle, reducing levels of estrogen in your body, preventing ovulation, and so reducing fibroids. However, they're effective only while you take them, and they can cause nausea, headaches, and irritability.

Progestin Although research doesn't yet indicate that synthetic forms of progesterone (progestin) can reduce fibroids, your doctor may recommend it to relieve symptoms, such as heavy bleeding (you'll probably be given a levonorgestrel (LNg) intrauterine device (IUD)) and pelvic pain. The drug can cause PMS-type symptoms such as bloating, moodiness, and pimples.

SURGICAL TREATMENTS FOR FIBROIDS

The most dramatic method of treating fibroids is surgery. However, before you allow your doctor to steer you down this route, please read the information in this box on each of the possible surgical techniques. I hope it'll enable you to make an informed choice about which treatment options are right for you. And remember, in at least half of all cases, fibroids cause no complications at all, meaning that you can simply leave them alone.

MYOMECTOMY

The operation to remove fibroids is called a myomectomy. The size of your fibroids and their position in your uterus will determine how a doctor performs your operation. For example, you'll be given a hysteroscopic myomectomy (using laser surgery) if your fibroids are growing on the inside of your uterus and are around 1in. or smaller. If your fibroids are on the outside of your uterus, you'll have an abdominal myomectomy. For this, the surgeon will make a small incision in your abdomen in order to remove the growths. In both cases you'll be given a general anaesthetic.

If you require a myomectomy, make sure you find a highly recommended specialist to perform it. Badly performed, a myomectomy can lead to significant blood loss, which may even require a full hysterectomy or may lead to the development of adhesions (scar tissue) that can, in turn, cause infertility.

If fibroids are stopping you from becoming pregnant, a myomectomy along with the natural approach to treatment (ideally for six months before you try for a baby) is by far the best way forward: The fibroids will be removed, and your body will be in ultimate balance for conception.

HYSTERECTOMY

The most extreme of all surgical techniques to treat fibroids is a hysterectomy. Doctors often take the approach that it's easier to remove the whole uterus than to perform a myomectomy to remove the individual fibroids. Please read my section on hysterectomy (pp.128–31) and make a calculated decision as to whether or not this is right for you. In most cases, it is not at all necessary to be so radical with the surgery. Fibroids

are usually perfectly treatable by other methods.

ENDOMETRIAL ABLATION AND RESECTION

If you don't want to conceive, and your fibroids are causing heavy periods, you may be offered an endometrial ablation and resection. In this procedure a surgeon inserts a laser or heated wire into the uterine cavity to destroy the tissue of the uterine lining. It's an irreversible treatment and will prevent a fertilized egg from ever implanting in your uterus.

NEW TECHNIQUES

There are two fairly new surgical techniques in the treatment of fibroids. Myolysis (laser ablation) is a technique in which the center of the fibroid is destroyed by a laser. This constricts the blood flow to the fibroid, causing it to shrink and die. The other technique, uterine artery embolization, injects tiny particles into certain arteries going into the uterus in order to "starve" the fibroids of a blood supply and so to shrink them. There is a risk of infection with this technique.

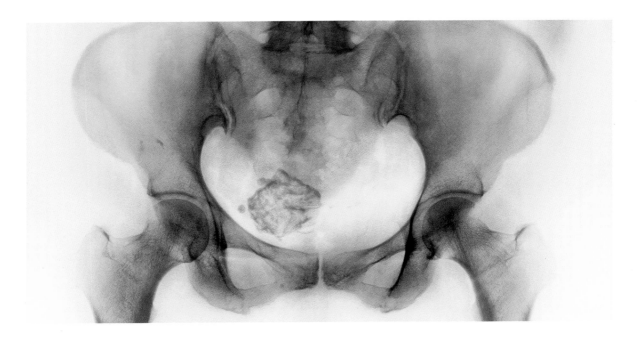

Above: X ray of a woman's pelvic region, showing fibroids (pink patches)

YOUR DIET

Ideally, you should use your diet to help control the growth of your fibroids, as well as to reduce the symptoms. Follow the dietary recommendations given here, and also the supplement advice from the section on heavy periods (see p.112). I've seen results using the natural approach to treatment (including the herbal remedies and self-help advice) within six months.

As fibroids are worsened by excess estrogen, follow the hormone-balancing diet (see box, p.57). In particular, pay attention to the following advice.

Avoid caffeine and limit bad fat Caffeine products increase menstrual flow and may worsen the symptoms caused by fibroids. In addition, one study, testing the effects of instant coffee on the reproductive system of mice, showed that the drink increased the likelihood of the mice developing fibroids. Saturated fats (found mainly in animal products, such as dairy and meat) block your body's ability to absorb essential fats, which it needs to beat fibroids, and they also increase estrogen levels in the blood. Women who eat more meat have a higher risk of developing fibroids than those who eat more green vegetables.

Boost fiber It's especially important to boost fiber because a fiber-rich diet helps eliminate unwanted estrogen from your body, through your bowels. Whole grains, such as brown rice, oats, and rye, and fresh fruit and vegetables, are great sources of fiber.

Increase phytoestrogen levels Phytoestrogen-rich foods boost your body's production of a protein called sex-hormone-binding globulin (SHBG), which controls how much estrogen is in your blood.

Love your liver Avoid any substance that compromises your liver function, such as alcohol, tobacco, and drugs (such as paracetamol and ibuprofen). You need your liver to clear "old" estrogens efficiently.

Buy organic If you suffer from fibroids, it's more important than ever to buy organic produce as much as possible. Pesticides in non-organic produce may contain xenoestrogens (see box, p.18), which can stimulate fibroid growth. Research shows that fibroids contain larger amounts of the pesticide DDT than any other tissue in the uterus.

HERBS

The following herbs will help reduce the fibroids. If you have heavy bleeding as a symptom, see the herbal advice on pages 112–13, too.

- AGNUS CASTUS (*Vitex agnus castus*) This herb has a good reputation for reducing excess estrogen in the body. You can take it throughout the month (even during your period) and on a long-term basis. Take 1 tsp. tincture in a little water, or 200–300mg in capsule form, twice daily.

- MILK THISTLE (*Silymarin marianum*) This liver tonic boosts your body's natural detoxification processes by helping to deactivate and excrete unwanted or "old" estrogen from your body. Take 1 tsp. tincture in a little water, twice daily; or 200–400mg in capsule form, daily.

OTHER NATURAL TREATMENTS

Homeopathy Homeopathic remedies will be unique to your physical and emotional symptoms, and you need to visit a qualified practitioner. The most common remedies a homeopath will prescribe for fibroids are Lachesis and Sanguinaria both in a 30c potency (twice daily), and they'll help control heavy bleeding if this is one of your symptoms.

Acupuncture In Traditional Chinese Medicine, practitioners believe that fibroids are a result of stagnant *qi* and blood through your uterus and liver (which flushes estrogens out of your system). See a practitioner who will aim to boost energy flow to your reproductive organs and optimize your liver function in order to treat fibroids.

Aromatherapy You can use aromatherapy to help balance your hormones, avoid stagnation in your uterus, and improve relaxation. Run a bath and add 2 drops each of the essential oils of ginger, which will boost your circulation; marjoram, which will ease constipation and uterus cramps, if these are among your symptoms; and rose, which has gentle hormone-balancing properties. As an alternative to using the oils in a bath, you could blend 6 drops of rose with 4 drops each of ginger and marjoram in 6 tsp. of sweet almond carrier oil and use it in a gentle abdominal massage, such as the massage on page 109.

SELF-HELP

I often find myself reminding my patients that fibroids are a benign condition that is not a precursor to cancer. So, unless your fibroids are adversely affecting your fertility or menstrual cycle, there's no need to panic about having dramatic treatment, such as surgery, to remove them. I think so much can be achieved by using natural methods and self-help.

Exercise Increasing the circulation to your pelvic region can help prevent or shrink fibroids, so any form of exercise that gets your heart beating faster and improves your circulation is good for this condition.

Burn excess fat Exercise and following the hormone-balancing diet will help you lose weight if you're overweight. As fibroids are estrogen-dependent and fat cells produce estrogen, making sure you're carrying as little excess fat as possible (within healthy guidelines) can help treat your condition. Check your BMI using the table on page 297 to see whether or not weight loss could help you. If you find that it could, use the techniques given on pages 300–301.

Make love It's possible, although unproven, that regular orgasms can help reduce fibroids—for exactly the same reason that exercise works. That is, orgasm increases the circulation to your pelvic region.

Endometriosis

Approximately 5 million women in the USA and 1.5 million women in the UK suffer from endometriosis. Not surprisingly, then, many of the women I see in my clinics have this chronic condition.

Endometriosis is characterized by cells from the endometrium (the lining of the uterus) that have migrated to form endometrial patches in other parts of the body—most commonly in the pelvic cavity (on the ovaries and cervix), but also more rarely in the bladder and bowel, lungs, heart, eyes, armpits, knees, or nasal passages (see box, opposite). A serious condition, it's most common in women aged over 30. Up to half these women will have fertility problems because of it.

SYMPTOMS

Pain in the pelvic region is the most striking and debilitating symptom of endometriosis and is not always confined to the lead up to and during your period. Some women experience pain all month. If the endometrial patches have migrated to your bowel or bladder, you may experience pain when you have a bowel movement or urinate. If you suspect you have endometriosis, keep a record of any pain you experience and see if it is cyclical—patterns of pain can help establish a diagnosis. You may also experience pain during intercourse (known as dyspareunia). This is one of the most common symptoms of endometriosis, so it's worth visiting your doctor if it applies to you.

Although pelvic and intercourse pain are the most identifiable symptoms, there are a number of others that in isolation may mean nothing, but together can indicate an endometriosis problem. Sadly, many women with endometriosis experience all of them, making this a truly debilitating condition. They include irregular and/or heavy periods, tiredness, lower back pain, digestive problems (such as bloating, diarrhea, and nausea) and difficulty in getting pregnant.

CAUSES

Doctors remain unclear as to exactly what causes endometriosis. Theories range from "retrograde menstruation," when endometrial blood sheds into the Fallopian tubes instead of out of the vagina, to problems with the immune system. No one has been able to say definitively which of the many theories is right, although probably, as with most things, a combination of factors lies at the root of the problem. We do know that the condition seems to run in families, and perhaps the most widely accepted explanation is that endometriosis is estrogen sensitive: The more estrogen you have in your system, the more susceptible you are. This would certainly explain an increasing trend for the condition in the modern world—if you delay having babies (as many women now do), you have more periods, so are exposed to more estrogen.

DIAGNOSIS

Doctors commonly under-diagnose endometriosis. For this reason, if your symptoms are cyclical and especially if you suffer from pain during intercourse and painful periods, insist your doctor tests you for the condition. The following are the most common methods of diagnosis your doctor will use.

Ultrasound Although an ultrasound scan is useful, it can't actually diagnose endometriosis. What it can

THE STAGES OF ENDOMETRIOSIS

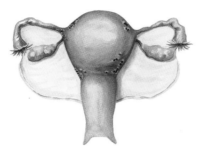

MINIMAL

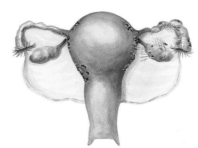

MILD

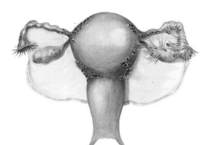

MODERATE

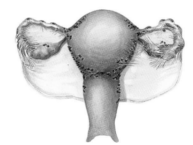

SEVERE

The blood you shed during your period is your endometrium, the lining of your uterus, which had been ready for a fertilized egg.

In endometriosis, however, patches of uterus-lining tissue exist outside the uterus. The endometrial cells that form these patches respond in exactly the same way to hormonal triggers as those in the uterine lining itself. This means that when your hormones trigger the stages of your cycle, all endometrium cells—even those outside your uterus—get the message to build up, break down, and shed away. But, for these patches, there's nowhere for the blood to drain, so the trapped blood causes the endometriosis symptoms.

There are four recognized stages of endometriosis. Stage I (top left) is known as "minimal" and is characterized by a small number of superficial endometrial patches within the pelvis. Stage II (top right) is called "mild." Here, the patches are more numerous, larger, and forming deeper into the "host" tissue. Stage III (bottom left) is "moderate." The patches are more numerous and deeper still, and have begun to form adhesions that literally "stick" the organs of the pelvic region together. Stage IV (bottom right) is "severe." This stage is characterized by dense, deep patches with adhesions that have completely blocked normal organ function.

show, however, is any abnormalities in the pelvic cavity, including any adhesions and cysts, which may be caused by endometriosis. An ultrasound can also pick up a condition called adenomyosis, in which patches of endometrium (uterine lining) are present in the myometrium, the uterus's layer of muscle tissue. Having adenomyosis is a strong sign that you have full-blown endometriosis and your doctor will probably send you for a laparoscopy.

Laparoscopy This is the gold-standard test for diagnosing endometriosis. You'll be given a general anaesthetic so that your doctor can use a harmless gas to "inflate" your abdominal cavity. Once your abdomen is inflated, your pelvic organs can be viewed easily using a laparoscope. This is a thin viewing tube your doctor inserts through an incision just below your navel. Using the laparoscope, he or she can see whether or not any endometrial patches exist in your abdominal cavity. If they do, the doctor can laser them off during the same procedure.

CONVENTIONAL TREATMENTS

The conventional way to treat endometriosis is to shut down your reproductive hormones using medication. This stops your periods, reducing the levels of estrogen in your body. Endometriosis is a complex condition and if anything your doctor says to you doesn't fit your experience or just doesn't make sense to you, don't be afraid to ask for a second opinion. (If you suffer from endometriosis, don't take HRT, which can make the condition worse.)

Danazol Because endometriosis grows in the presence of estrogen, giving you a weak, male hormone to take effectively stops ovulation altogether, shutting off your body's estrogen supply. Bear in mind that any male hormone may have the effect of giving you "male" symptoms, notably acne, facial hair, weight gain, and a deeper voice. Nausea, rashes, headaches, and moodiness may also occur.

The contraceptive pill If you take the Pill "back to back," without breaking for a withdrawal bleed, you can reduce the impact of endometriosis.

Gonadotrophin-releasing hormone (GnRH) analogues These drugs put you in a temporary state of menopause, shutting down your estrogen supply. Your doctor will prescribe them as an injection, nasal spray, or implant (which goes just under the skin).

Diathermy or laser surgery If drug treatments aren't successful, your doctor may advise you to have diathermy (the use of intense heat) or laser surgery to burn off the endometrial patches. A doctor performs the procedure during a laparoscopy (see left) with the aim of removing as much endometriosis as possible and freeing up any organs that have fused together with adhesions (endometrial scar tissue).

Hysterectomy As an absolute last resort, your doctor may offer you a hysterectomy. However, unless your ovaries are removed as well as your uterus, the patches are likely to grow back elsewhere in your body because your ovaries will continue to make estrogen. Most doctors agree that, although endometriosis affects the uterus, the uterus itself isn't the problem.

YOUR DIET

The general consensus is that excess estrogen plays a significant role in the spread of endometriosis, so it's important you follow the hormone-balancing diet (see box, p.57). In particular, steer clear of saturated fat (see p.26) entirely. Studies show that women who eat meat once a day are twice as likely to have endometriosis compared with those who eat less red meat and more fruit and vegetables. In one study, women with the highest intake of red meat increased their risk of developing endometriosis by 80 to 100 percent; those with the highest intake of fresh fruit and vegetables reduced the risk by about 40 percent. Choose foods rich in unsaturated fats such as nuts, seeds, and oily fish.

As part of the hormone-balancing diet, you should reduce your intake of caffeine, which has a diuretic effect on the body, depleting valuable reserves of vitamins and minerals that are essential for hormone balance. It's worth noting that studies show women who drink more than two cups of coffee a day have an increased risk of endometriosis. Supplement instead with herbal teas and dandelion coffee (dandelion is known for its beneficial action on the liver, which helps rid the body of excess estrogen).

SUPPLEMENTS

If you suffer from endometriosis, supplements can help in two main ways: to try to combat the condition by reducing excess estrogen and at the same time to relieve the symptoms. Use the following in combination, and don't forget to take into account what's already in your daily multi-vitamin and mineral supplement.

■ B-COMPLEX (containing 25mg of each B-vitamin, daily) The B-vitamins help the liver deactivate excess estrogen and help create beneficial prostaglandins, which are anti-inflammatory. Vitamin B1 can significantly reduce the intensity of period pains.

■ VITAMIN C with bioflavonoids (1,000mg, twice daily, as magnesium ascorbate) This antioxidant can help your body destroy endometrial patches. Bioflavonoids help relax smooth muscle and to prevent inflammation.

■ VITAMIN E (400iu, daily) Vitamin E is especially helpful for period pains and also heavy bleeding, two of the main symptoms of endometriosis.

■ MAGNESIUM (300mg, daily) Your uterus is a muscle, and magnesium is a muscle relaxant to help ease symptomatic pain. Take it as a citrate.

■ ZINC (15mg, daily) This nutrient is important for hormone balance and for the conversion of fatty acids to beneficial prostaglandins.

■ OMEGA-3 FATTY ACIDS (1,000mg fish oil containing at least 700mg EPA and 500mg DHA, daily) Your body needs these to produce beneficial prostaglandins to ease inflammation and cramps. (Use flax seed oil if you're vegetarian.)

HERBS

While the changes in your diet and to your supplement regime take effect, herbs can help normalize your hormone levels and also help you cope with specific symptoms of endometriosis. (Use the herbs listed on page 103 to ease period pain.)

Herbs are powerful medicines, but they're also more subtle in their action than pharmaceutical drugs. For this reason, initially try a combination of herbal remedies and your normal pain medicines. Very gradually reduce your medication until your body is using the herbs alone to deal with your symptoms (how long this takes will vary from woman to woman). With any luck, and by following the nutritional and supplement advice to restore balance, too, you should ultimately be able to eliminate your reliance on the herbal remedies as well as the drugs.

Take the herbs listed below for between three and six months. If you see no improvement in your symptoms in that time, consult a qualified herbal practitioner who can treat your unique constitution.

■ AGNUS CASTUS (*Vitex agnus castus*) This herb is especially helpful in enabling your body to produce good amounts of progesterone, which can offset excess estrogen. Take 1 tsp. tincture in a little water or 200–300mg in capsule form, twice daily.

■ DANDELION ROOT (*Taraxacum officinale*) Important herb for healthy liver function. Take 1 tsp. tincture in a little water, twice daily or 200–400mg in capsule form, daily.

■ ECHINACEA (*Echinacea purpurea*) Weak immunity may cause endometriosis. Supplement with this great immunity booster. Take it for ten days on, three days off, ten days on, and so on. Take 1 tsp. tincture in a little water, two or three times daily; or 300–400mg in capsule form, daily.

■ MILK THISTLE (*Silybum marianum*) This liver tonic can help keep the liver in peak condition for detoxifying the body of "old," excess estrogens. These can recirculate and target endometrial patches, encouraging growth. Take 1 tsp. tincture in a little water, twice daily; or 200–400mg in capsule form, daily.

YOGA FOR ENDOMETRIOSIS

It's well known that endometriosis is made worse by stress and tension, so the restorative, calming effects of yoga may do much to ease your symptoms. It can also boost circulation to your reproductive organs. Wear loose, comfortable clothes and practice on a mat or doubled-over towel for at least ten minutes a day. Never strain.

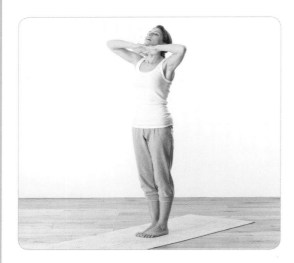

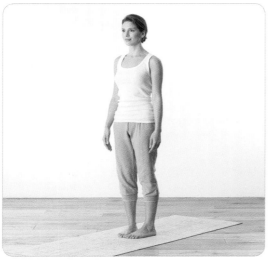

ENERGIZING BREATH (LEFT, TOP)

Stand, feet together. Link your fingers and place them under your chin. Put your elbows together. Inhale through your nose for a count of five. As you do so, raise your elbows out to the sides as high as possible, opening your palms but keeping your fingers together. Feel the breath at the back of your throat. Tilt back your head. Exhale completely through your mouth. Bring your elbows and palms together and lift your head. Repeat once more.

MOUNTAIN POSE (LEFT, BOTTOM)

Stand with your feet together so your big toes are touching and your heels are slightly apart. Relax your arms by your sides. Spread and lengthen your toes, make sure your kneecaps are facing forward and keep your pelvis balanced over your legs. Continue to lengthen upward, stretching your spine and opening your chest. Drop your shoulders and lengthen the back of your neck. Hold this pose for one minute. Relax, then repeat once more.

SIDEWAYS STRETCH (OPPOSITE, TOP)

Stand straight with your legs hip-width apart and your toes facing forward. Inhale and lift your right arm in the air. As you exhale, gently bend over to the left side, sliding your left hand down your left leg. Don't strain. Breathing normally, try to hold the

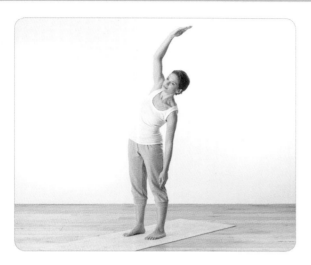

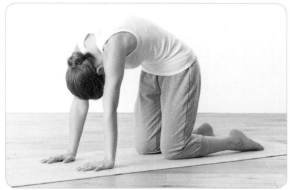

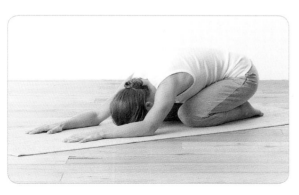

position for a count of five, or ten if you feel strong enough. Inhale and return slowly to an upright position. Exhale and slowly lower your arm and relax. Repeat on the other side. Practice the whole sequence five times altogether.

THE CAT (LEFT, CENTRE)

Position yourself on your hands and knees, ensuring your weight is distributed evenly. Point your fingers forward. Inhale slowly, pull in your stomach muscles, and curve your back towards the ceiling to create an arch. Tuck your chin into your chest and hold for a count of five. Exhale slowly as you relax your spine and bring your head back to its normal position. Continue exhaling as you reverse the arch of your spine, pulling your head back to look upward. Inhale again as your move your head, neck, and spine back to the starting position. Keep your movements slow and never strain. Practice the whole sequence five times altogether.

CHILD'S POSE (LEFT, BOTTOM)

Kneel on a mat on the floor and sit back on your heels so your heels are directly underneath your bottom and your knees point forward. Pull your knees apart slightly and keep your toes together to form a V-shape with your thighs. Roll your spine downward, folding your upper body over your thighs with your arms extended loosely in front of you. If possible, touch the floor with your forehead (separate your knees a little more if need be, but keep your bottom in contact with your heels). Relax for a count of 20 or as long as you're comfortable. Slowly roll back upward to a sitting position.

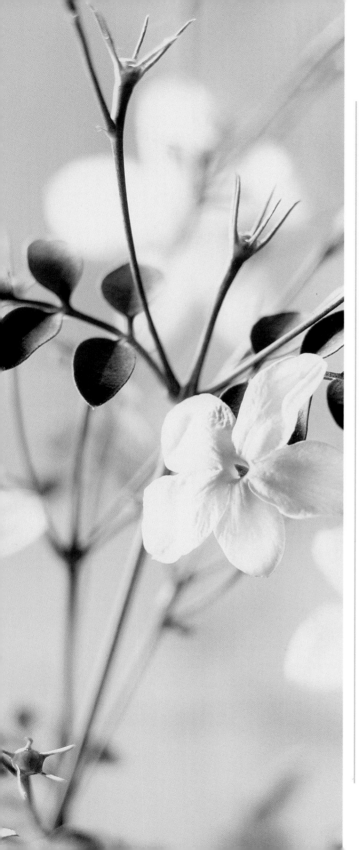

OTHER NATURAL TREATMENTS

Homeopathy To reduce pain in the lower abdomen, homeopaths usually prescribe Lachesis 30c and Calcarea 30c (each taken twice daily).

Acupuncture The acupuncture points commonly associated with endometriosis are found on the ears, abdomen, wrists, feet, legs, and back. Your practitioner will treat these and other points relevant to your particular constitution.

Aromatherapy Regular abdominal massage with aromatherapy oils can help ease the cramping associated with endometriosis. Use the technique described on page 105, with a therapeutic aromatherapy blend of 15 drops of any combination of the following essential oils in 6 tsp. sweet almond oil: clary sage, Roman chamomile, marjoram, jasmine, and rose absolute. Alternatively, put one or two drops of each oil in a warm bath and soak in it for 20 minutes to soothe the pain.

SELF-HELP

Use towels Tampons can contain dioxins (environmental estrogens) and hamper the flow of blood from your body. Use unbleached, organic cotton towels.

Optimize your weight Fat manufactures estrogen, and studies show that women who are overweight generally have more estrogen in circulation. Follow the guidelines on pp.296–301 to optimize your weight.

Exercise Increasing circulation to the pelvic region through exercise helps ease period pain, balance hormones, and reduce stress. If your condition is so severe that aerobic exercise is out of the question, yoga is an excellent alternative (see pp.122–3).

Relax Stress can worsen the pain of endometriosis, and some experts believe it can even trigger the condition. Regular meditation can help women sleep better, ease stress, and cope with pain (see pp.50–51).

Left: Jasmine (*Jasminum officinale*)

Preventing uterine cancer

Uterine cancer (also known as endometrial cancer) forms in the lining of the uterus, usually in the mucus-secreting cells, and is the fourth most common cancer among women.

If you go through menopause after the age of 52, or your periods begin before the age of 12, you may be at a higher risk of developing uterine cancer than women who do not. Menstrual problems and irregularities, such as heavy bleeding and absent periods, not having children, taking certain estrogen-rich medication, obesity, high blood pressure, and a family history of breast cancer, ovarian cancer, and colon cancer are all also considered risk factors for the disease.

The good news is that although some of these, such as a family history of the disease, are out of your control, there are plenty of risk factors you can influence. Do your best to lose weight (see pp.300–301) if you're overweight, take steps to reduce your blood pressure if necessary, and try to balance your hormones naturally, rather than relying upon hormone-related medication (although always talk to your doctor before switching from conventional to natural medicine). The hormone-balancing diet (see box, p.57) and the supplements and herbal remedies recommended for absent periods (see pp.107–8) will help you do this. In addition, quit smoking, reduce your alcohol consumption, and get regular exercise—all of which will help minimize risk.

Abnormal bleeding is one of the most common early symptoms of uterine cancer, so please check with your doctor if your menstrual bleeding is unusual or heavy, or occurs between periods or after menopause. Other symptoms include lower back pain and abdominal pain. A watery, blood-tinged discharge may also occur, followed by vaginal bleeding. As endometrial cancer is most common in women over the age of 50, I strongly advise women past this age to have an annual pelvic ultrasound scan that can detect any unusual growths or masses in your uterus (if you can't get this done locally, contact my clinic; see p.320).

Caught early, most cases of uterine cancer can be completely successfully treated, and treatment will almost always prolong life.

ENDOMETRIAL HYPERPLASIA

Irregular periods, heavy periods, and prolonged bleeding (heavy bleeding for more than seven days) can all be symptoms of endometrial hyperplasia, the thickening of the uterine lining. Estimates are that between one and four percent of women with mild hyperplasia will, in time, develop uterine cancer. This statistic rises to more than 20 percent if the hyperplasia is advanced. Because the condition poses such a serious threat to your health, talk to your doctor about conventional treatment. Take the medication he or she offers to shed the uterine lining or have surgery to remove it. Also take the nutritional supplements listed for absent periods (p.107). You can take the herbal remedies, too, but only if you've had surgery, NOT if you're taking medication to shed your uterine lining.

Prolapsed uterus

Your uterus is held in place by a series of muscles and tissues. When these become weak or slack, your uterus may "drop" into your vagina—this is known as a prolapsed uterus.

A prolapsed uterus feels like a hard lump on the outside of your vagina, particularly when you stand up. Some women also experience symptoms of lower back pain, stress incontinence, dragging sensations in the abdomen, constipation, and painful sex.

Anything that weakens your body's supporting tissues makes prolapse more likely; for example, falling levels of estrogen at menopause, or smoking. Difficult and prolonged labors also increase the risk, as do constipation, chronic coughing, being overweight, and a lot of heavy lifting.

CONVENTIONAL TREATMENTS

Your doctor will diagnose a prolapsed uterus by giving you an internal examination or perhaps an ultrasound scan. He or she may offer the following treatments.

Pessary For a minor prolapse, your doctor may fit a ring-shaped polythene pessary to lift your uterus and hold it in place. You'll need to change the pessary every three to 12 months.

Vaginal cones A vaginal cone, which is inserted like a tampon, contains weights that you "hold" inside your vagina using your pelvic floor muscles. You do this for a certain amount of time each day. In this way you strengthen the muscles that hold the uterus in place.

Surgery It's possible to have surgery to re-suspend your uterus back into its normal position, but the most common surgical solution your doctor will offer you is hysterectomy (see pp.128–31). I urge you to try all the alternatives before you decide to have your uterus removed—this should be only a last resort.

If your prolapse is so severe that structures protrude from your body, then you should try nutrition, herbal remedies, and natural treatments alongside surgery. If your prolapse is mild, before considering surgery, try the natural approach alone, along with pelvic-floor exercises (see box, opposite) and/or vaginal cones, for six months. Hopefully, in this time you can correct the problem without invasive medical intervention.

YOUR DIET

Prolapse is not strictly a hormonal condition, but it can get worse around menopause, when hormone levels dip, so I recommend you follow my hormone-balancing diet (see box, p.57) to keep your body in the best possible condition. In particular, eat plenty of fiber to prevent constipation (straining can worsen prolapse), and stock up on whole grains and flax seeds. Eat five portions of fruit and vegetables daily. It's important to keep up your fluid intake to prevent constipation, too. However, don't overdo it, and make sure you empty your bladder frequently (a build-up of pressure in your bladder can also strain your pelvic floor).

Foods rich in vitamin C, bioflavonoids, and vitamin A help strengthen the uterus's supporting structures. This is because they provide an abundant supply of collagen, a protein that maintains the integrity of ligaments and bone. Eat plenty of onions, parsley, legumes, citrus fruits, berries, and grapes and drink green tea.

SUPPLEMENTS

Supplement your multi-vitamin and mineral with the following (accounting for what's in your multi, too).

- VITAMIN A (25,000iu, daily) This vitamin helps the body produce collagen (see left). Take it as beta-carotene.

HERBS

Take the following herbs in a combined tincture (equal parts of each herb). Put 1 tsp. of the combined tincture in a little water and take it two or three times daily. If you prefer to take capsules, take 300mg of each herb (organic where possible), twice daily.

- DONG QUAI (*Angelica sinensis*) This herb increases circulation to the uterus, nourishing it and keeping it generally healthy.

- HORSETAIL (*Equisetum arvense*) Horsetail contains flavonoids, which can help strengthen connective tissue in the uterus.

- FALSE UNICORN ROOT (*Chamaelirium luteum*) and LADIES' MANTLE (*Alchemilla vulgaris*) These herbs are excellent for strengthening weak muscles in the pelvic floor.

- RED RASPBERRY LEAF (*Rubus idaeus*) This herb contains fragrine, an alkaloid that gives tone to the muscles of the pelvic region, including those of the uterus.

OTHER NATURAL TREATMENTS

Homeopathy Sepia 30c, Pulsatilla 30c, or Belladonna 30c are all commonly prescribed for prolapse, along with other constitutional remedies. Take each twice daily to relieve the dragging, downward pressure in your lower abdomen.

Acupuncture An acupuncturist will often aim to raise what is termed "sinking spleen *qi*." Doing this is said to help raise the organs that have prolapsed.

Osteopathy An osteopath helps realign your muscles and skeleton in general, while also identifying and helping to rectify inappropriate muscle patterns that may be making your prolapse worse.

SELF-HELP

Aromatherapy massage Massage your abdomen daily with either rosemary or black pepper essential oil. This helps ease any pain in your pelvic area and stimulates circulation to the uterus. Add 14 drops of one of these essential oils to 6 tsp. sweet almond carrier oil. Put a few drops of the blend into the palm of your hands and massage your abdomen using the technique on page 105. (You can combine the oils if you prefer— use 7 drops of each oil in the same amount of carrier.)

Stay healthy It's important to optimize your weight so that you avoid unnecessary strain on your muscles and ligaments. Refer to pages 296–301 as to how to get your weight right for your build. In addition, try to keep coughs at bay. If you develop a cough, treat it promptly to avoid the pressure it places on your pelvic floor.

PELVIC-FLOOR EXERCISES

Pelvic-floor exercises (or Kegel exercises) can strengthen the muscles in your vaginal wall, helping prevent prolapse. Before you try the exercise, check you can recognize your pelvic muscles: Next time you to go the bathroom, squeeze to stop the flow of urine. The muscles you use to do this are your pelvic muscles. Practice the following several times a day.

1 Slowly contract the muscles of your pelvic floor. Hold for a count of two (as your muscles strengthen work up until you can hold a count of ten). Release. Repeat ten times. When you've finished rest for one minute before going to step 2.

2 As quickly as you can, tighten and release your pelvic-floor muscles about 30 times.

Hysterectomy

Hysterectomies are among the most common surgical procedures given to women: 600,000 a year are performed in the USA alone. But, are these operations necessary, or simply the easiest option to offer?

A hysterectomy is a surgical procedure in which a surgeon removes some or all of a woman's reproductive organs. You probably have friends who have had a hysterectomy, but would you know what do to if your doctor recommended one for you? First of all, I want to make clear that from the evidence I have seen, and see every day, that the majority of hysterectomies are unnecessary. For example, they are commonly recommended to cure heavy periods, fibroids, endometriosis, prolapse, and pelvic inflammatory disease (PID)—all of which can often be well treated using the natural approach and other forms of conventional medicine. A hysterectomy does provide a permanent solution to all of these problems—but, unless you have uterine or ovarian cancer, or you have given birth and this has led to complications, it's not always the only solution.

If you take only one piece of advice from this book, let it be this: Please consider all the alternatives before you make the radical step of having some or all of your reproductive organs removed. Ask your doctor for justifications, alternatives, and consequences. Ask for a second, third, and fourth opinion. Ask yourself questions (see box, left), too. Don't take anything at face value and take your time until you're convinced that a hysterectomy is the right choice for you. In most cases, there's no immediate hurry to make a decision.

ABOUT THE PROCEDURE

A hysterectomy is major surgery that requires a lengthy stay in the hospital, incisions, general anaesthetic, and painful days and weeks afterwards. It can also trigger sudden and unexpected physical, sexual, and psychological changes. You'll no longer be able to have children. If you have your ovaries removed (and sometimes even if you don't), you'll have to deal overnight with the symptoms of menopause. You may also experience urinary incontinence and weight gain. All these changes are the result of declining estrogen levels.

If a hysterectomy *is* the option that's right for you, consider what type you should have. The following are the four types of surgery available. As a rule of thumb, try to have as little removed as possible.

YOUR DECISION CHECKLIST

Ask yourself the following questions. If you answer no to any, could it be time to reconsider?

- [ ] Have I had my last child?

- [ ] Do my symptoms affect my daily life?

- [ ] Have I tried all the natural alternatives?

- [ ] Am I ready to deal with the symptoms of sudden, early menopause?

- [ ] Is my life at risk without this procedure?

AREA REMOVED DURING SURGERY

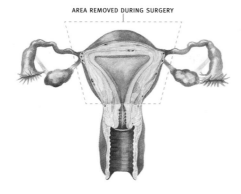

SUB-TOTAL ABDOMINAL

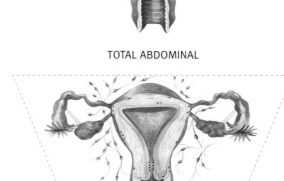

TOTAL ABDOMINAL

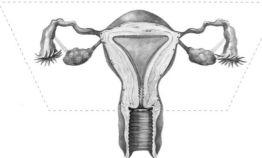

TOTAL WITH BILATERAL SALPINGO-OOPHORECTOMY

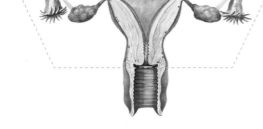

RADICAL ABDOMINAL

Sub-total abdominal hysterectomy

This represents the least invasive version of a hysterectomy, as it removes only your uterus, allowing you to keep the rest of your reproductive organs. As your cervix is left in place, you'll have a reduced risk of vaginal prolapse (where the inside of the vagina moves outside the body—sort of turning itself inside out). Intercourse is likely to continue to be pleasurable.

Total abdominal hysterectomy

For this type of hysterectomy, surgeons remove both your uterus and cervix. It will take you at least three months to recover. The surgery may make it harder for you to reach orgasm. As your cervix is removed during this procedure, you won't need to continue to have Pap smears, and you're less likely to get any immediate menopausal symptoms because your ovaries will have been left intact (see p.130).

Total abdominal hysterectomy with bilateral salpingo-oophorectomy

In this technical-sounding version of the abdominal hysterectomy, you'll have not only your uterus and cervix removed, but your ovaries and Fallopian tubes, too. If you hadn't already reached menopause, you'll be given hormone replacement therapy (HRT) immediately after your operation, and you'll need to take it in the long term. This is because removing your ovaries plunges you suddenly into menopause (see p.130). So, the younger you are when you have the surgery, the longer you'll have to take HRT. You should expect to stay on HRT until you're around 50 years old.

Radical abdominal hysterectomy

The most extensive form of hysterectomy, this removes not only all your reproductive organs, but also your cervix, the tissue at the top of your vagina and your pelvic lymph nodes. A doctor should offer it only to treat a condition such as cervical cancer. The surgery can damage your bladder, urinary tract, and bowels. You'll need at least three months to recover.

Non-surgical procedures

Some kinds of hysterectomy can be performed without the need to make an incision in your abdomen.

Vaginal hysterectomy Unless your uterus is large, your surgeon may be able to remove your uterus and cervix through an incision inside your vagina, rather than in your abdomen. The procedure and recovery time are quicker than in abdominal hysterectomy.

Laparascopically assisted vaginal hysterectomy In this highly complex procedure, a keyhole surgeon uses a laparascope to look into your pelvic cavity and then cuts away your uterus and cervix, removing them through your vagina.

THE EFFECTS OF LOSING YOUR OVARIES

If you're still menstruating when you have a hysterectomy that removes your ovaries, too, you'll go into menopause right away. It's important to understand exactly what this means before your surgery, so you are as emotionally prepared as you can be.

During a "natural" menopause, your ovaries gradually reduce the amount of estrogen they produce over a number of years. When your ovaries are removed during surgery, that supply of estrogen is cut off suddenly. In some cases, this can be a shock to your system both physically and emotionally. If you're older than 50 when the surgery's performed, you'll already have naturally lower levels of estrogen in your body. Even if you haven't already gone through menopause, in these circumstances you may experience fewer, if any, symptoms of immediate menopause (hot flashes and night sweats, mood swings, and so on), and your doctor may take no further action. However, if you're under the age of 50, your doctor may prescribe you HRT, which you'd need to take until you reach 50, when you'd have gone through menopause naturally.

I'm often asked if keeping your ovaries will prevent an early menopause. Although it's more likely you'll stave off menopause if your ovaries remain intact, changes in the blood supply to your ovaries following surgery mean that you're at an increased risk of entering menopause within five years of your hysterectomy. However, I firmly believe that keeping your ovaries and using natural techniques to hold back menopause will help you feel healthier for longer.

ARMING YOUR BODY AND MIND

A hysterectomy is a serious operation. I urge you to get yourself as fit as possible before you go in for surgery, so that you'll cope better with the surgery itself and also speed your recovery. Use the following to help your body—and mind—bounce back.

HYSTERECTOMY AND TYPES OF HRT

A woman with menopausal symptoms who has gone through a natural menopause will usually be offered HRT combining both estrogen and progestin. (Estrogen alone would increase her risk of uterine cancer because it builds up the lining of the uterus.) However, after a hysterectomy, the threat of uterine cancer no longer exists, so your doctor will probably offer you estrogen-only HRT. To find out what this means for your body, and how you'll be given the drugs, turn to page 249.

YOUR DIET

The dietary recommendations, especially eating plenty of fruit and vegetables and cutting out caffeine, in the first part of this book (see pp.24–9) will help boost your health and your immune system, so you're less likely to get an infection after the surgery. (Infection is a risk factor in any surgical procedure.) You'll be given a cocktail of medication while you're in the hospital—from the anaesthetic you'll have when you go into surgery, to painkilling medication after it. Your liver is charged with eliminating all these toxins from your system, so try to avoid alcohol from the moment you hear you're having surgery, and give your liver some downtime before it has to do some serious work.

SUPPLEMENTS

Supplements are an excellent way to ensure that your body has full stocks of the nutrients it needs to bounce back as quickly as possible. Take a daily dosage of 1,000mg of immunity-boosting vitamin C (with bioflavonoids), 30mg zinc citrate, and 1,000mg aged garlic capsules. Take a good probiotic (see box, p.33), too, as it helps build up the healthy bacteria in your gut, which form part of your immune system. The probiotic also offsets the negative effects on your gut of any antibiotics you're given. Find a probiotic (see p.320) that contains at least ten billion bacteria in each capsule.

HERBS

To help protect yourself against post-operative infection, especially while you're in the hospital, take echinacea (*Echinacea purpurea*). A potent immunity-booster, this herb has been proven to increase the activity of the body's killer T-cells, white blood cells that stave off infection. Begin taking it as soon as you have a date for your surgery, but take it in a pattern of ten days on, one week off, ten days on, and so on. Studies show that the herb is more effective when you don't take it continuously. Use echinacea tincture (take 1 tsp. in a little water, three times daily) or take it in capsule form (300–400mg, twice daily).

OTHER NATURAL TREATMENTS

Homeopathy Visit a homeopath both before and after surgery so he or she can give you individualized remedies to speed the recovery process. As a start, you could take Arnica 30c several times daily in the week leading up to your operation.

Aromatherapy Essential oils can help ease pain and encourage healing and restful sleep after your operation. Try spritzing some lavender and German chamomile in your hospital room, or put a few drops on your pillows or forehead before you sleep. In addition to promoting relaxation, lavender has antibacterial qualities, which can help fight infection—try adding a few drops to your nighttime bath.

SELF-HELP

Vitamin-E oil If you're having surgery that requires an incision, check with your doctor for contraindications, and if he or she is happy, apply vitamin-E oil directly to your skin both before and after the operation. The oil boosts wound-healing and reduces the risk of scarring. Simply pierce a vitamin-E capsule (or use a few drops of pure vitamin-E oil from an oil bottle) and rub the oil into the wound site (or the place where the incision will be made), twice daily.

Managing your emotions It's difficult to predict how you'll feel after a hysterectomy because each woman responds in her own unique way. However, it's important to be ready for some kind of reaction because having a hysterectomy is a life-changing experience. While some women feel instantly healthier and rejuvenated, others feel that a significant part of them has been stolen away. This loss is like any other, and it's important to work through the grief process by expressing it verbally and having an outlet for your emotions. You may consider counseling, but, before your operation, try to line up a close friend or loved one who'll be ready to listen to you without judging you after your surgery, and to offer you support when you need it.

YOUR CERVIX

The lowest portion of your uterus, your cervix provides the gateway to all your reproductive organs. Taking care of your cervix is vital not only for the cervix itself, but for the rest of your reproductive system, too.

Your cervix provides a passageway between your vagina and uterus. Its beneficial mucus secretions (see p.15) protect all your reproductive organs from the harmful pathogens (bacteria, viruses, and other infective microbes) that exist outside your body.

WHAT CAN GO WRONG?

Like every part of your body, it's perfectly likely that your cervix will remain healthy throughout your reproductive life. However, as with all other parts of your body, your cervix is also susceptible to some forms of disease. Specifically, the dangers for the cervix are abnormal cell growth (which has the potential to lead to cancer), general infection, and sexually transmitted disease (STD; see pp.148–51).

One common problem is cervicitis, or inflammation of the cervix. This condition is usually caused by some kind of irritation to the cervix (such as wearing a tampon for too long), or by a vaginal infection or an STD. In most cases, it can be cleared with the use of antibiotics. More serious, however, is a condition known as cervical dysplasia, which is the name doctors have given to abnormal changes in cervical tissue. The condition itself does not have any symptoms, but it is considered precancerous—left untreated it can lead to an early stage of cervical cancer known as "cervical carcinoma in situ." For this reason, it's vital that you have a regular Pap smear (see p.135). Other problems for your cervix include harmless cervical polyps (tongue-like projections that grow out from the cervical opening or os) and benign cervical cysts.

TAKING CARE OF YOUR CERVIX

Your cervix is a critical part of your reproductive system, so keeping it healthy is of paramount importance. Here are a few simple self-help tips to help prevent problems and guard your cervical health.

Review your diet Follow my hormone-balancing diet (see box, p.57) because studies show that drinking too much alcohol, being overweight, and eating a diet rich in refined foods, saturated fats, and sugar can affect your hormonal health and all aspects of your physical health, including the health of your cervix.

Eat plenty of B-vitamins Found naturally in green and yellow vegetables and citrus fruits, B-vitamins are crucial for cervical health because a deficiency, in particular of folic acid, can increase the risk of abnormal cell changes in your cervix. If you're taking the Pill, taking supplements of folic acid is especially important because the Pill increases the rate of cell division in your cervix, which may lead to abnormalities. As well as eating plenty of B-rich foods, take a daily B-complex supplement that contains 400µg folic acid and 25mg each of most of the other B-vitamins.

Take burdock root This herbal remedy (Latin name, *Arctium lappa*; see p.132) is known to help prevent or even reverse precancerous changes in the cervix. Herbalists believe that it's most effective when used fresh, but the active constituents can still work if you use it dried. If you're concerned about cervical

YOGA FOR YOUR CERVIX

Yoga's Tailor's pose is beneficial for cervical health because it helps keep your cervix flexible and improves circulation generally to the pelvic region. Practice the posture in a quiet place where you'll be undisturbed. Wear loose, comfortable clothing that won't restrict your movement. If the pose hurts your ankles against the floor, put a folded towel beneath them for cushioning.

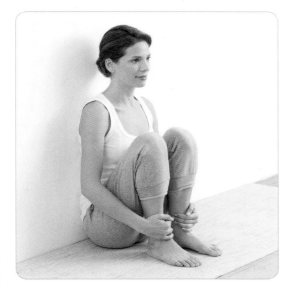

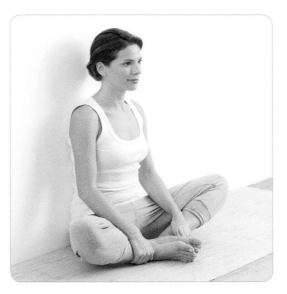

1 Spread a mat or blanket on the floor so you can sit on it with your back against a wall. Make yourself comfortable and put your legs straight out in front of you. Bend your knees and draw back your feet, bringing them as close to your body as possible.

2 Allow your knees to gently fall outward until you feel a stretch in your inner thighs. Bring the soles of your feet together. Gently hold your ankles but try to keep your back straight against the wall (if you can't keep your back straight and hold your ankles, hold your calves instead). Don't bounce your knees, simply rest in the position. Breathe deeply, in through your nose and out through your mouth, for as long as you feel comfortable.

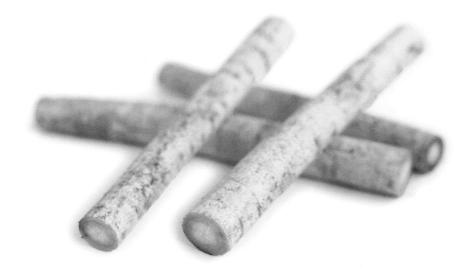

ABOVE: Burdock root (*Arctium lappa*)

cancer, take burdock root either as a tincture (1 tsp. tincture in a little water, two or three times daily) or in capsule form (500–700mg, daily). Or, burdock root makes a good hot decoction, which can provide a healthy alternative to caffeine-rich tea and coffee. To make the decoction, simmer 2 tbsp. finely sliced fresh burdock root in 4 cups water for ten minutes (keep the lid on the pan). Let it cool, then strain. Take one cup of the liquid, twice daily. (You can store the remainder in a sealed container in the refrigerator for 24 hours.)

Be vigilant As well as making sure you have regular Pap smears, you need to look out for any unusual symptoms, such as painful intercourse, odd-smelling discharge, unusual dryness or an increase in discharge (that isn't linked to your usual hormonal fluctuations), bleeding after intercourse, unexpected bleeding, and persistent pelvic pain. Report any of these to your doctor immediately.

Practice safe sex Using a condom can help prevent some STDs that affect the cervix (such as HPV, the human papillomavirus, which causes genital warts). Above all, it's vital that you get to know your partner's sexual history before you have intercourse.

Quit smoking Smoking cigarettes increases your risk of dysplasia—the cervical cell changes that can lead to cancer. If you smoke, quit.

Don't douche I recommend that you avoid douching because it can affect the consistency and protective benefits of cervical mucus; it may even damage the cervix itself. Bathing and showering are fine, but other than those, the vagina does a fine job keeping itself clean without intervention.

Take care of your well-being Last, but by no means least, adopt a healthy lifestyle. Stress and lack of exercise both have a negative effect on all the cells in your body, including those of your cervix. Practice the yoga Tailor's pose (see box, p.133) every day as part of a regular exercise plan to improve the health of your cervix and help you unwind.

Cervical tests

In the mid-20th century Georgios Papanikolaou, a Greek doctor living in New York, developed the "Pap" test—a way to discover mutations in the cells of the cervix with the aim of detecting cervical cancer.

More than 60 years on, most women of childbearing age will have had at least one cervical test in their lifetime. By inserting a small instrument called a speculum into the vagina, a doctor is able to retrieve a small number of cells from the surface of the cervix. Traditionally, these are smeared onto a glass slide (giving us the common phrase "Pap smear" for the procedure), but nowadays they are often deposited into an alcohol solution (see below) and then sent to a laboratory for examination. A scientist can then look for signs not only of actual cervical cancer, but also of STDs (see pp.148–51) and cervical dysplasia, which are both risk factors for cervical cancer.

WHAT HAPPENS TO YOUR PAP SMEAR?

If you've had a traditional Pap smear, a trained lab technician examines the cells under a microscope and grades them according to the degree of abnormal changes. If the lab finds significant changes, your doctor may recommend you have a colposcopy (see right).

In recent years the accuracy of Pap smears has come under scrutiny, with many women receiving incorrect smear analyses. Some women have been told that their smears are abnormal, when in fact they're normal; others that their Pap smears are normal when the cells on the slide show a problem.

The truth of the matter is that the process of analyzing Pap smears is repetitive and tiring. Doctors are now increasingly using a test where the scraped cells from the cervix are placed in an alcohol solution, which filters out cellular debris from the scrape and enables the technician to light up abnormal cells with a fluorescent dye. Scientists are also trialing computer cell screening, which has the benefit of relieving some of the margin for human error but does still require on-screen analysis by human eye.

Even though Pap smears aren't 100 percent accurate all the time, they can still catch 60 to 85 percent of all abnormalities—giving you a chance to get early treatment, if necessary.

WHAT YOUR TEST RESULTS MEAN

If a Pap smear shows mild or moderate cervical cell changes, your doctor should arrange HPV testing. HPV stands for human papillomavirus, the virus that causes genital warts. We know that HPV is also responsible for nearly 100 percent of abnormal cervical cell changes in women, to the point that it may be said to be a cause of cervical dysplasia. If your HPV test comes back negative, you should have another smear and another HPV test in six months. If the second HPV test shows up negative again, your cervical abnormality has not progressed and typically your doctor won't offer you any further treatment because your risk of developing cervical cancer is negligible.

If, however, the HPV test is positive, your doctor will advise you to have a colposcopy, which provides a more thorough analysis of the changes to your cells. In order to perform the colposcopy your doctor will inject a small amount of acetic acid (essentially, vinegar) into your vagina, which has the effect of forcing the cells of your cervix to fill with water, making them no longer translucent. The colposcope itself is positioned outside your vagina and shines a bright light onto the cervix. Abnormal cells appear white through the colposcope, allowing your doctor to detect them.

However, many women who have the HPV virus never experience any cervical dysplasia because their immune system keeps the virus in check. Nevertheless, as you get older, particularly once you're over the age of 30, the virus poses an increasingly greater risk of causing cervical dysplasia, making it essential that you regularly visit your doctor for a Pap smear.

Many women are diagnosed with mild cell changes that never develop into cancer or cause any problems. In the great majority of cases, abnormal cell growth returns to normal. On the following pages, we'll look at what happens when a Pap smear reveals that you do have cervical cancer, as well as ways to arm your body against cervical cancer in the first place.

CLASSIFICATION OF CELL CHANGES

CIN stands for cervical intraepithelial neoplasia, and it's an international system of classification to grade the severity of an abnormal Pap smear. It's a measure of the number of new abnormal cells on the surface of your cervix.

- CIN I: Mild abnormal cell growth.
- CIN II: Moderate abnormal cell growth.
- CIN III: Severe abnormal cell growth (known as "carcinoma-in-situ"). Although severe, the abnormal cells are still on the surface of the cervix. Left untreated, they could spread below the surface and invade other pelvic organs. The problem is then invasive cervical cancer.

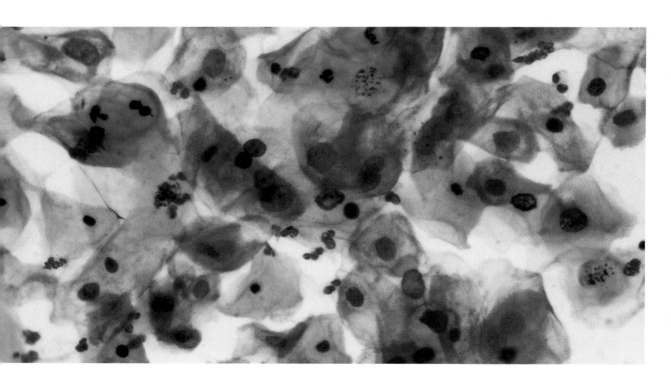

Above: Cervical cells in a Pap test

Preventing cervical cancer

Being told you have abnormal cells on your cervix can be extremely frightening. But it doesn't necessarily mean you have cervical cancer—and there's plenty you can do to prevent cervical cancer.

Around 370,000 cases of cervical cancer are diagnosed in the world each year. The main risk factor for the disease is the human papillomavirus (HPV). Anything that increases your risk of contracting this virus is itself a risk factor for cervical cancer. This includes early sexual activity (young cells may be more susceptible to the cervical damage the virus may cause) and poor immunity. In addition, smoking is a separate major risk factor because nicotine triggers damage to cervical cells.

SYMPTOMS AND DIAGNOSIS

If you experience any bleeding after intercourse, or if you have bleeding between periods and a continuous vaginal discharge, I urge you to see your doctor right away. Ask for a Pap smear to rule out cervical dysplasia—remember that harmless cervical erosion and cervical polyps can cause bleeding between periods, too, so don't assume the news will be bad. Your doctor will perform a colposcopy (see pp.135–6) to establish whether or not you have abnormal cell growth on your cervix, and, if you do, he or she will order a biopsy to establish whether or not the cells are cancerous.

CONVENTIONAL TREATMENTS

After a diagnosis of abnormal cell changes, your doctor will offer you the treatment that's most appropriate for the extent of the abnormalities. The following aim to prevent cervical dysplasia becoming cervical cancer.

Diathermy The CIN grading that categorizes the cell changes in your cervix refers to cells on the surface of the cervical tissue. A doctor can destroy these abnormal surface cells quickly and easily using heat (diathermy), giving you just a local anaesthetic. Although you may bleed for up to three weeks afterwards, this is a highly effective technique, and it's unlikely that abnormal cell changes will recur. Afterwards, I would strongly advise you to have six-monthly cervical tests, eventually spreading them out to yearly when your doctor says it's okay to do so. Laser surgery (burning cells off with a laser) and cryosurgery (freezing them with a small probe) are also suitable treatments for outer-surface cervical abnormalities.

Cone biopsy Sometimes it might be necessary to cut away the affected cells in your cervix rather than destroying them with heat. This is called a cone biopsy, and a doctor will often choose this method of treatment if he or she can't see the cells clearly. Performed under local or general anaesthetic, a cone biopsy is so-called because your doctor uses a heated loop to extract a cone-shaped piece of tissue from your cervix. (The cut-away tissue is cone shaped because the part that's removed closest to the vagina is wider than the tissue taken from the junction of the cervix, following the natural shape of the neck of the vagina.)

Cone biopsy is both a treatment and a diagnostic technique. The abnormal cells are cut away (and it's unlikely you'll have a recurrence) as a method of treatment but are then sent to a laboratory for further analysis. You may have some bleeding for up to three weeks after the procedure while the tissue is healing.

Vaccine A vaccine is now available to young girls to try to help prevent them from developing cervical cancer. It's normally given to girls around ages 11 to 12 and aims to protect them against becoming infected with HPV (see p.135). The vaccination is extremely controversial because it reduces the risk of a girl contracting genital warts, and therefore (the argument goes) could lull girls into a false sense of security and encourage promiscuity. Some reports suggest that the vaccination can have a number of unpleasant side-effects, including nausea, muscle weakness, fever, dizziness, and numbness. More worryingly still, some doctors have reported instances of girls developing paralysis, convulsions, and sight problems after they'd being given the vaccine. As a result, I don't recommend this vaccine to any of my patients, or their daughters.

YOUR DIET

Nutrition plays a crucial role in helping to prevent cervical dysplasia, and the right balance of nutrients may even, according to some studies, reverse abnormal cell changes altogether.

First and foremost, boost your intake of immunity-boosting antioxidants, in particular beta-carotene (which the body uses to make vitamin A), which research shows can be significantly deficient in women with cervical cancer. Orange vegetables and fruits are a sure sign of good beta-carotene content, so stock up on carrots, sweet potatoes, and cantaloupe, among all the other brightly colored fruit and vegetables you see. In addition, leafy greens such as broccoli, kale, and cabbage are all good vegetable sources. Other important antioxidant nutrients are vitamins C (in citrus fruits, green beans, and so on) and E (also found in leafy greens, as well as nuts and seeds), and the minerals zinc (in legumes, nuts, and whole grains) and selenium (fish and shellfish, grains, and garlic).

In addition, pile your plate with foods rich in folic acid (leafy green vegetables, yellow vegetables, and citrus fruits). An important B-vitamin, folic acid has been shown to slow the mutation of abnormal cells.

SUPPLEMENTS

The following supplements are specifically targeted at helping your body fight HPV and cervical dysplasia, which may lead to cervical cancer. Take a daily multivitamin and mineral (see p.320), adding in extra supplements of the nutrients below if the amounts in your multi don't meet the following requirements.

■ B-COMPLEX (containing 25mg of each B-vitamin, daily) Research shows a strong link between a deficiency of vitamin B6 and cervical cancer: Between a quarter and a third of women with cervical cancer lack sufficient levels of this important nutrient. Remember, the B-vitamins work as a team, so always choose a B-complex supplement, rather than an individual supplement. The exception can be folic acid (see below).

■ VITAMIN C with bioflavonoids (500mg, twice daily, as magnesium ascorbate) Studies indicate that women with cervical dysplasia often have low levels of vitamin C. This vitamin is both a powerful antioxidant (and so helps prevent abnormal cell changes) and a general immunity-booster (so can help your body fight off forms of infection).

■ FOLIC ACID (800μg, daily) Amazingly, even though a deficiency in folic acid may not show up in a blood test, it will show up on a cervical scrape because a lack of folic acid results in abnormal cell changes in your cervix. If you're on the Pill, its especially important to take folic acid.

■ SELENIUM (200μg, daily) and ZINC (50mg, daily as zinc citrate) These antioxidants are crucial for maintaining the health and function of all your body's cells.

■ CAROTENES (50,000iu, daily) We already know that beta-carotene is a crucial nutrient in the prevention of cervical cancer, but other carotenes are important, too. Tomatoes and other red fruits and vegetables (such as red bell peppers) contain a carotene called lycopene. Some experts believe that lycopene may be more powerful than beta-carotene in helping to prevent or reverse cervical dysplasia. If you take a supplement, you can be sure to be benefiting from a full range of different carotenes and all their positive effects.

HERBS

The world of herbs offers several powerful antivirals. Because we know that most cervical dysplasia is caused by a virus (HPV; see p.135), we can harness the power of these herbs against this disease. The dosages I've given are for using each herb individually. Ideally, you would want a combined effect, and it would be better to mix the herbs together in equal measures and take 1 tsp. of the combined tinctures in a little water, twice daily.

■ ASTRAGALUS (*Astragalus membranaceus*) Studies show that astragalus is an effective antidote to a number of different viruses. It also grows best in selenium-rich soils, so may help boost your selenium levels, too. (Selenium is an important antioxidant; see opposite.) Take 1 tsp. tincture in a little water, twice daily; or 500–900mg in capsule form, daily.

■ CAT'S CLAW (*Uncaria tomentosa*) This herb helps increase the activity of white blood cells in the body (to fight the HPV virus), and also has strong antioxidant properties, making it anti-carcinogenic. Take 1 tsp. tincture in a little water, twice daily; or 500–900mg in capsule form, daily.

■ ECHINACEA (*Echinacea purpurea*) This powerful antiviral herb can help your body fight HPV. Studies show that echinacea is more effective if you take it with short breaks. So, take it for ten days on, then break for a week, then resume for ten days, then break again, and so on. Take 1 tsp. tincture in a little water, three times daily; or 300–400mg in capsule form, twice daily.

■ GOLDENSEAL (*Hydrastis canadensis*) Immunity-boosting goldenseal has a strong antimicrobial action and may even help reduce or eliminate cell abnormalities in the cervix. Take 1 tsp. tincture in a little water, twice daily; or 300–600mg in capsule form, daily.

■ THUJA (*Thuja occidentalis*) Because HPV causes genital warts and thuja is effective against genital warts, it stands to reason that this powerful antiviral herb can help fight HPV. Take 1 tsp. tincture in a little water, twice a day; or 500–900mg in capsule form, daily.

SELF-HELP

Practice safe sex In the great majority of cases, cervical dysplasia is a sexually transmitted disease—it's extremely rare for virgins to have it. So, unless you're in a permanent relationship, always use condoms during intercourse and don't sleep with a man unless you know his sexual history. Unfortunately, condoms won't protect you from contracting HPV entirely because the virus also lives on skin cells around the genitals. So, avoid sleeping with a partner whom you know has genital warts (and don't be afraid to ask) and try to limit the number of sexual partners you have.

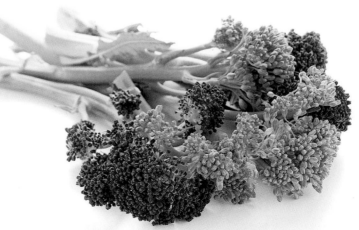

BROCCOLI FLORETS are a rich source of beta-carotene.

YOUR VAGINA

Your vagina is a good barometer of your overall reproductive health. If you keep your vagina healthy, you'll be making good headway in keeping the rest of your reproductive system healthy, too.

Your vagina plays host to a finely balanced ecosystem of good bacteria (called lactobacilli), which helps maintain the vagina as an acidic environment (which itself keeps infection at bay) and constantly fights off unhealthy bacteria. Scrupulously clean, with a self-regulating system for fighting bacteria, the vagina, when it's healthy, can be cleaner than your mouth.

Although some women simply have lower levels of healthy bacteria in their vagina than others, and are therefore more at risk of infection, there are a number of things that can upset this otherwise healthy ecosystem. These include multiple sexual partners, vaginal infections, and antibiotics that wipe out all bacteria (whether they're good or bad).

Under normal circumstances, your vaginal walls excrete an acidic mucus to keep unhealthy organisms at bay. When the ecosystem is disturbed, the vagina overproduces its mucus in an attempt to maintain cleanliness. This results in an unhealthy discharge. Changes in vaginal discharge can often indicate not only an infection but general hormonal imbalance, or even a cyst.

WHAT HAPPENS WHEN THINGS GO WRONG?

The most common kind of vaginal infection is a yeast infection, also called thrush (see pp.144–7). However, general vaginal infections (see opposite) and sexually transmitted diseases (see pp.148–51), such as chlamydia and gonorrhoea, are also conditions that can seriously impact the health of your vagina.

HOW TO TAKE CARE OF YOUR VAGINA

The most important thing you can do for a healthy vagina is to practice good hygiene, which keeps the beneficial bacteria flourishing. Clean the entrance to your vagina regularly, so discharge can't build up and attract unhealthy bacteria. I don't advise douching. "Flushing" water into the vagina upsets its pH balance, making it too alkaline and prompting it to kill off healthy bacteria, and many douches contain perfumes or soaps that can irritate the vaginal lining. Clean your vagina simply by rinsing with plain water. For the top ten tips on keeping your vagina healthy, see page 143.

PELVIC INFLAMMATORY DISEASE

This term (abbreviated to PID) is used to describe any infection in the reproductive organs. The infection may occur not only in the vagina, but also in the ovaries, Fallopian tubes, and uterus. The symptoms of PID can be similar to those of many vaginal infections (see opposite), but these symptoms are likely to be much more severe. It's also likely they'll be accompanied by fever. PID can be life-threatening, so see a doctor immediately if you think you may have the condition.

Vaginal infections

Your vagina is a warm, moist environment—and a perfect breeding ground for unwanted invaders. Vaginal infections result when your vagina's protective mechanisms malfunction for some reason.

TYPES OF VAGINAL INFECTION

If a woman comes to see me with a vaginal infection that isn't thrush, it's usually one of two types. The first, and most common, is bacterial vaginosis (BV). This is caused by an overgrowth of "unhealthy" bacteria within the vagina, itself the product of increased alkalinity in the vagina's ecosystem (see opposite). Unprotected sex, having multiple sexual partners, using an intrauterine device (IUD) for birth control, douching, and using vaginal deodorants are all ways in which you can upset the acid–alkaline balance in your vagina.

The second type is a condition called trichomonas vaginalis. This is a sexually transmitted condition in which an infected partner passes a tiny parasite (called a protozoan) into the vagina during intercourse.

SYMPTOMS

BV may show no symptoms at all, although some women do experience a greyish or yellow discharge that may also have a foul, fishy smell. You may find that the discharge is more noticeable after sexual intercourse. Intercourse may become painful (around the vagina), and you may have a slight burning when you pass urine. Trichomonas vaginalis may also have no noticeable symptoms, or you may have general symptoms of soreness around your vagina and a fishy, discolored discharge, which is often frothy.

Any of these symptoms should prompt an immediate visit to your doctor (as long as this is not at the same time as your period), especially if you're trying for a baby (BV can cause miscarriage). Your doctor will take a swab from your vagina and send it off for analysis. If the test comes back positive for either infection, your doctor may want to screen your partner, too.

CONVENTIONAL TREATMENTS

Both illnesses are treatable using prescribed medication, so you must visit your doctor.

Antibiotics Doctors commonly prescribe doxycycline or clindamycin for BV. These drugs can cause nausea, vomiting, and other gastrointestinal disturbances.

Antimicrobials The medication metronidazole is an antimicrobial that efficiently eliminates anaerobic bacteria. It can treat both BV and trichomonas vaginalis.

YOUR DIET

Eating a healthy, balanced diet, such as that outlined on pages 24–9, will help keep your body's acid–alkaline balance in check. In addition, try to eat more plain, organic live yogurt, which contains beneficial bacteria. (You could apply plain yogurt topically to your vagina, too.) Avoid fruit yogurts and probiotic drinks, as these are sugar-laden. For the same reason, avoid alcohol for the duration of your infection. Anything that contains sugar encourages unhealthy bacteria to grow. In addition, alcohol lowers your immunity.

Pack your diet full of vegetables that are rich in beta-carotene, which your body uses as vitamin A and will help boost your immunity. Yellow, orange, and red fruits and vegetables are all rich sources.

SUPPLEMENTS

Supplementation can strengthen the internal structures of your body to prevent the spread of infection and boost immunity. Take the following for the course of your infection and for four weeks after you've recovered. Account for what's contained in your daily multivitamin and mineral when supplementing.

■ B-COMPLEX (containing 25mg of each B-vitamin, daily) Vitamin B helps the formation of healthy cells to replace the infected ones.

■ VITAMIN C with bioflavonoids (1,000mg, twice daily, as magnesium ascorbate) This helps strengthen body structures and boost immunity.

■ VITAMIN E (400iu, daily) This is a potent immunity booster. If you're sore around your vagina, open a vitamin-E capsule and gently rub in the oil.

■ ZINC (30mg, daily) This powerful immunity booster encourages faster healing.

■ PROBIOTICS (containing at least ten billion organisms per capsule; one capsule daily) Help your vagina recolonize its good bacteria by taking a supplement. If you're taking an antibiotic, then take the probiotic at a different time of day. If you like, when you take the oral probiotic, use a vaginal pessary containing beneficial bacteria at the same time for added effect.

HERBS

Many herbs help the body attack bacteria as well as boost the immune system. Take the following during infection. With the exception of garlic, combine the tinctures in equal measures and take 1 tsp. of the combined tincture in a little water three times daily; or take 300mg of each individual herb daily, until the infection has gone.

■ BARBERRY ROOT BARK (*Berberis vulgaris*) This remedy contains an alkaloid called "berberine," which research shows can be effective against bacterial and fungal infections.

■ ECHINACEA (*Echinacea pupurea*) and MYRRH RESIN (*Commiphora molmol*) Both these herbal remedies have strong antimicrobial effects and so are useful in the fight against any infection. Use echinacea in your combined tincture intermittently (one week on, one week off) for the best effects.

■ GARLIC (*Allium sativum*) Garlic has highly effective antibacterial properties. Take garlic supplements (1,000mg, daily) when you're fighting infection to give your immunity a boost. Aged garlic is the best form to take.

■ MARIGOLD (*Calendula officinalis*) Marigold is both healing and antimicrobial.

OTHER NATURAL TREATMENTS

Aromatherapy Tea tree essential oil has strong antimicrobial and antifungal properties. Combined with apple cider vinegar, which helps restore the acid–alkaline balance of the vagina, tea tree essential oil makes a therapeutic addition to a bath. Use 5 drops tea tree in three cups apple cider vinegar. Swirl the mixture into a warm bath and relax in the water for 20 minutes or so. Repeat nightly or every other night until your infection has gone.

SELF-HELP

Follow all the guidelines in the box opposite to keep your vagina healthy. In addition, to give yourself the best chance of a speedy recovery, try the following:

Quit smoking Smoking can increase the chances of a simple vaginal infection turning into something more serious such as pelvic inflammatory disease (PID; see box, p.140).

Visit your doctor Don't be tempted to think that your infection is simply a bout of thrush, and try to resist any inclination to simply go to the pharmacy to buy over-the-counter medication for a yeast infection. If you have any of the symptoms given on page 141, see your doctor for a diagnosis. Once you have your diagnosis, you can use all the natural treatments given here, but it's also important to take any medication that your doctor recommends. Remember that vaginal infections can lead to serious complications (such as infertility) if they're left untreated.

THE TOP TEN WAYS TO KEEP YOUR VAGINA HEALTHY

1 USE WATER Use only water to keep your vagina clean and avoid all perfume soaps and deodorants, which can irritate the vaginal lining.

2 WIPE FRONT TO BACK Always wipe from front to back after urination or having a bowel movement to minimize the risk of unhealthy bacteria entering your vagina.

3 USE A CONDOM Minimizing the number of sexual partners you have is the best way to protect your vagina. However, if you do have multiple partners, use condoms to minimize your risk of getting an STD.

4 STAY AWAY FROM SUGAR Unhealthy bacteria thrive on sugar, so a low-sugar diet starves them into submission.

5 STAY AWAY FROM MUCUS-PRODUCING FOODS Red meat, refined grains, and dairy products (except yogurt with active cultures; see 7, below) can send the mucous membranes of your vaginal walls into overdrive, altering the acidic environment you need to keep infections at bay.

6 BOOST YOUR BETA-CAROTENE Converted to vitamin A in the body, beta-carotene is essential for your immunity. Good sources include carrots, sweet potatoes, and apricots, as well as any other brightly colored, orange, or yellow fruits or vegetables, and leafy greens, such as broccoli, kale, and spinach.

7 BOOST THE GOOD BACTERIA Eat plenty of organic yogurt with active cultures, which is rich in healthy bacteria. Alternatively (or additionally), take a probiotic supplement containing at least ten billion beneficial bacteria per capsule (one capsule daily), especially if you're also taking antibiotic medication.

8 AVOID ALCOHOL Alcohol encourages yeast growth in the vagina, which can lead to a yeast infection (sometimes called thrush; see pp.144–7). Alcohol is also full of sugar and puts strain on your liver, which needs to work at full pelt to detoxify your system.

9 REVIEW YOUR WARDROBE Cotton underwear can help your vagina "breathe" and so prevent heat and sweating, which can encourage the growth of unhealthy bacteria. Tights, swim suits, exercise clothing, or jeans worn for long periods of time can also create excess heat and dampness, which cause unhealthy organisms to flourish. Avoid wearing underwear at night and, if you think your laundry detergent or fabric softener is causing irritation to your vagina, change it immediately.

10 CHANGE YOUR SANITARY PROTECTION REGULARLY If you use tampons, make sure you change them at least every four hours and try to use organic cotton tampons, which are less likely to leach chemicals into your vagina. If you use sanitary towels, change them every three hours, or more frequently if your period is particularly heavy.

Yeast infections

Also known as thrush, vaginal yeast infections occur in an estimated 75 percent of all women at some point in their lives. They're probably among the most common infections I'm asked to treat.

Your body contains billions of different organisms, most of them essential to health, and many perfectly harmless. One of these normally harmless organisms is the fungus *Candida albicans*, which in a healthy body is kept in check by billions of beneficial bacteria. However, if an imbalance occurs, in particular in the body's natural acid–alkaline balance, levels of beneficial bacteria fall and organisms such as *Candida albicans* begin to thrive. When the *Candida albicans* fungus takes over, the result is a vaginal yeast infection.

The most obvious sign that you have a yeast infection is a sticky, white discharge from your vagina, not associated with your usual menstrual cycle (its yeasty smell will give it away). Itching, and soreness during lovemaking and urinating are also tell-tale signs.

Consider your lifestyle or other factors that might have led to the condition. Thrush often occurs if you're run down, under stress, taking antibiotics or hormone medication (such as the Pill or HRT), or if you're pregnant. However, even if all the pieces of the jigsaw fit and you think you almost certainly have a yeast infection, it's important to visit your doctor to confirm the diagnosis and rule out anything more serious, including cervical cancer.

CONVENTIONAL TREATMENTS

Your local pharmacy will be able to sell you any number of antifungals to treat a yeast infection. Although it's perfectly commonplace to buy antifungals in this way,

I wouldn't recommend it. The symptoms of yeast infection can also be the symptoms of other vaginal infections (see pp.146–7), and you must make sure you take the right treatment. Always visit your doctor. Although he or she may prescribe you with the very thing you'd have bought anyway, at least you'll know that you're treating your condition properly.

Oral treatments You may be a given single-dosage oral treatment, which will contain fluconazole, an antifungal. The benefit of this form of treatment is that it takes only one dose to treat the problem. However, side-effects include mild nausea, abdominal pain, diarrhea, flatulence, and rashes.

Creams and pessaries Topical treatment is one of the easiest ways to overcome a vaginal yeast infection. Your doctor may prescribe an antifungal cream, which you rub onto your vagina, or a course of pessaries, which you insert into your vagina. Always finish the course otherwise the yeast overgrowth can easily take hold again.

YOUR DIET

Your body already has a yeast overload, so try to keep out all foods that contain yeast or are made using it—from bread to Champagne. In addition, the levels of good bacteria in your vagina are in part estrogen-dependent. This means that it's crucial you get your hormones in balance by following the hormone-

YEAST INFECTIONS are also known as candidiasis.

balancing diet (see box, p.57). In particular, try to cut out sugar in all its forms, such as that added to foods and drinks, as well as sugar in cakes, candy, and other refined foods. While you have the yeast infection, it's better to avoid fruit juice, which is high in fruit sugar and low in fiber. Sugar is food for yeasts and bacteria, so a diet that is high in sugar can only hamper your body's attempts to overcome an infection.

A good food to eat if you suffer from a yeast infection is organic yogurt with active cultures. This yogurt is an important source of beneficial bacteria that can help overcome yeast overgrowth. You can apply it topically to your vagina, too, if you like.

Garlic contains a compound called allicin, which research shows has known antimicrobial and antifungal properties and even, specifically, can help the body fight candida overgrowth. Raw garlic provides the greatest therapeutic benefit, so chop it finely into salad dressings or chew on a raw clove each day. (Alternatively, you can take it as an herbal supplement. Take 1,000mg aged garlic, daily.)

SUPPLEMENTS

Account for the contents of your multi-vitamin and mineral when using the following supplements.

■ BETA-CAROTENE (25,000iu, daily) Many women with thrush are deficient in this nutrient.

■ ZINC (30mg, daily) A potent immunity booster, zinc is often deficient in women with thrush. Take it as zinc citrate.

■ FOS (10g, daily) All fruits and vegetables contain the water-soluble fiber fructooligosaccharides (FOS), which is a pre-biotic—a food source that promotes the growth of friendly bacteria in your system. You can sprinkle the supplement form of this important nutrient on food.

■ OMEGA-3 FATTY ACIDS (1,000mg fish oil containing at least 700mg EPA and 500mg DHA, daily) Omega-3 oils are antifungal.

■ PROBIOTICS (containing at least ten billion organisms per capsule; one capsule daily) This supplement actively fights infection by recolonizing your body with good bacteria. Vaginal pessaries that contain probiotics work well, too.

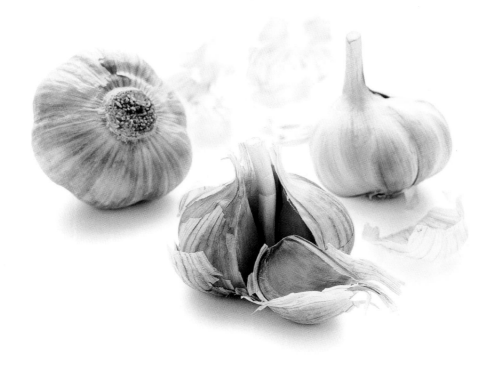

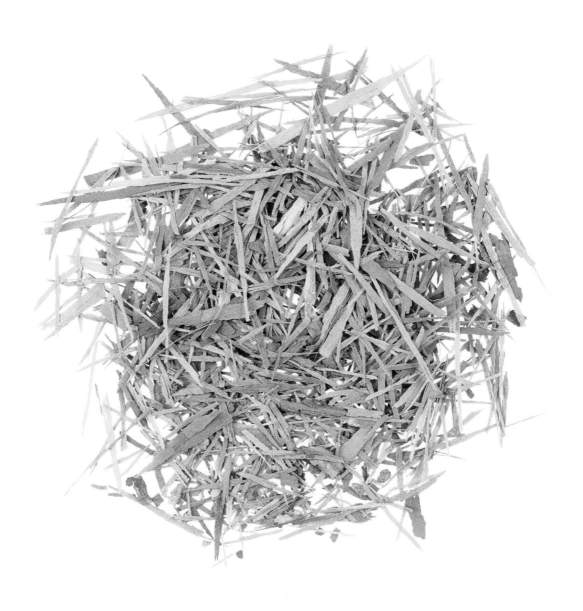

HERBS

Make up a combined tincture using equal parts of the following herbs and take 1 tsp. in a little water, two or three times daily; or take 300mg of each of the herb in capsule form, daily. You could add in herbs from the vaginal infections section, too, if you like (see p.142). Take the combination to overcome a bout of thrush and also to prevent a recurrence.

■ ECHINACEA (*Echinacea purpurea*) This immunity-boosting essential has been proven to reduce the number of attacks of candida infection in women who are prone to the condition.

■ GOLDENSEAL (*Hydrastis canadensis*) This herb activates the body's white blood cells giving it potent immunity-boosting powers. An active constituent called "berberine" specifically provides it with antifungal and antibiotic actions. In all,

goldenseal is an important remedy for yeast infections.

■ PAU D'ARCO (*Tabebuia impetiginosa*) The inner bark of this herbal remedy has potent antifungal properties. When you buy your remedy, make sure it is whole-bark pau d'arco you're buying, and not any isolated or extracted compounds from other species (check the Latin name to be sure) or just the outer bark. Remedies made using the whole bark will not give side-effects.

OTHER NATURAL TREATMENTS

Aromatherapy There are several essential oils that are good to use if you suffer from thrush. The best is tea tree essential oil, which is both antifungal and soothing. Use up to five drops in your bath. Alternatively, to soothe the vagina (especially if you have itching, inflammation, and soreness), add up to ten drops each of the essential oils of lavender and bergamot in a warm bath. (This blend will also help fight the infection and act as a preventative.) Relax in the water for 20 minutes or so. Repeat this bathing routine every night during an infection if you find it helps. Finally, you could try adding a few drops (between four and six drops) of cistus essential oil to your bath. This warming, musky oil helps soothe inflammation.

SELF-HELP

Use salt Adding a handful of sea salt to your bath-water or washing yourself in a salt solution (1 tsp. salt in 2 cups water) can help soothe irritation and itching in the vagina.

Hang loose If you want to overcome—or prevent—a yeast infection, your vagina needs to be able to "breathe." Man-made fibers, such as nylon, encourage heat and sweating, which in turn creates a breeding ground for yeast fungi. Always wear cotton underwear and avoid wearing nylon tights as much as you can. When you do wear them, make sure you choose a pair with a cotton gusset. In addition, always get out of your exercise clothes as soon as you've finished exercising. Finally, make a habit of sleeping "commando."

Use sanitary towels If you suffer from thrush, avoid using tampons and opt for sanitary towels instead. Towels allow menstrual blood to flow naturally out of the vagina, which is healthier and cleaner than tampons (these keep the blood trapped inside you). However, don't use towels on days when you don't have your period, as the plastic strip at the bottom prevents air from circulating properly around your genitals.

Avoid perfume Perfumed soaps and bubble baths can alter the natural acid–alkaline balance of your vagina, helping fungal microbes to thrive. In addition, avoid powders and feminine hygiene products that can cause irritation. If you like to use a special scent, pick a favorite essential oil and add a few drops of it to your underwear after you've put it on.

Get your partner checked out If you suffer from recurrent bouts of thrush, be aware that your partner may have thrush as well, with or without the symptoms. For this reason, it's important for him or her to be tested and treated, too. If your partner isn't treated, and does have the infection, you'll simply pass it backward and forward between you.

Opposite: Pau d'arco (*Tabebuia impetiginosa*)

Sexually transmitted diseases (STDs)

Chlamydia, gonorrhoea, hepatitis B, genital herpes, HIV, genital warts, and syphilis—these are all names of STDs, conditions that are transferred from one person to another through sexual contact.

In 2006, the USA clocked up more than a million new cases of chlamydia, and the numbers for all the other STDs were rising, too. The figures are staggering—and scary—because these illnesses can at best cause problems with fertility and at worst shorten life. If you believe you may have contracted an STD, it's absolutely essential that you see your doctor immediately. The reasons why will be obvious once you've read what each STD is and what it does to your body. (Note that STDs are sometimes referred to as STIs, which stands for sexually transmitted infections.)

TYPES OF STD
Chlamydia A bacterial infection, chlamydia is most common in women under the age of 25. It's dangerous because 75 percent of infected women and 25 percent of infected men have no symptoms at all—which means that many carriers have no idea that they have the disease. This allows chlamydia to progress unhindered inside the body and also permits those infected to go on passing it on to others. Those who do show symptoms can have abnormal discharge, pain during urination and sex, and general pain in the lower abdomen. In women, the condition commonly affects the uterus and Fallopian tubes. Left untreated it can lead to pelvic inflammatory disease (PID; see box, p.140). Because it inflames the lining of the uterus and destroys the cilia (hairs) that move the egg along the Fallopian tubes,

IN THE USA more than 500,000 people contract gonorrhoea annually.

chlamydia can cause infertility. Happily, when it's diagnosed early enough, it can be successfully treated with antibiotics.

Gonorrhoea Another bacterial infection, gonorrhoea can invade the cervix, uterus, throat, rectum, bones, or eyes, causing pelvic pain, discharge, bleeding, and painful urination. If you have gonorrhoea in your eye, you may become sensitive to light. It can also spread to the Fallopian tubes, and it can cause PID, but its long-term implications for fertility are less severe than for chlamydia. Your doctor will diagnose gonorrhoea usually using a urine test, or a swab from an infected area. The disease can be treated with antibiotics.

Hepatitis B The word "hepatitis" means inflammation of the liver; hepatitis A, B, and C are liver inflammations caused by a virus. The hepatitis-B virus is transmitted by sexual contact (and infected needles) and, in extreme cases, can cause liver cancer. You may suffer flu-like symptoms or a gastric upset, although almost half of all cases of hepatitis B show no symptoms at all. Your doctor will give you antiviral drugs to treat the illness, but eventually the condition should go away on its own. If you think you're at high risk of contracting hepatitis B, consider being vaccinated against it.

Genital herpes Caused by the herpes simplex virus (the same virus that causes common cold sores), genital herpes is spread by skin-to-skin contact at the affected area with an infected person. The virus causes blisters that burst to form painful ulcers around the genitals. The blisters often cause pain on urination and are usually preceded by flu-like symptoms and sometimes a headache for around a week. In most cases, you'll recover in a few days without treatment—but as with cold sores, the virus lies dormant and may flare up again, usually if you're stressed or run down. Tell-tale signs of an attack are numbness or tingling in the buttocks or at the backs of the thighs. If you're in late pregnancy and contract the virus, it can cause brain damage in your unborn baby and even fatality. Your doctor or gynecologist will recommend that you have a Caesarean section to prevent the baby from coming into direct contact with the sores during a vaginal birth.

HIV First recognized in 1984, the human immunodeficiency virus (HIV) causes AIDS (auto-immune deficiency syndrome) and is the world's sixth leading cause of death among young men and women. Although modern treatments can prolong a relatively healthy, normal life, the virus is almost always fatal. It's transmitted mostly through unprotected sex and by an infected mother to her unborn baby. The only way to protect yourself against sexually transmitted HIV is to use condoms. If you're infected, your doctor will offer you antiviral treatment aimed at prolonging your life and relieving the symptoms of your illness.

Genital warts Genital warts are caused by the human papillomavirus (HPV), which is a known cause of cervical cancer (see pp.135–6). (If you contract genital warts, you must visit your doctor for regular Pap smears.) When warts develop, they tend to appear on the outer genital area or in the vagina, on the cervix, in the anus, and sometimes in the throat. In most cases the warts heal by themselves, but if you feel they're unsightly or they're affecting your self-esteem, talk to your doctor about removing them using freezing,

cutting, or burning, or applying a chemical cream or fluid to reduce their growth. Bear in mind, though, that these are not cures, merely treatments for the symptoms—the virus remains permanently in your body.

Syphilis A bacterial infection, syphilis is completely curable through the use of antibiotics. In its harmless, early stages it may simply give you painless sores in the genital area, usually two or three months after you've caught the disease. However, in its advanced stages, syphilis can invade and damage the heart, eyes, bones, brain, and nervous system—in very rare cases, even resulting in death. If you're pregnant and have syphilis, you'll pass the infection on to your unborn baby.

HOW TO SAFEGUARD YOURSELF

Be aware of the signs If you experience any abnormal vaginal discharge, abdominal pain or discomfort, bleeding between periods or after sex, genital itching, blisters or ulcers, painful sex, or painful urination; or if you have any other symptoms that show abnormalities of your vagina, uterus, or cervix, I can't stress how important it is to see your doctor immediately.

Get tested Some countries, such as Sweden, routinely screen for chlamydia, and as a result cases are much lower than elsewhere in the world. If no such screening program exists where you live, ask your doctor for a test at any time. Remember chlamydia often shows no symptoms, so I would recommend you get tested if you have a new partner. Also have a routine Pap smear (for cervical abnormalities) every three years—unless you know you have HPV, in which case you must follow the advice of your doctor as to when you need to be retested.

Use barrier contraceptives If you embark on a new sexual relationship, use condoms until you know your new partner has been tested and given the all clear for all STDs. Don't take his or her word for it—remember that STDs are often without symptoms. If your

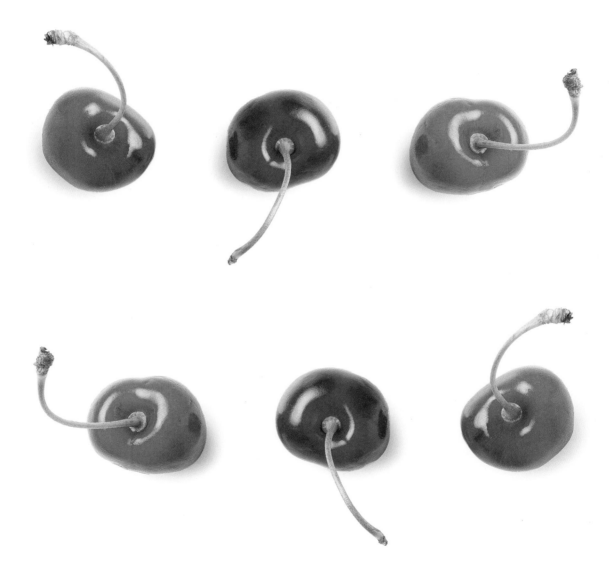

partner refuses to wear a condom, consider using a female condom. This was designed to give women greater control over their sexual health. It consists of a polyurethane sheath with two rings; a small springy ring that fits around the cervix, like a diaphragm, and a larger ring that remains outside the vagina through which the penis can enter.

Boost your immunity Follow my guidelines for a healthy, balanced diet (see pp.24–9), which will improve the overall health of your reproductive system and boost your immune system. Eat plenty of antioxidant-rich fruits, vegetables, and whole grains, as well as other foods rich in immunity-boosting nutrients such as beta-carotene, folic acid, and flavonoids. Proanthocyanidins are especially powerful antioxidants (much more powerful than the antioxidants in vitamins C and E) and help improve heart health and circulation. They strengthen the connective tissues in the body, helping create strong barriers against infection. You can find them in berries, cherries, and grapes.

Be sex smart Remember that oral sex isn't necessarily safe sex—you can still get herpes, gonorrhoea, syphilis, hepatitis, and HIV by practicing oral sex. Get your partner checked out before you become intimate.

HOW TO HELP YOURSELF IF YOU'VE BEEN INFECTED

Please don't wait to see if you think you've been infected. Visit your doctor immediately, because the longer you wait, the greater the risk to your long-term health and well-being.

If your doctor prescribes you medication, it's important that you take it as he or she has prescribed it for you. However, using complementary medicine alongside conventional medicine, can help ease symptoms and speed recovery.

Use your diet Follow the hormone-balancing diet (see box, p.57) and read up on how to safeguard the health of your vagina (see box, p.143). Boost your immunity with lots of fruits and vegetables (see left), and sprinkle raw, chopped garlic into salad dressings.

Boost the good bacteria The antibiotics your doctor may prescribe you will not only kill off the bad bacteria in your system but the good bacteria, too. For this reason, it's important to supplement with a probiotic. Take a probiotic supplement daily that contains at least ten billion beneficial bacteria per capsule.

Keep checking Even once the medication has cleared up your symptoms, visit your doctor for a follow-up appointment. Insist that he or she tests you for the disease again, especially if you've been diagnosed with chlamydia, gonorrhoea, or syphilis. You need to make sure that you've completely cleared the infection before you stop taking medication. You should also make sure that the infection has gone before you have intercourse again—even with a long-term partner.

Talk before you try If you're preparing or planning to get pregnant and have been diagnosed with an STD, avoid intercourse until you've talked to your doctor. Certain STDs can be transmitted to the fetus during childbirth, or even while still in the uterus. If you're pregnant already, ask your doctor what treatment you can be given, if any, and find out whether it might be better for you and your baby to have a Caesarean delivery instead of a vaginal birth.

Don't feel guilty So many women I see feel that contracting an STD makes them somehow dirty or bad. You may have been a little impulsive or reckless, but you have no need to feel any shame or guilt. You just need to get yourself treated to minimize the risks to your long-term health, and to learn from your mistakes. Don't feel bad about letting any past partners know about your illness, either. Only if you tell them can they get themselves tested, and stop passing it on to others if they have it.

Cystitis

The female anatomy, which is so complex and clever in so many ways, also makes us more prone to bladder infections, known medically as cystitis and sometimes called urinary tract infections (UTIs).

A woman's urinary anatomy is much more compact than a man's: the female urethra (the tube from the bladder through which you pass urine) is considerably shorter and much closer to the anus. This "geography" makes it much easier for bacteria to pass into the woman's bladder, causing an infection that inflames the bladder lining. This then leads to the classic cystitis symptom of feeling a frequent, urgent need to go to the bathroom, even if there's very little urine actually inside the bladder itself. What urine you do pass usually stings the sore and inflamed lining of your urethra on its way out. In severe cases of cystitis, your urine may be tinged with blood. You may also feel nauseous, headachy, or feverish and have lower abdominal pain.

CAUSES

Although bacteria are always the direct cause of cystitis, doctors categorize the condition in two ways—infectious and non-infectious (or bacterial and non-bacterial). Neither is more common than the other.

Infectious cystitis This occurs when bacteria (usually E-coli bacteria, although not the same E coli that causes food poisoning) reach the bladder and irritate the lining, causing inflammation. It's perfectly normal for E coli to exist in the bowels and, because the opening to the urethra is especially close to the anus in a woman's body, it's easy for the bacteria to pass from one to the other. In the bladder, however, they begin to multiply, irritating the bladder lining and causing pain, inflammation, and infection.

Hormone levels may be responsible, too. During menopause, low estrogen levels can lead to thinning of the vagina tissue, which means that bacteria can more easily pass through to the urinary tract. Reduced estrogen can also make the urethra and lining of the bladder thinner, drier, and more likely to get infected. During pregnancy, high levels of progesterone relax the muscles in the bladder and the ureter (the tube that goes from the kidney to the bladder), slowing down urine flow. This means that bacteria have more time to multiply, giving infection the opportunity to set in.

Non-infectious cystitis This kind of cystitis is usually the result of too much or aggressive lovemaking, which bruises the bladder; it isn't usually the direct result of an infection. Although non-infectious cystitis triggers the symptoms of cystitis by itself, it also makes you more susceptible to a secondary bacterial infection. Wearing a sanitary towel for too long; constrictive underwear, tights or trousers; cosmetic irritants, including soaps and bubble baths; vibrations from riding a horse or motorcycle; spicy foods, caffeine, and alcohol; dehydration; and chlorine in swimming pools can all also cause non-infectious cystitis.

CONVENTIONAL TREATMENTS

Infectious cystitis can spread from the bladder to the kidneys, and a kidney infection is a serious condition that can lead to permanent kidney damage. For this reason, it's crucial that you visit your doctor at the first sign of a cystitis infection.

Antibiotics Your doctor will prescribe antibiotics for infectious cystitis, which will relieve symptoms quickly and clear the infection usually within a week. Any antibiotics will destroy not only the unhealthy bacteria in your system, but the healthy ones, too. So, be aware that you'll need to take extra probiotic supplements (see below) to replenish stocks.

YOUR DIET

Eating healthily, according to the guidelines on pages 24–9, will help boost your immunity and encourage your body to overcome infectious cystitis. In particular, pay attention to the following, which help kill off the bad bacteria, as well as restore balance in your system.

Avoid acidity Acidic foods and drinks, such as tea, coffee, alcohol, sugar, meat, spicy foods, and undiluted citrus juices, can trigger cystitis. If you're prone to the condition, try to avoid them. If you're overcoming a cystitis infection, eliminate them from your diet completely. Stick to water (and lots of it) instead.

Drink barley water Barley water makes a great anti-inflammatory agent for the urinary system. Put 4 cups water in a pan and bring to a boil. Add ¼ cup whole barley and simmer for 20 minutes. Pour in the juice of one lemon and simmer for a further ten minutes. Remove from the heat and allow to cool. Pour out a cupful and sip it over the course of the day. You can store any leftover barley water in an airtight container in the refrigerator for up to 24 hours.

Eat yogurt Organic yogurt with active cultures contains beneficial bacteria (probiotics) that help recolonize your system with good flora. This is especially important if you've been taking antibiotics.

Avoid all sugar Sugar is the favorite food of bacteria and will only worsen your infection. Cut it out of your diet altogether during a bout of cystitis—in all its forms, from sweets to fruit juices.

KEEP A FOOD DIARY

Some, but not all, women with cystitis find that certain "healthy" foods aggravate their condition. These foods include strawberries, potatoes, tomatoes, spinach, and rhubarb. If you're prone to attacks of cystitis, keep a food diary to see if a particular food triggers the infection. Every day, write down everything you eat and drink, making a note of any symptoms. Keep the diary for at least three months. If you think you find a culprit, avoid that food for two weeks, then reintroduce it to see if the cystitis returns. If it does, you know that food is a trigger and you can stop eating it altogether.

Drink cranberry juice As long as it's unsweetened, and wholly natural, cranberry juice will help overcome cystitis because cranberries are high in substances called proanthocyanidins. These prevent the E-coli bacteria from attaching themselves to the mucus lining of the bladder and urethra. If the bacteria can't attach, they can't multiply, and this means they simply get washed away in your urine. You can use cranberry juice as a preventative if you're prone to bouts of cystitis. However, to reiterate, do make sure that it is unsweetened *natural* cranberry. Or, you could take a powdered cranberry supplement, or eat handfuls of the fresh fruit if you prefer.

Eat garlic A wonderful natural medicine, immunity-boosting garlic helps eliminate the E-coli bacteria, along with others indicated in cystitis. Raw garlic is much more effective than cooked, so chop it finely and sprinkle it over salads or into dressings; or eat whole cloves if you can bear to. Alternatively, take garlic as a supplement (1,000mg aged garlic, daily).

SUPPLEMENTS

Take the following during a bout of infectious cystitis.

■ VITAMIN C with bioflavonoids (500mg, four times daily) Studies show that vitamin C can prevent E coli from multiplying and taking hold. Take it as magnesium ascorbate, which is less acidic than ascorbic acid.

■ BETA-CAROTENE (25,000iu, daily) The precursor to vitamin A, beta-carotene is a potent antioxidant that can help your cells to fight infection.

■ ZINC (30mg, daily) This is another important antioxidant that can help fight against an infection.

■ BROMELAIN (500mg, three times daily between meals) A natural enzyme, bromelain has anti-inflammatory properties for your bladder. You can use it to help treat non-infectious cystitis, too.

■ PROBIOTICS (containing at least ten billion organisms per capsule; one capsule daily) The amount of beneficial bacteria in yogurt with active cultures is quite low, so for the best defence against infection, eat yogurt *and* take a supplement. You can also use lactobacillus vaginal pessaries during an infection.

HERBS

Combine the tinctures of each of these herbs in equal parts, then take 1 tsp. of the combined tincture in a little water two or three times daily (or, take a 300mg capsule of each herb, twice daily) from the first signs of infection until it has gone.

■ CORN SILK (*Zea mays*) Add this herb if you have urinary-tract pain.

■ ECHINACEA (*Echinacea purpurea*), GOLDENSEAL (*Hydrastis canadensis*) and UVA URSI (*Arctostaphylos uva-ursi*) These herbs are all general antiseptics.

■ HORSETAIL (*Equisetum arvense*) This herb treats

problems with the kidneys and urinary tract. It is anti-inflammatory, antibacterial, and diuretic.

■ YARROW (*Achillea millefolium*) Yarrow is anti-inflammatory and helps fight infection. As well as taking yarrow as part of your blended tincture, you could drink it as a lukewarm infusion, four times daily.

OTHER NATURAL TREATMENTS

Homeopathy I've seen good results with homeopathic treatment for cystitis. Ideally, you should see a practitioner, who'll prescribe remedies according to your individual constitution and symptoms. However, generally he or she will prescribe Cantharis 30c (twice a day) for burning, cutting pains and a non-stop need to urinate; or Belladonna 30c (twice a day) for a burning sensation with little clots of blood in bright-red urine (see a doctor if there's blood in your urine).

Aromatherapy Dilute 15 drops of sandalwood essential oil in 6 tsp. warmed sweet apricot oil, place a few drops on your hands, and massage your abdomen (see box, p.105); or add 3 drops of bergamot, 5 drops of sandalwood, and 2 drops of tea tree essential oils to your bath and bathe in the infused water for 20 minutes each evening until your infection has gone. These oils have a strong affinity for the genito-urinary tract, making them valuable in the treatment of cystitis.

SELF-HELP

Alkalize your urine There's nothing worse than the burning sensation that occurs as you pass urine when you have cystitis. This is a result of your urine being extremely acidic. You can help neutralize this acidity by dissolving 1 tsp. bicarbonate of soda (baking soda) in about 2 cups warm water. Drink the mixture. Do this twice daily. (Note: Don't use this remedy if you suffer from epilepsy.)

Go when you need to go Holding on to your urine puts a strain on your bladder, worsening a bout of cystitis. Use the bathroom always as soon as you feel the need to urinate.

Take a shower A shower is a much more hygienic form of washing than a bath. So, if you're prone to bouts of cystitis, opt for showering rather than bathing. (Although, you can still use the aromatherapy bath to ease your symptoms once you have the infection.)

Opposite: Cranberry juice (see Your Diet, p.153)

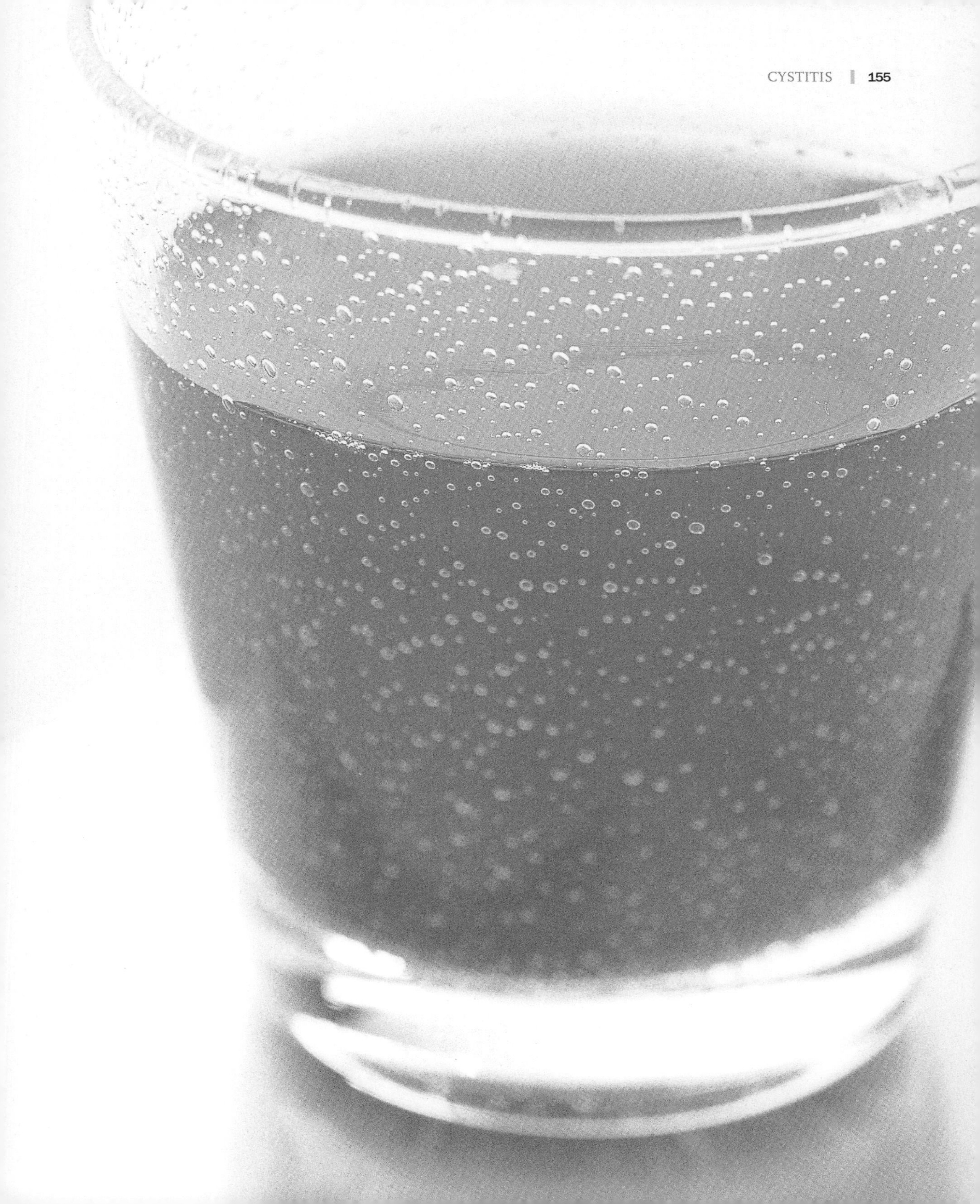

Painful sex

Sex is a natural part of a loving relationship, and it has a number of health benefits, too. Painful sex, on the other hand, is not normal or healthy. Indeed, it may be a symptom of another, underlying problem.

As well as being pleasurable, sex has several positive effects on the body, including encouraging the release of "feel-good" hormones, improving posture, improving relaxation and fitness levels, and even reducing the risk of heart disease. In short, regular sex is good for your body and your mind. However, these benefits can only occur when the sex is comfortable and enjoyable for both partners. If you experience pain around or in the vaginal or pelvic area during intercourse, you suffer from painful sex and it's a condition you should aim to treat, just like any other.

If you do experience painful sex on a regular basis, remember it's *never* a part of normal sexual intercourse. Don't be anxious about telling your partner because he may have no idea unless you talk about it. All the natural therapies recommended on pages 158–9 can offer relief, but painful sex is usually a sign that something else is wrong, so you first need to seek advice and treatment from your doctor.

CAUSES

Vaginal infection Yeast infections (see pp.144–7) and those caused by bacteria (see pp.141–3) can show no symptoms, but they can make sex painful, because the infection inflames the mucous lining of the vagina walls, so the rubbing motion of the penis causes stinging. Genital warts (see p.149) also cause painful sex.

Vaginal irritation The marketplace teems with products that can irritate the delicate lining of your vagina. Among them are contraceptive foams, creams, or jellies, latex diaphragms and condoms, vaginal deodorant sprays, laundry detergents, and bath and shower products. Scented tampons, wearing unscented tampons for more than four hours at a time, and wearing panty liners or pads when you're not menstruating can also cause irritation. Follow the advice in the box on page 143 for how to keep your vagina healthy, and avoid irritants as much as you can. (However, don't stop using condoms—barrier-method protection is essential if you don't know your partner's sexual history.)

Vaginal dryness Sexual arousal causes the walls of the vagina to excrete mucus that lubricates the vagina, keeping intercourse pleasurable and pain-free. When there isn't enough lubrication, sex can be painful. Lack of foreplay or feeling nervous or tense about having sex are the most common causes of reduced lubrication. If you're anxious about sex, it's really important to talk to your partner; or if you can't talk to him, talk to a friend or doctor about your concerns. Never do anything you aren't comfortable doing.

Alternatively, vaginal dryness may occur during the years preceding menopause, when your estrogen levels begin to fall, resulting in changes in your production of vaginal mucus. If your dryness is caused by hormonal changes such as these, find a natural lubricant that is free from petrochemicals, parabens, glycerine,

THE MEDICAL TERM for painful sex is "dyspareunia."

silicone, and other irritants. I recommend "Yes Pure Intimacy," which is available worldwide, to the women who come to my clinic (see p.320).

Vaginal tightness This can occur when you feel tense or are not fully relaxed when vaginal penetration occurs. It may happen even when you've produced enough lubrication. If you're only just embarking on your first sexual relationship, your tightness may be because your hymen is still unstretched. This last problem will improve over time.

Vaginismus This serious condition causes strong, involuntary spasms in the muscles of the vagina that often make penetration impossible, even by a finger or tampon. Vaginismus usually results from some sort of psychological trauma associated with intercourse or penetration. I strongly advise that you talk to your doctor about your fears and concerns so he or she can guide you accordingly. One possible (conventional) solution is vaginal dilation. For this procedure, your doctor will give you a dilator, a penetrative device that you insert into your vagina. At first, the dilator will probably be about the circumference of a small finger. Over time, you use bigger dilators until you're using one that has a circumference similar to that of a penis. Don't feel rushed through the process—make sure your doctor works at your pace, so you're comfortable with every step.

Vulvodynia This chronic (ongoing) condition causes a burning and/or stinging sensation of the vulva (the

HOW TO RESTORE INTIMACY

Letting things bother you can be disastrous for all aspects of a relationship, including in the bedroom. It's important to talk issues through with your partner, and for your communication to be open but respectful. With any luck, once communication is easy, intimacy will be, too.

MAKE TIME TO TALK There's no point trying to have a serious conversation when you're waiting for guests to arrive, or while the kids are still up. Set aside talk time and respect it. Turn off all phones and unplug the TV. Put some gentle music on, if you like.

TAKE TURNS Agree before you begin that you'll each have a chance to talk. Don't interrupt each other: listen and, when it's your turn, respond. Not only does this prevent a verbal tug of war, it gives you time to reflect on your responses so they're more considered and conciliatory, rather than knee-jerk or defensive.

OWN YOUR FEELINGS Talk to your partner with "I" statements, such as "I have a problem with ... ," or "I feel that ...." Don't say "You do/don't do this ... ," which apportions blame and puts your partner on the defensive.

MAKE A DATE When you've both said all you need to, end your conversation positively by making a date. Schedule some time for the two of you to do something you both enjoy together. This might be a walk in your favorite park, a quiet supper together, or a hike in the hills. Try to make it something that's conducive to conversation. You might both enjoy the movies, but unless you go for dinner afterwards, movies don't present an optimum chance for talking. Establish some physical contact: hold hands as you walk or over the table as you dine.

genital area that includes your clitoris, labia, and vaginal opening), making sex extremely painful and uncomfortable. Your doctor can make a diagnosis only when he or she has ruled out other conditions that cause vulva pain, such as yeast infections and STDs, and will probably prescribe you anti-inflammatories and anti-histamines to help control the symptoms.

Constipation The wall of your vagina is sensitive to compression. If, during penetration, it's squashed between two hard objects, such as the man's erect penis and a stool in your colon, you'll have pain.

Other causes Deep, thrusting penetration can cause pelvic pain, which is no more normal or acceptable than vaginal pain during sex. Labor problems that tear the ligaments supporting the uterus, botched abortions, violent intercourse or rape, hysterectomy, infections of the cervix or uterus, PID (pelvic inflammatory disease; see box, p.140), ovarian cysts, fibroids, and a retroverted uterus (see box, p.13) are all potential causes of pelvic pain during intercourse. Please see your doctor and talk through your symptoms so he or she can treat you appropriately.

YOUR DIET

A healthy diet rich in fruits, vegetables, and whole grains (see p.24–9) ensures you're getting enough fiber to keep your bowel movements regular. Although this may seem unconnected, regular movements not only help balance your body systems (by making sure that old hormones are finding their way out of you) so you're in prime health, but they also prevent painful sex as a result of constipation (see above).

As well as making sure your diet is healthy, it's important to drink plenty of fluids. Aim for six to eight glasses of water a day. This will encourage lubrication (your body needs water to make vaginal mucus) and prevent constipation. To keep track of how much you're drinking, fill two or three glass bottles with your daily water intake and empty them by the end of the day.

SELF-HELP

Make time for foreplay If you don't become sufficiently aroused during intercourse, you may have trouble lubricating properly. Talk to your partner about what turns you on, and make sure you have plenty of time to get in the mood for lovemaking.

Shed the baggage If you feel any anger or resentment towards your partner, you'll find it hard to be intimate, and even harder to become aroused. Try not to let any problems in your relationship fester or accumulate—deal with them as they come along. Use the techniques in the box on page 157 to help you get your relationship back on track.

Believe you're beautiful Poor body image can inhibit arousal in much the same way as difficulties within a relationship. Large, small, round, or long, your partner thinks you're sexy—it's why he or she was attracted to you in the first place. Sometimes something as simple as a little light exercise every other day can make you feel better about yourself. As soon as your body image improves, so will your willingness for intimacy. If things are really bad, consider seeing a counselor to talk through your body issues.

Take a post-pregnant pause If you've had an episiotomy or vaginal tear during childbirth, sensitive scar tissue can make penetration difficult or painful. Wait at least six weeks after the birth of your baby before you have intercourse.

Find the right doctor If you find it hard to talk to your doctor or your doctor can't find anything physically wrong with you, be persistent and get a second, third, or fourth opinion until you find a doctor who has an understanding of your condition and will offer you the right guidance and help.

Keep healthy Have an annual gynecological exam to make sure you don't have endometriosis, fibroids, yeast infections, or STDs. Then, follow my guidelines for a healthy vagina in the box on page 143.

Keep a diary If you often experience painful sex, it might be sensible to keep a record for a few months of when it occurs and under what circumstances. This will help you find out if it occurs at a certain time of the month, in a certain position, when thrusting is deep, when there isn't enough foreplay, or when your partner

withdraws. The more insight you can gain into the problem, the more likely you are to resolve it.

Abstain from pain If you know you'll experience pain during intercourse, don't think you have to keep it to yourself. Talk to your partner about the many other ways to be intimate and to have sex without the need for penetration. Work together to find a solution that makes sex enjoyable for both of you.

YOGA FOR GREAT SEX

On a physical level, yoga can increase blood flow and thus sensation to your genital and reproductive organs. On a more subtle level, it eases irritability and helps you to develop an awareness of sensation, improving arousal and so reducing intercourse pain.

This yoga pose, named Wide Straddle Forward Bend, helps open up the hips, giving you greater flexibility and making you more sensitive to arousal. Wear loose-fitting clothes and find a space where you'll be undisturbed. You can practice it as often as you like.

Sit on the floor with your back straight and your legs stretched straight out in front. Imagine a cord pulls you upward from the top of your head; feel your spine lengthen. (Take care not to arch your back.) Sitting up straight, slowly open your legs wide until you feel a slight stretch in your inner thighs. Keep your kneecaps pointing upward and flex your toes so they point towards the ceiling. Once you feel balanced, slowly walk your hands along the floor in front of you. Lean your torso forward, folding down from your hips and keeping your spine and neck straight. Go only as low as is comfortable; don't strain your back. Hold the stretch for five to ten complete breaths, then walk your hands back up to the sitting position.

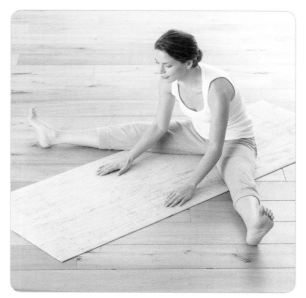

YOUR LEGS

I think there's not a woman I see who, if asked, wouldn't say she wanted long, smooth legs like a Barbie doll. Taking care of your legs, whatever their shape, is really about taking care of your whole body.

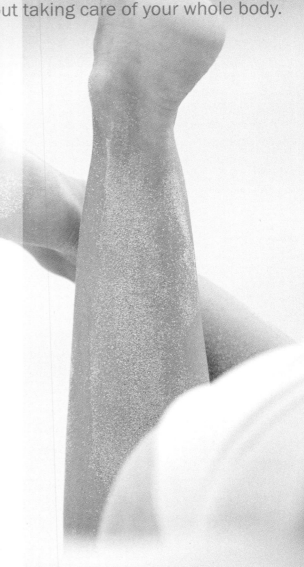

As you age, the muscle tone, shape, and skin condition of your legs (and the rest of your body) can start to deteriorate. But just as it's possible to improve the health of all your internal body systems, so it's possible to optimize the health of the parts you can see on the outside. Start off by eating healthily, according to my guidelines on pages 24–9. Then, try to make sure you exercise regularly (see below). Although healthy eating and regular exercise are essential in the quest for beautiful legs, another crucial step in your leg health is to avoid or minimize problems that can make your legs look unattractive. In this section, I want to look at how to overcome two of the most common conditions that can make legs appear both unsightly and unhealthy: cellulite and varicose veins (and spider veins).

THE TOTAL LEG WORKOUT

Combining cardiovascular exercise to get your heart rate a little above normal (such as brisk walking, cycling ,and jogging) with muscular exercise (such as toning exercises and weightlifting) will help your legs to keep their shape. Make sure you exercise each of the muscle groups in your legs in turn. Exercise your buttock muscles using leg lifts (on all fours, raise each leg in turn) to give yourself the appearance of longer legs. Then, exercise the quadriceps (front thigh muscles), hamstrings (rear thigh muscles), calves, and Achilles' tendons (in the ankles). Squats and raising and lowering on tiptoes will give you a good, all-around leg workout. Take time to stretch all these muscle groups before and after exercising, too, to keep your legs long-looking.

Cellulite

Cellulite is caused by clumps of unmetabolized fat, water, and trapped waste under your skin that push up against surrounding fibrous tissue and harden into the telltale dimpling.

If you have poor blood flow to your connective tissues, they will swell and stretch apart, allowing fat to bulge through, giving you cellulite. Poor lymph flow, toxicity in your system, heredity factors, hormonal imbalance, lack of sleep, smoking, stress, and over-exposure to the sun also play a part in causing this condition.

YOUR DIET

Follow my hormone-balancing diet (see box, p.57), which will help combat the free radicals and tissue damage that cause cellulite. In addition, try to make your diet rich in lecithin, a nutrient that can help repair tissue cells in your skin to prevent fat deposits coming to the surface. Lecithin-rich foods include eggs, apples, peanuts, and cruciferous vegetables.

SELF-HELP

Get moving! Exercise is one of the best ways to shift cellulite because it boosts blood and lymph circulation, encourages sweating to remove waste materials, and restores a slim subcutaneous fat layer. Aerobic exercise that raises your heart rate combined with gentle toning is best. Aim for 30 minutes of aerobic exercise daily, and 30 minutes toning three times a week.

Brush your body Dry body brushing—also called skin brushing—helps break up fatty deposits, aids lymphatic drainage, and stimulates circulation. Skin brushes are available from most good pharmacies and are best used first thing in the morning, before you shower. See box, below, for the technique.

CELLULITE BODY BRUSHING

Overall it should take between three and seven minutes to "body brush" your entire body. Importantly, remember always to brush towards your heart.

1 Use firm, rhythmic strokes to brush the sole of your right foot. Then brush over the top of your foot towards your ankle. Move to your lower leg; cover the whole surface. Brush from your knee to the top of your thigh. Brush your buttock area up to your waist. Repeat on your left leg.

2 Brush at the top of your buttocks and move upward. Brush the whole of your back up to your shoulders. Brush your right arm, paying particular attention to the area around your armpit. Repeat on your left arm. Finish by brushing gently over your throat and neck.

Varicose veins

Lumpy and permanently extended purplish veins, varicose veins typically appear on the calves of your legs. They can cause pain, aching, throbbing, ankle swelling, restless legs, and night cramps.

When leg veins are healthy, the valves within them open to let blood flow through and then close smoothly to prevent that blood from draining back down towards the feet. Over time, from constant use and aged vein tissue, the valves stretch and become less efficient. This means blood begins to fill up and stagnate in the veins, eventually leading to pain and distension. This in turn can lead to complications such as ulcers, and swelling and inflammation in other veins.

WHO GETS VARICOSE VEINS?

Experts believe that two thirds of women suffer from varicose veins, probably because of fluctuating hormone levels throughout a woman's life. Many women develop varicose veins when they're in their twenties or thirties. But it's not until they reach their forties and fifties, when the veins have worsened and are painful, that many seek treatment.

Pregnancy, standing still, or sitting with your legs crossed for long periods, constipation, weight gain, and heredity can all cause varicose veins. Other causes include lack of exercise, a poor diet, and hormonal shifts before a period or around menopause.

CONVENTIONAL TREATMENTS

Your doctor may recommend any of the following, depending upon the severity of your symptoms.

Support stockings Elastic support stockings compress the veins but can appear even more unsightly than the veins themselves. If you need lots of support, your doctor can prescribe compression stockings, which exert pressure on the vein walls and force the blood from smaller to larger veins.

Sclerosing fluid Your doctor may suggest injections of sclerosing fluid to irritate the lining of the vein. This prevents blood flow through the vein, destroying it.

Surgery This is a same-day surgery to remove the veins or tie them off, but it can take up to three weeks to recover. You may still develop new veins, although this is less likely if you have sclerosing fluid injections, too. In order to optimize the chances of permanently becoming varicose-vein free, follow the natural health guidelines opposite.

SPIDER VEINS

Spider veins form when tiny blood vessels close to the skin's surface break or dilate to form pinkish-reddish "constellations." Many women hate them, but they're not as serious as varicose veins and pose less of a health risk. However, they can cause your legs to ache if you stand for a long time. Your doctor may advise sclerosing fluid (see above) or laser surgery to remove them, but natural treatments will also help.

YOUR DIET

Follow my guidelines for a healthy diet on pages 24–9 and make sure you eat plenty of fiber and drink enough water every day because straining and constipation can increase pressure on your leg veins. Foods that are especially helpful for varicose veins include berries, cherries, grapes, buckwheat, and onions.

HERBS

A daily dose of butcher's broom (*Ruscus aculeatus*) and horse chestnut (*Aesculus*) may reduce any swelling. Combine tinctures of both in equal parts and take 1 tsp. of the blend in a little water once a day on an ongoing basis. Or, take 300mg of each herb once a day.

OTHER NATURAL TREATMENTS

Aromatherapy The following is one of my favorite aromatherapy treatments for varicose veins. Add 2 drops marigold (calendula) essential oil to 3 tsp. witch hazel and gently rub the blend over your varicose veins at the end of every day.

SELF-HELP

Keep moving At least 30 minutes of exercise a day should become a priority because moving keeps your blood circulating and stops it from stagnating in the vein. Brisk walking every day for 20 or 30 minutes is all you need, but try if you can to do your walking on mud or grass instead of pavement because hard pavement puts pressure on your legs and may make vein swelling worse. If you need to stand for long periods, tighten and relax your calf muscles frequently. When sitting down keep your back straight and avoid crossing your legs, and try not to sit for more than an hour at a time.

Quit smoking Studies show that varicose veins are more common in women who smoke.

Put your feet up Elevating your legs will ease pain. Rest your legs on a footstool at home and against the wall or on a shelf when you sit at your desk at work.

YOGA FOR VARICOSE VEINS

This is Corpse pose, which helps free up blood flow in the legs.

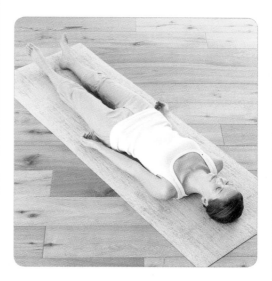

1 Sit, legs straight out in front of you, back straight. Lean back to rest on your elbows. Breathe in and out through your nose.

2 Slowly lower your back to the floor, arms by your sides. Gently stretch your legs away from you, then relax them. Allow them to fall open naturally. Turn your palms upward. Consciously relax your shoulders downward, away from your ears.

3 Close your eyes and breathe steadily in through your nose and out through your mouth. Stay like this for as long as you feel comfortable, focusing on your breath if your mind gets distracted.

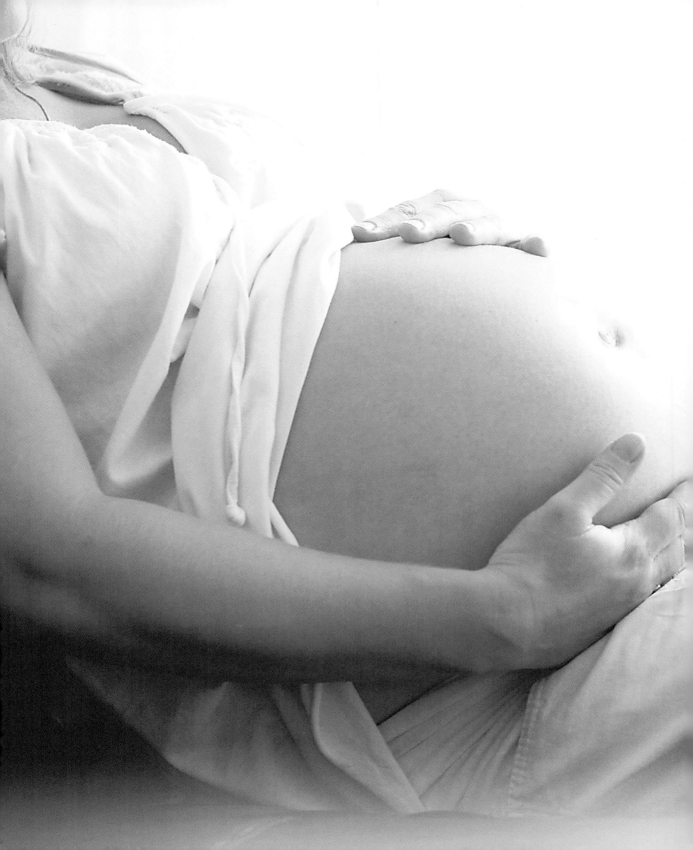

Conception, pregnancy, and birth

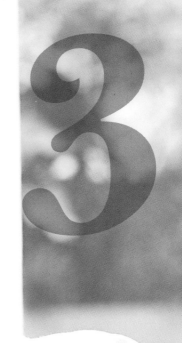

The decision to try for a baby can be a hugely exciting one, filled with the magic of creating new life. However, for many of the patients I see, it can also be a time of great uncertainty. This isn't just because getting pregnant isn't always as easy as most people think. If you do get pregnant, things are going to happen to your body that can be quite frightening if you aren't prepared for them.

In my opinion, it's crucial that you know how to get yourself into good health before you conceive. We know that if you take steps to improve your health, you'll not only get pregnant faster but also increase your chances of having an easy pregnancy, a smooth labor and birth, and a healthy baby. As well as telling you how you can take these steps, this chapter explores why infertility is increasing and what to do if getting and staying pregnant may be a problem for you.

MAKING BABIES

The process of conception and birth may have existed since humankind first walked the Earth, but it doesn't alter the fact that growing a new life is still in many ways a complete and utter miracle.

Natural conception occurs when a man's sperm enters a woman's body during intercourse and then fertilizes an egg that's making its way down her Fallopian tube. For conception to occur, an egg must be fertilized within 24 to 36 hours after ovulation, but, happily, sperm can live for up to 72 hours inside a woman's body. So, if you want to make a baby, the best time to have sex is from 72 hours before to 36 hours after you ovulate. For most women, ovulation occurs around 14 days before their period starts (see also p.94). For example, if you have a 28-day cycle, you probably ovulate on day 14 (count the first day of your period as day one), so you're most fertile between days 11 and 15. If you have a 32-day cycle, you probably ovulate on day 18, so you're most fertile between days 15 and 19.

THE SIGNS OF PREGNANCY

The fertilized egg makes a six-day journey through the Fallopian tube to the uterus. By the time it arrives, it has become an embryo, a ball of dividing cells carrying genetic material from both of you. This embryo then settles into the lining of your uterus.

During this time you may experience a missed period (one of the first signs of pregnancy), although some women do continue to experience a little monthly bleed at around the time they would have had periods. Other changes include fatigue, nausea, tender breasts, frequent urination, unusual food cravings, and an aversion to coffee, tea, or alcohol. If you want to confirm your pregnancy, you can buy a test from a pharmacy. If the first test is negative, but you still feel pregnant and

have missed a period, wait a week and test again. If the test is still negative, but you still haven't had a period, I'd encourage you to see your doctor.

WHAT'S YOUR DUE DATE?

The average time a woman is pregnant is 280 days, so to work out your due date, take the first date of your last period, go forward nine calendar months, then forward one more week. Although this will give you a due date, bear in mind that a perfectly normal pregnancy can last anywhere between 37 and 42 weeks, so the date is just a guide—in the end, nature will take its course.

THE STAGES OF PREGNANCY

The first three months of your pregnancy are called the first trimester. By the third month, your baby has typically grown to 2½in. long, and it's called a fetus. If you suffered from morning sickness, you may notice that it eases as the 12-week milestone passes.

Months four to six are called the second trimester. You may find that you feel less tired and notice swelling in your lower abdomen. By month five, you may feel fluttering sensations—a sign your baby is kicking and moving. He or she is now around 13in. long.

The final three months of pregnancy are called the third trimester. You may find the weight of the baby, amniotic fluid, uterus, placenta, and extra fat quite burdensome now. By the end of month nine, your baby will weigh around 7 to 9lb. and be completely formed. He or she should settle into the birth position, and the head should engage ready for delivery.

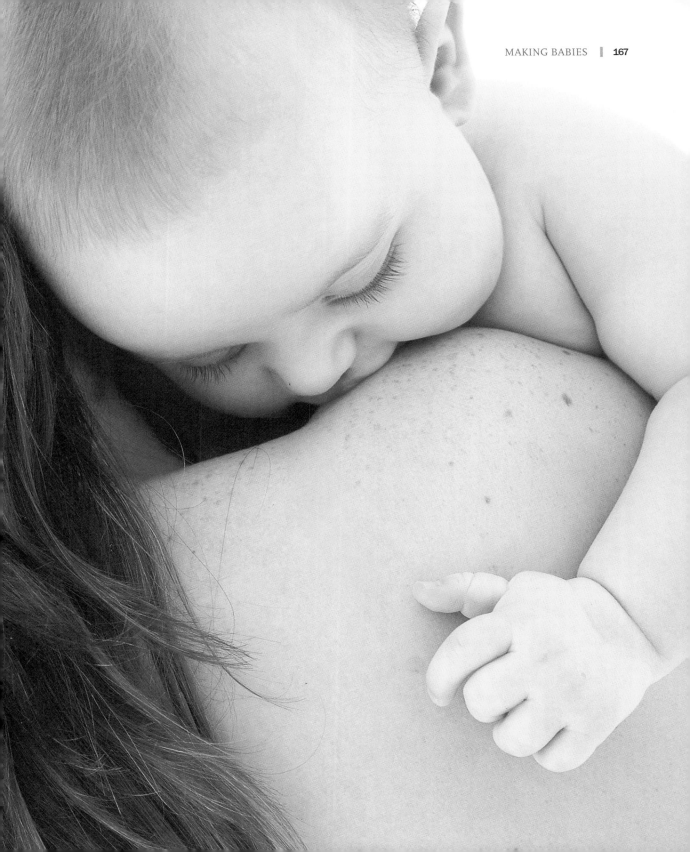

Pre-conception care

I recommend that all my patients (both male and female) follow a three-month health plan before trying for a baby. This boosts fertility and encourages a healthier pregnancy, delivery, and baby.

In suggesting a three-month period of pre-conception care, my aim is to encourage you to look at all the different aspects of your lifestyle, such as your diet (including the supplements you take), levels of exercise, living environment, and stress levels. You aren't just making it easier to get pregnant and have a healthy baby—a good pre-conception care plan may also help determine your child's health in adult life because research shows that what happens around the time of a baby's conception and during pregnancy can increase or decrease the risk of heart disease, high blood pressure, and diabetes later on in that baby's life.

YOUR THREE-MONTH PRE-CONCEPTION PLAN

Your reserve of eggs was established in your body before you were born, so the number of eggs you had at birth was already set in stone and there's nothing

QUALITY CONTROL FOR SPERM

Never forget: getting pregnant takes two. In couples who find it difficult, one third of problems can be attributed to the man, one third to the woman, and one third to a combination of both.

A number of diet and lifestyle factors can have a negative effect on a man's fertility. The following are the most important steps your partner can take to maximize the quantity and quality of his sperm.

REDUCE ALCOHOL Alcohol affects the liver, which clears out "old" hormones, and it may cause the man to accumulate small amounts of the "female" hormone estrogen. Alcohol also blocks the body's ability to absorb certain nutrients, including zinc, which is crucial for male fertility.

QUIT SMOKING Chemicals in tobacco can damage DNA in sperm, which nature is then more likely to reject for fertilization. If fertilization did occur, damaged sperm may increase your likelihood of miscarriage.

STAY COOL Hot baths, tight underpants, and heat in general disrupt the manufacture of sperm in the testes. Sperm production takes place at 89°F, but our normal body temperature is 98.6°F, which is why the testes are on the outside of a man's body (unlike a woman's reproductive organs, which are inside). Anything that heats up the sperm, or even brings the testes closer to the body (such as driving for long distances), can reduce sperm count.

you can do to change it. However, by following my pre-conception plan for three months, you do have control over the quality of those eggs.

It takes a woman approximately three months to mature the egg that will be ready for ovulation each month, and it takes the man around three months to produce a batch of sperm. Three months is the magic number also because it takes that long for your body to eliminate completely certain fertility-limiting toxins and increase its levels of crucial nutrients that boost fertility, as well as for you to break your unhealthy lifestyle habits and turn them into healthy ones. How you both live during that three months—how you eat, what levels of fitness you attain, how many toxins you're exposed to, and so on—can make a significant difference to the quality of the egg you're maturing and all the sperm your partner's body is busy making.

The three-month pre-conception plan is made up of five simple steps.

STEP ONE: EAT WELL

Perhaps the most important thing you can do to boost your chances of conceiving and having a healthy baby is to eat a healthy diet—this isn't a diet in the sense of weight loss but in the sense of improving the nutrients you put into your system so that you can balance your blood sugar and maintain a healthy weight, both of which make an invaluable contribution to optimizing your levels of fertility hormones.

Before conception (and throughout your pregnancy), your aim should be to include a good variety of foods with sufficient intake of carbohydrates, fiber, and essential fats, healthy amounts of protein, and lots of water. Make your diet rich in fruit and vegetables; whole grains, such as wholewheat pasta, brown rice, and wholegrain bread; lots of good-quality protein from organic nuts, seeds, fish, eggs, and legumes; and a supply of "good fats," including extra-virgin olive oil, hemp seeds, and fish oils (eating two servings of organic salmon a week and a handful of nuts and seeds a day will help). Following are the nutrients you need to know about. Some help prepare your body to conceive, others to optimize the health of your developing fetus. All are important for both you and your partner.

Drink fresh and pure Aim for at least six to eight glasses of water a day, more if you're exercising. Diluted fruit juice, herbal teas, and, of course, water all count towards your fluid intake, but you should avoid carbonated soft drinks, tea and coffee because they unsettle your blood-sugar levels and deplete your body of valuable fertility-boosting nutrients. Tea and coffee are also diuretic, so will dehydrate you.

Boost fertility vitamins Make sure you eat plenty of foods rich in vitamins B6, C, and E, and folic acid. Several studies show that B6 is essential for hormone balance and fertility. Eggs, bananas, peanuts, mushrooms, oats, soy, sunflower seeds, salmon, mackerel, and lentils are particularly good sources of vitamin B6. Vitamin C can help trigger ovulation and, along with vitamin E, may help keep you fertile for longer and improve the quality of your eggs. Vitamin C is found in fruits and vegetables, particularly citrus fruits, berries, green vegetables, such as Brussels sprouts, and cauliflower. Vitamin E plays a beneficial role in egg production. Food sources include seeds, nuts, egg yolk, oily fish, and broccoli. Folic acid is critical to your baby's health—not just in the earliest days of pregnancy but before you even conceive. You'll find it in leafy green vegetables, citrus fruits, nuts, legumes, and whole grains. Vitamin A (or beta-carotene) is a crucial vitamin for male fertility. Brightly colored fruits and vegetables are high in beta-carotene.

Boost zinc Zinc is essential for conception—in fact, severe zinc deficiencies can impair fertility in both men and women (a man needs it to make the head of the sperm hard so it can penetrate the egg for successful fertilization). Get the required amount (about 15mg a day) by eating plenty of almonds, fish, beans, yogurt, oats, corn, eggs, peas, and whole grains.

Eat more magnesium Studies show that a deficiency in magnesium can adversely affect a woman's fertility. To boost your intake, eat plenty of nuts, vegetables, brown rice, eggs, and sunflower seeds.

Stock up on manganese Good levels of the mineral manganese may help boost the quality of a man's sperm and will help prevent birth defects in newborns, improve the general health of the baby, and prevent behaviour problems later in life. The best food sources of manganese include whole grains, seeds, leafy green vegetables, green beans, sweet potatoes, onions, strawberries, bananas, apples, and eggs.

Raise levels of selenium Like zinc, selenium appears to be essential for sperm production (tests show that the concentration of selenium in a man's body is highest around the testes). In women, selenium deficiency has been linked to an increased risk of miscarriage. Good food sources include eggs, nuts, broccoli, and garlic.

Boost calcium If you're trying to get pregnant, calcium is important because it's needed for your baby's teeth, bones, and nervous system. You can get calcium from dairy products (choose organic, full-fat products, rather than skim), but bear in mind that there are plenty of other, non-dairy sources of calcium. These include fish such as salmon; fruits and vegetables such as oranges, prunes, and leafy green vegetables; sesame seeds; almonds; legumes; and whole grains.

Feast on good fats Saturated fats found in animal meat and trans fats found in processed food are harmful—they can cause hormone imbalance and so reduce fertility. Essential fats, on the other hand, which are found in nuts, seeds, and oily fish, play a crucial role in hormone balance and fertility and the development of a healthy baby. Scientists have found that they're vital for the formation of a growing baby's brain, eyes, and nervous system.

Don't forget the supplements A good multi-vitamin and mineral designed for enhancing fertility acts like an insurance policy because your food may not always contain all the nutrients that you need (see p.32). Also, when you're aiming to boost fertility in only three months, a supplement can help optimize the levels of nutrients in your system in the shortest time possible. According to researchers a good-quality, specially formulated fertility multi-vitamin and mineral supplement may double your chances of getting pregnant and help you produce better quality eggs. The fertility supplements I use in my clinic are called Fertility Plus for Women and Fertility Plus for Men and are available online (see p.320).

STEP TWO: MANAGE YOUR WEIGHT

A certain amount of body fat is vital to maintain your menstrual cycle. If you dip under that amount and lose too much weight, this can disrupt hormonal balance and stop you from ovulating. On the other hand, if you gain too much weight, this can also interfere with ovulation because excess fat causes an imbalance in the ratios of your reproductive hormones. For a man, being overweight can affect male fertility, reducing both the quality and quantity of sperm.

If you're over- or underweight, I recommend you aim to get back to a healthy weight during the three-month plan. To see if you're a healthy weight for your height, refer to my guidelines on page 297. If you find that you're overweight, remember the best way to lose weight isn't to diet but simply to eat healthily and increase the amount you exercise.

If you find that you're underweight and you need to gain weight, rather than lose it, don't be tempted to reach for cookies and junk food to increase your calorie intake. Try to resist these foods—although they fill you up and will help you gain weight, they prevent you eating the more nutritious fertility-boosting foods that you and your baby need. Instead, aim to eat plenty of healthy, fresh foods at every meal and have a small snack mid-morning and mid-afternoon.

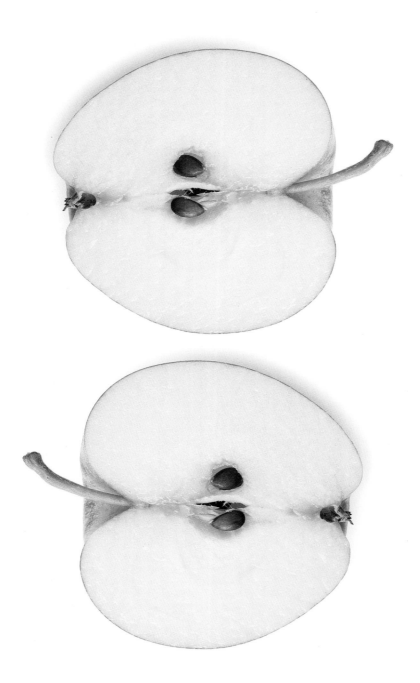

STEP THREE: BE FIT AND WELL

Becoming as fit and as well as you possibly can involves you and your partner exercising regularly, for at least 30 minutes a day, because regular exercise encourages hormonal balance, which in turn boosts your fertility. As well as eating healthily and exercising regularly, you and your partner also need to find a qualified, experienced healthcare professional to work with to ensure that you're both free from infections and any sexually transmitted diseases (see pp.148–51), such as chlamydia, which can limit your fertility and put the health of your future baby at risk.

STEP FOUR: DE-STRESS

Chronic stress increases your body's levels of the stress hormone cortisol. In order to make cortisol, your body uses progesterone, robbing it from its other function of playing a part in your fertility cycle (see box, p.19). Also, stress is thought to interrupt the proper functioning of the hypothalamus in the brain, which triggers the pituitary gland to release fertility hormones. High levels of cortisol are also associated with blood-sugar imbalance and weight gain—both indicated in reduced fertility.

Moreover, stress adversely affects sex drive in both men and women (owing to the effects of cortisol on the production of male hormones, also known as androgens, which boost libido): If you're not enjoying sex or having too little of it, you're less likely to get pregnant.

Being stressed can increase your risk of having a stillborn baby, too. A study from the University of Denmark of almost 20,000 women suggests that women who are stressed, anxious or lacking self-esteem in the last three months of their pregnancy are more likely to suffer stillbirth. The increased risk may be down to raised levels of stress hormones cutting the blood supply to the placenta—and so the oxygen supply to the fetus. Other studies show that stress triples the risk of miscarriage in the first weeks of pregnancy

PRE-CONCEPTION CONTRACEPTION

If you're planning to try for a baby, it's really important that in the three-month pre-conception period you use a form of contraception that allows your cycle to return back to normal as soon as you stop using it.

Many women instinctively opt for the contraceptive pill, but it isn't always the best choice. When some women come off the Pill, their fertility gets a boost and they conceive quickly, but for others there's no kick-start in ovulation and their ovaries lie dormant for many months, or even years. Some women I've treated have not had a period for three years after coming off the Pill. In addition, the Pill depletes the body of certain nutrients, including several B-vitamins and folic acid (see above), and upsets the balance of others, including depleting fertility-essential zinc.

Natural family planning—learning to recognize what time of the month you're fertile—seems to work for some couples, but it isn't foolproof, even for women with regular cycles. In particular, natural family planning isn't a good choice if you've suffered from irregular or absent cycles (as in many women with PCOS; see pp.83–7).

Because you can't predict how your body will react to the Pill, and natural methods aren't reliable, I recommend, dur-ing the pre-conception period, you use a barrier method of contraception, such as a condom or diaphragm, which will be effective but won't manipulate your hormones.

and that children from stressed pregnancies are more likely to be hyperactive and have emotional problems, as well as suffering from stress themselves.

Use the techniques on pages 309–11 to reduce the levels of stress in your life. Try to make sure you make time for you and your partner. Make a date once a week to do something fun together that has no time-limit—a long walk in the sunshine, or a lazy day in the garden, or watching some DVDs. Often only simple, small changes to your routine can help the pressure lift away.

STEP FIVE: DETOX YOUR LIFESTYLE

As with nearly everybody in today's society, you've probably been exposed to all sorts of petrochemicals, heavy metals, and other toxins over your lifetime, from cigarette smoke, traffic fumes, and the pesticides and preservatives used on and in food. Some of these substances can act as hormone mimics or disrupters—and for women who are trying for a baby, this is really bad news. Toxins can also affect the quality and the quantity of your partner's sperm.

Quit smoking The first thing to address, if you haven't already, is smoking. According to a report in February 2004 by the British Medical Association, smoking damages the reproductive system in both men and women and increases the risk of miscarriage in women (passive smoking increases miscarriage rates, too). Other research has linked smoking to an increased risk of birth defects, such as spina bifida and cleft palate. Research from the University of Idaho suggests that the toxic chemicals in cigarettes can cause negative changes in DNA that are passed down via the sperm to future generations.

Drink less alcohol Studies show that as little as one drink a day can affect fertility in both men and women, so my advice is for you both to stop drinking altogether in the pre-conception period—and, for you, throughout any ensuing pregnancy.

Avoid environmental toxins No pre-conception care plan would be complete without taking into account the effect on your body of hormonally active substances (xenoestrogens; see box, p.18) in the environment. There's no need to become paranoid, though, as in most cases healthy eating, regular exercise, and following the common sense precautions in the box below are enough to reduce your risk of toxic overload. Remember that it's important for your partner to follow these guidelines, too.

HOW TO TACKLE THE TOXINS

- Choose organic food where possible, but if the fruit or vegetables are not organic, either wash them thoroughly or peel them.
- Cook in stainless steel, cast iron, or glass cookware instead of aluminum. Avoid nonstick pans because the coating may be carcinogenic.
- Store your food in glass or china, rather than wrapping it in plastic wrap. Avoid heating foods in plastic containers. Fatty foods are particularly at risk because xenoestrogens are lipophilic, meaning they're drawn to fat.
- Use a water filter, either a pitcher one or one plumbed in under the sink.
- Ask for white fillings at the dentist rather than amalgam ones, which contain mercury.
- Look for "natural" household cleaners and for products to put on your skin, such as natural deodorants and moisturizers, to significantly reduce the toxic load in your environment and on you and your partner. Natural products are now widely available in supermarkets.
- Keep plants in your home because they help absorb toxins from the environment.

Egg donation

The process of having children is often not as natural or straightforward as we think it should be. For some couples, egg donation provides a precious lifeline to parenthood.

Even in the healthiest couples, with no fertility issues whatsoever and hormones perfectly in balance, pregnancy rates are only one in four for every cycle. So, it's easy to see why many couples don't get pregnant the first time round, nor the second, nor may be even the 12th. If you're under the age of 35, follow my pre-conception plan and give yourself nine to 12 months to conceive. If you haven't conceived by then, consult your doctor. If you're over 35, follow my pre-conception plan, but see your doctor as soon as you begin trying for a baby, so that you waste no time if there's a problem. If it turns out that your eggs are not suitable for fertilization or that you're age is preventing pregnancy, you may want to consider egg donation. If successful, this process will enable you to experience pregnancy just as if conception had been natural.

WHO IS EGG DONATION FOR?

Diet, supplements, and lifestyle changes can work miracles in some cases of infertility, but not all. Sadly, some couples simply can't have their own children because the woman's body cannot or does not produce viable eggs. (Fertility problems aren't always down to the woman—but problems with sperm are covered on pages 178–9.) Egg donation is often an option if you've gone through a premature menopause or were born without functioning ovaries (a condition known as Turner's syndrome), or if your ovaries are resistant to stimulation by the pituitary hormones (known as "resistant ovarian syndrome"). You may also benefit from egg donation if you've had a poor ovarian response to hormonal stimulation in the past; or you may consider it because you've lost ovaries as a result of disease, surgery, or treatment for cancer, or because you've inherited a genetic condition you don't want to pass on to your children.

You may also find egg donation beneficial if you're older, possibly over the age of 40, because your own eggs may no longer be of the best quality, which means that donor eggs will give you a better chance of achieving pregnancy. The same is true if you've undergone several IVF cycles without success.

WHO DONATES THE EGGS?

If you're considering fertility treatment using donor eggs, it's important to understand the process that brings the precious eggs to you and to know what the options are for where those eggs come from. Unfortunately, and for obvious reasons, eggs are a lot less easy than sperm to collect—there are risks attached to both ovarian stimulation (whereby the donor's ovaries are stimulated to mature more than one egg in a cycle; see p.176) and egg collection—so it's understandable why donors are hard to find. As a result, many couples wait for several years to receive donor eggs; some even end up going abroad.

EVEN THE MOST fertile women have only a 25 percent chance of conceiving in each cycle.

Unknown donors

Most clinics prefer to recruit donors who are not known to the woman receiving the egg. One source of donor eggs is women who've already had families and who are considering sterilization. Doctors may ask these women to consider using fertility drugs to stimulate their ovaries before the operation, so egg collection can take place at the same time as the sterilization. A few women may decide to undergo the process simply because they already have a family of their own and want to help couples less fortunate than themselves.

In some cases, a woman undergoing in-vitro fertilization (IVF; see pp.183–4) may offer to donate some of her eggs, in order that, in return, she doesn't have to pay for that IVF cycle. This can have emotional repercussions for the donor if she doesn't get pregnant but the woman she donated her eggs to does.

Growing awareness of how genetic origins affect a person's future health means that, today, in some countries, such as the UK, children born as a result of egg donation can, when they reach the age of 18, find out the identity of their genetic "parents." In this case, the donor would have to be prepared to one day discover that she did, in fact, have a genetic child. Under present rules, donors can still remain anonymous in the USA, Australia, and most European countries. Ensure that your consultant tells you about the law in your own country before you consider donor insemination (or becoming a donor).

Known donors

If you have a family member or friend who is willing to donate her eggs to you as a "known donor," you're incredibly lucky. However, it's important that both you and the donor understand the arguments both for and against this approach. On the positive side, you can have every confidence about where the egg has come from and, if your donor is a family member, such as a sister, you know that your baby will have a similar genetic blueprint to you. The donor can know that she is giving you the most precious thing anyone can give.

On the negative side, there's a real possibility that the donor would, in time, feel that she has maternal rights over decisions regarding the child's upbringing (bearing in mind that it's likely a known donor will see your child grow up). The risk of emotional turmoil can be very great, and it's important that you both undergo some form of counseling before giving this enormous gift to, or receiving it from, a loved one.

THE DONOR'S HEALTH

Commonly, egg donors must have reached a certain age, usually older than 21 but younger than 35. The lower limit ensures that a woman can legally enter into a contract; while the upper limit reflects the fact that older women respond less well to fertility drugs. There's also a chance that an older woman's eggs will be abnormal, making pregnancy less likely or increasing the risk of a birth defect. Some donor programs prefer to use donors who've already given birth or already successfully donated eggs. The belief is that these women are more likely to be fertile, and it's easier to anticipate their feelings about having genetic offspring born to someone else. Remember that, in some parts of the world, a baby conceived from someone else's egg will one day have a right to find out who his or her genetic "mother" is.

A woman who wants to become an egg donor may need to undergo several medical assessments before she is accepted. These include a physical and gynecological examination, a medical history, and questions about her family's medical history, including any hereditary diseases she may be susceptible to. She'll have blood and urine tests, and a psychological evaluation, and she'll be screened for diseases such as hepatitis B and HIV. If she withholds any information and, as a result, a child is born with a hereditary disease or a disability she should have known about, she may be legally liable. She'll also have an opportunity to discuss her rights and responsibilities. A donation will not occur unless the donor is accepted, matched with a recipient, and has given her written consent.

THE EGG-DONATION PROCESS

If you're thinking of receiving an egg from a donor, understanding the process of donation will help you feel part of the miracle of your baby's life and also enable you to support the person donating, if she is known to you. Equally, if you're thinking about becoming an egg donor yourself, it's important to know that, if you're accepted and want to go ahead with the process, it's time-consuming and requires utter commitment. For example, during the donation cycle, you'll:

- be given medication for a couple of weeks, and have several blood tests and ultrasounds
- be responsible for arranging your work or home schedule to fit with the demands of the egg-donation process
- be required to refrain from drinking alcohol, smoking cigarettes, and using illegal drugs
- not be able to use any prescription or non-prescription drugs without permission
- be expected to abstain from unprotected intercourse during specific weeks of the treatment
- have to sign consent forms that leave the fate of your eggs entirely up to the recipient—you have no say about what happens to them

WHAT DRUGS WILL THE RECIPIENT AND THE DONOR HAVE TO TAKE?

Both you and the donor will be given drugs (often the contraceptive pill) to synchronize your cycles. The donor will then be given drugs to stimulate the release of more than one egg at ovulation (to maximize the egg "harvest"), and you'll be given other drugs to make sure that your uterus lining is ready as soon as the eggs are retrieved. The timing is important because once the donor's eggs are harvested, mixed with sperm and fertilized, your uterus has to be ready for implantation, just as it would be if you had conceived the baby naturally.

The second drug given to the donor is a daily hormone injection to encourage her ovarian follicles to grow and her eggs to mature. Then, finally, she'll be given another hormone injection to complete the egg-maturation process. Usually, the donor can perform the injections herself, at home. Sometimes, she may even be given the hormones by mouth, rather than injection, although this practice tends to be less common.

Some women experience mild side-effects while taking these drugs, including hot flashes, feelings of depression and irritability, headaches, and sleeplessness. The side-effects usually disappear once the second drugs are given, and they're not a cause for concern. However, very rarely (in about one percent of cases), the woman's response to the fertility drugs is excessive and a large number of eggs develop, causing her ovaries to swell. This condition is known as ovarian hyperstimulation syndrome (OHSS) and in severe cases it can be fatal. Nausea and vomiting, abdominal pain and swelling, and shortness of breath are all signs of this condition. The donor may also feel weak and faint and notice a reduction in urine output. These are serious complications and will require urgent hospital treatment. Some doctors believe that fertility drugs also increase the risk of ovarian cancer, however, as yet, there is no firm evidence to support this theory.

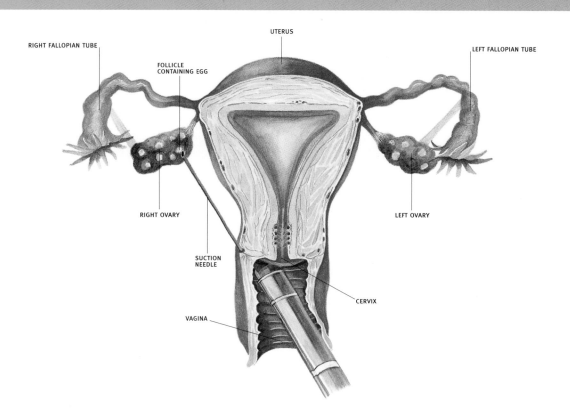

RIGHT FALLOPIAN TUBE

UTERUS

LEFT FALLOPIAN TUBE

FOLLICLE
CONTAINING EGG

RIGHT OVARY

LEFT OVARY

SUCTION
NEEDLE

CERVIX

VAGINA

COLLECTING THE EGGS

Once an ultrasound detects that the donor's eggs are mature enough, they may be collected from her ovaries in one of two ways. The first is by ultrasound probe. In this procedure (see illustration, above), she'll usually be given a sedative, or occasionally a general anaesthetic, so doctors can insert a needle through the wall of the vagina and into the follicles of the ovaries to remove the eggs. An ultrasound probe guides the way. If the donor is having only a sedative, she may ask for painkilling drugs to take before the procedure, as it can be uncomfortable.

The second method is by laparoscopy. In this procedure, the woman will be given a general anaesthetic, and a surgeon will make a small cut just below her navel so that he or she can insert a laparoscope (an instrument for looking into the abdomen) and then, separately, a hollow needle to remove the eggs. Following a laparoscopy, the donor may experience some abdominal pain, similar to the discomfort of a painful period. However, the pain usually disappears in a short time.

Once the eggs are harvested, they are mixed with sperm so fertilization can occur.

Sperm donation

Every year in the USA more than 30,000 sperm-donor insemination children are born, while in the UK approximately 13,000 donor insemination cycles are carried out.

The practice of donor insemination has been around for more than 100 years. The introduction of intracytoplasmic sperm injection (ICSI; where the sperm is injected directly into the egg) and surgical sperm retrieval (where immature sperm can be obtained from the testes) have helped some men with poor sperm to father their own children.

WHO IS DONOR INSEMINATION FOR?

By far the most common group of people seeking this form of treatment is couples who wish to have a child but are unable to do so because the male partner has poor sperm or no sperm in his semen. Perhaps he has had a vasectomy or has suffered testicular damage as a result of chemotherapy or radiotherapy for the treatment of cancer. Alternatively, he may be unable to ejaculate normally (for example, he may have a condition called retrograde ejaculation in which the semen ejaculates "backward" into the bladder instead of out through the urethra); or he may suffer another irreversible factor that affects his fertility.

Another group of people who may use this treatment is couples who wish to have a child but are concerned that the male partner may pass on a serious or life-limiting inherited disease, such as hemophilia, Duchene's muscular dystrophy, or an incurable sexually transmitted disease, to the new baby. Single women and lesbian couples who wish to have a child may also use sperm donation.

DONATED SPERM IS frozen and stored in liquid nitrogen.

WHO DONATES SPERM?

In some countries, such as the USA, sperm donors are paid, but in the UK most sperm donors are altruistic volunteers who are paid only reasonable expenses. Students or men who already have a family and want to help others are often good recruits. In some cases, however, a couple may wish to use a "known" donor—often a relative of the partner so the baby will be genetically related to its father. As with egg donation, this carries with it many emotional issues. It's really important that any known donor and the couple he is trying to help are fully aware of the responsibilities of all parties to each other. They both must also agree on the influence the donor will or will not have into the future. As with egg donation, the baby may in time have a right to discover who his or her genetic "father" is (see box, opposite), so it's important that you're all emotionally prepared for this eventuality, however far in the future it seems.

Typically, sperm donors are aged between 18 and 45 years old and are healthy men of normal intelligence and fertility with no history of mental disorders or genetic or inherited diseases. Sperm donors undergo blood tests and genital examination, including checking for urethral discharge, genital warts, and ulcers. The clinic will typically contact the potential donor's doctor (with the donor's permission) to see if there are any medical reasons to preclude him from donation. You should be aware that not all fertile men necessarily

IDENTIFIABILITY—THE OFFSPRING'S RIGHTS

The UK's Human Fertilisation and Embryology Authority (HFEA) maintains a register detailing information about sperm donors. This is intended as a safeguard against inappropriate sexual relationships between children sharing the same (genetic) father.

Once they reach the age of 18, children conceived by sperm donor have the right find out the identity of their donors. The right extends to the children's parents, the couples who received the sperm in the first place, too. This is a dramatic shift in the law. Up until April 1, 2005, sperm donors remained anonymous, and recipient couples received only basic non-identifying information. With growing awareness of the impact of genetic origins on a person's long-term health, the British government lifted the need for anonymity.

It's interesting to note that, in 1985, Sweden was the first country to lift the lid on donor identity, enabling every child to know his or her genetic father.

Not only the UK, but also Australia has followed suit. In the USA, donors can still remain completely anonymous. Fertility clinics in the States are concerned that, without the right to anonymity, donors would become increasingly hard to find and their numbers would dwindle (this is exactly what's happened in the UK). However, some US fertility clinics offer "open" donors, who've agreed that their genetic offspring may contact them when that child reaches 18 years of age.

---

make suitable sperm donors. This is because sperm donors must have high numbers of motile sperm to compensate for the fact that some will die in the freezing process. A normal semen analysis can pick up levels of sperm motility, as well as looking at the overall count and the number of normal sperm. The screening process itself may take anything up to six months.

If a man is accepted as a sperm donor, he's required to sign legal forms giving consent that his sperm samples may be stored for up to ten years and may be used to treat other people. In addition, a clinic will make notes about the donor's physical appearance (such as his build, and skin, eye, and hair color), so that a couple can select sperm that match their own physical characteristics.

WHAT HAPPENS TO THE SPERM?

Once a donor has given his sperm, it is screened and tested in a laboratory to ensure that all is well, and then it's mixed with a preservative solution used in freezing (known as a cryopreservative), divided into several different vials, sealed, frozen in liquid nitrogen, and stored at temperatures of −320°F. The sperm can remain safely frozen for up to ten years.

Each batch of sperm is carefully catalogued and labelled to ensure that clinics can match it easily to the requirements of suitable recipients.

USING THE SAME DONOR AGAIN

If you're successful as a result of donor insemination, you may want to try for a second child with the same donor. This is generally not a problem as the clinic will have a record of the donor and should have access to more of the donor's sperm. In general, donor sperm is not used for more than ten live births. (The same is true for donor eggs.) This helps avoid the remote possibility that two children born as a result of clinics using the same donor might wish to marry.

Assisted conception

From in-vitro fertilization to gamete intra-fallopian transfer (with the wonderful acronym GIFT), assisted conception techniques have enabled thousands of infertile couples to have children.

In my practice, I've found that, in the great majority of cases, making positive changes to aspects of diet and lifestyle can work wonders to improve a couple's chances of conceiving naturally. However, sometimes nature has entirely different ideas, and there'll always be couples for whom the only way into parenthood is assisted conception.

No matter how you're going to conceive (whether naturally or using assisted conception), you should always put into place my three-month pre-conception care plan (see pp.168–73). These fertility-boosting recommendations won't just increase the likelihood of success through assisted conception, they'll also give you the best possible chance of giving birth to a healthy baby, who goes on to live a healthy life.

FERTILITY DRUGS FOR WOMEN

When you make the decision to undergo assisted conception, your doctor will prescribe you a series of medications to help maximize the chances of success. On the opposite page, I've listed the fertility drugs your doctor is most likely to offer you. Some will stimulate ovulation, and some will suppress it in order to control its timing. Make sure you're fully informed about the effects of the drugs you're taking before you begin any fertility treatment.

STRESS LEVELS AND ASSISTED CONCEPTION

Once you've made the decision to go for assisted conception, you need to be aware that your treatment program can be incredibly stressful, both emotionally and physically. Not only will your body be bombarded with fertility drugs, you'll face the emotional roller coaster of highs and lows that goes with the whole process.

As you embark upon your journey, try to keep a sense of perspective. The average success rate for assisted conception techniques, such as in-vitro fertilization (IVF), is only 25 percent, which is lower than much of the hype might suggest. Try to carry on with your life as normally and as happily as possible. Research shows that women who feel anxious as they undergo IVF can produce almost a fifth fewer eggs and have fewer of them fertilized than their less-stressed counterparts. Do all you can to keep stress under control by following the tips on pages 309–11 and also by making the most of natural therapies, such as acupuncture and massage (see p.47 and pp.48–9).

To stimulate ovulation

■ CLOMIPHENE CITRATE This drug triggers the surge of luteinizing hormone (LH), which prompts ovulation. In women who don't ovulate, clomiphene citrate results in ovulation for approximately 80 percent of cases, with a live birth rate from this treatment alone of 40 to 50 percent. The dosage of clomiphene will vary depending on how you respond in terms of ovulation, but it's usually 150mg three times a day. If the dosage is too high, the drug can affect your cervical mucus, making it hostile to sperm; a high dosage can also increase your risk of miscarriage should you become pregnant.

You'll be asked to start taking clomiphene at the beginning of your cycle, usually over the course of five days. If you haven't become pregnant after five or six cycles, the treatment isn't working and your doctor shouldn't encourage you to keep taking the drug. Be aware that studies show taking clomiphene for 12 or more cycles can increase your risk of ovarian cancer.

There is some evidence to show that, when taken with an insulin sensitizer, such as metformin, clomiphene significantly increases the chances of ovulation and pregnancy. In addition, some research suggests that using estrogen supplementation with clomiphene, to encourage the lining of the uterus to thicken, increases pregnancy rates.

■ HUMAN MENOPAUSAL GONADOTROPHINS (hMG) If you've tried clomiphene but have been unresponsive to it, your doctor may suggest you next try hMG. This class of drugs (which includes both follicle-stimulating hormone—FSH—and LH and is given by daily injection) stimulates the ovaries to grow a number of follicles in each cycle and in this way increases the chances that ovulation will occur.

■ HUMAN CHORIONIC GONADOTROPHIN (hCG) The placenta naturally produces this hormone during pregnancy. When it's taken as a fertility drug (by injection a few days before ovulation), it can increase the number of eggs the ovary releases. It's successful at kick-starting ovulation in 90 percent of the women who take it; while the pregnancy rate from using hCG is about 15 percent per cycle. It is often used with intra-uterine insemination (IUI; see pp.182–3).

■ BROMOCRIPTINE or CABERGOLINE If the reason you don't ovulate is because your body overproduces the hormone prolactin (a doctor will perform a blood test to confirm this), you may be asked to take bromocriptine or cabergoline to lower the levels of prolactin in your system. Prolactin prevents ovulation by stopping the release of both FSH and LH by the pituitary gland. The drug is taken by mouth.

To stop ovulation

■ GONADOTROPHIN-RELEASING HORMONE (GnRH) AGONISTS GnRH agonists are normally used during IVF and intracytoplasmic sperm injection (ICSI) treatments (see pp.183–4 and 186, respectively). During your cycle, a surge of LH from your pituitary gland triggers your body to release an egg from one of your ovaries. GnRH agonists cause your pituitary gland to release its reserves of LH, preventing this surge and so stopping ovulation.

■ GONADOTROPHIN-RELEASING HORMONE (GnRH) ANTAGONISTS GnRH antagonists have a similar effect to GnRH agonists in that they stop ovulation. They suppress the production of LH, giving no LH surge, so ovulation can't happen.

The main difference between the two drugs is that agonists exhaust your store of LH, whereas antagonists block its production. Both drugs have the same aim: to enable a fertility specialist to time egg collection or insemination accurately, without the risk that you'll ovulate spontaneously (and so have to abandon that cycle of IVF).

The other difference between the two drugs is the speed with which they work. Agonists can take up to a week to stop ovulation, whereas antagonists work in a matter of hours. Whether your doctor chooses to use a GnRH agonist or antagonist depends on the protocol the clinic is using for that particular IVF cycle, and this can vary from woman to woman.

FERTILITY DRUGS FOR MEN

If your partner's semen analysis has identified problems with his sperm, your doctor or fertility specialist may recommend that he takes certain drugs to correct the problem. The following are those drugs most commonly recommended for men.

■ CLOMIPHENE, TAMOXIFEN OR TESTOSTERONE Low sperm count is the most likely cause of male infertility, and a doctor may offer any of these three drugs in the hope that it will increase sperm production. Clomiphene and tamoxifen are anti-estrogens, so they make your partner's body release more FSH and LH and produce more testosterone. Men as well as women produce both FSH and LH from the pituitary gland. Your partner's body needs FSH for sperm development, and it's thought that higher levels of FSH may also improve sperm production. A man needs LH for the production of testosterone, so a drug form of LH is suggested for men with low testosterone levels. However, as yet, there is no evidence to say that either approach will definitely boost numbers of sperm.

■ HUMAN CHORIONIC GONADOTROPHIN (hCG) and/or HUMAN MENOPAUSAL GONADOTROPHINS (hMG) If your partner's blood tests show that he has low levels of LH (needed for the production of testosterone) and FSH (needed for sperm maturation and development), a doctor may prescribe either hCG (LH) or hMG (a mixture of LH and FSH) to see whether adding either or both of these hormones back improves sperm count and quality. Your partner's response to the drugs would be monitored over a period of three months.

■ CORTICOSTEROIDS In approximately ten percent of cases, male infertility results from the man's own immune system releasing antibodies that attack the sperm

as they're produced. A semen analysis can test for these antibodies, and, if they're found, a doctor may prescribe your partner with a course of corticosteroids to suppress the immune system. Be aware that, as yet, there's no firm evidence as to the reliability of this treatment, and side-effects include weight gain, bloating, rashes, and insomnia.

■ BROMOCRIPTINE or CABERGOLINE In women, high levels of prolactin in the system prevents ovulation (see p.181); in men, however, it causes impotence and lack of sex drive. A blood test can confirm high prolactin levels, which are then lowered using either of these drugs. Your partner's dosage will depend upon the precise prolactin measurement, and doctors will monitor his response.

ASSISTED-CONCEPTION TECHNIQUES

If triggering ovulation and/or stimulating sperm production alone aren't successful for you, your fertility doctor may suggest that you take the next step and try an assisted-conception technique, such as one of those that follow here. It's a wonderful thing that some couples do go on to conceive and have healthy babies using these techniques, but I try to encourage all my patients to bear in mind that assisted-conception methods are not a cure-all, and they do not work for everyone. This shouldn't necessarily discourage you—after all, positive thinking has great power in these situations—but the emotional roller coaster and turmoil of failed attempts can be hugely stressful for both partners, and

for their relationship, and it's important to be realistic. In the USA in 2007, the success rate for women under the age of 35 was 39.9 percent and for women over 40 only 11.7 percent. In 2004, the success rate in the UK for IVF was 27.6 percent for women under the age of 35 and ten percent for women aged over 40.

Intra-uterine insemination (IUI)

As the name might suggest, the aim of IUI is to get your partner's sperm closer to your eggs than you can achieve through normal sexual intercourse. A fertility specialist will use a catheter to place the sperm directly into your uterus at exactly the time you're expected to ovulate. This positions the sperm so they're ready to

WHY DO PEOPLE OPT FOR ASSISTED CONCEPTION?

This pie chart shows the various reasons why couples opt for assisted conception techniques such as IVF (see below). Some couples may have both a male-factor and a female-factor fertility problem (for example, low sperm motility and blocked Fallopian tubes) and therefore the categories can overlap. What I want you to know is that you aren't alone—and also that, even though it's the woman who "gets pregnant" and the woman who carries the baby, in a third of cases, a problem with the man's sperm prompts couples to go for assisted conception. Problems with the Fallopian tubes account for one-third of assisted-conception cases, with ovulatory dysfunction taking up one-fifth. However, please remember that, in a loving relationship neither of you should apportion blame. Amazingly, in 6 percent of all couples who opt for IVF treatment, no cause will ever be found. This is why it's so crucial that if this is the case for you, you follow my preconception care guidelines, so that one day it may just happen—as I'm proud to say, I have seen time and again.

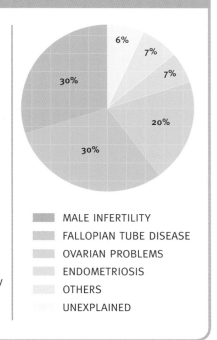

- MALE INFERTILITY
- FALLOPIAN TUBE DISEASE
- OVARIAN PROBLEMS
- ENDOMETRIOSIS
- OTHERS
- UNEXPLAINED

travel up the Fallopian tubes just as your ovary is releasing an egg. Your doctor may suggest that you take a fertility drug, such as hCG (see p.181), to assist ovulation during your IUI treatment, but generally this assisted-conception technique is less invasive and less expensive, and you need fewer drugs, than with IVF or ICSI (see below).

In my opinion, throughout the world, doctors don't offer IUI enough. So, if you fulfill the following conditions, and you're confident that your partner has healthy sperm, I urge you to try it as a first course of action. It is most suitable for women who are under the age of 35 with a diagnosis of unexplained infertility, which means there isn't any medical or physical reason why you can't get pregnant. IUI is also suitable if your cervical mucus is blocking the entry of sperm, but it is not suitable if you have blocked or damaged Fallopian tubes, nor is it suitable if you're over 40 because, generally, the overall success rate (ten to 15 percent for each attempt) for the treatment becomes too low.

In-vitro fertilization (IVF)

By far the most popular and well-known assisted-conception procedure, IVF is commonly known as the "test tube" technique. This slightly glib term belies a highly intricate process in which your eggs are mixed with your partner's—or a donor's—sperm in a petri dish in order to stimulate fertilization and produce embryos. Once the embryos are formed, they are transferred into your uterus. Embryo transfer usually happens three days after egg collection, but sometimes this time gap can be longer—around five to six days. In these cases, the fertility clinic is waiting for the embryo to develop into what's called a blastocyst. The blastocyst is in a more advanced stage of development, in which the bundle of dividing cells is more ready to attach to the wall of the uterus. Doctors may use this procedure if there are a large number of successful embryos in the petri dish. It permits the doctors to select for transfer those cell bundles most likely to successfully implant. Transferring the embryos or blastocysts is a simple procedure in which a soft, fine catheter is passed through the cervix and the cell-bundles are simply deposited in the uterus.

Although originally designed for women with Fallopian-tube damage, IVF is now used for couples with a wide range of fertility problems, including abnormal sperm, ovulation problems, endometriosis, and unexplained infertility. Bear in mind that there is a long run-up to the point at which the embryos are placed in your uterus, and both you and your partner will need to have a number of different tests (blood tests for hormones, ultrasound scans, semen analysis, and so on) ahead of the IVF treatment. You'll also need to follow the clinic's protocol concerning the use of fertility drugs and be monitored to make sure you're responding as you should. The risk of multiple births, not surprisingly, increases with IVF treatment, which is why the law in the UK permits the transfer of only two embryos in any one treatment cycle for women under the age of 40, and no more than three in women over 40. In the USA, there are no laws limiting the number of embryos transferred during IVF. However, the Society for Assisted Reproductive Technology and the American Society for Reproductive Medicine recommend that fertility clinics transfer only two embryos to women under 35, up to three embryos to women between the ages of 35 and 37, four to women who are aged between 37 and 40, and no more than five to women over the age of 40.

Natural IVF or mild IVF

In standard IVF, fertility specialists use drugs to stimulate your ovaries to produce eggs, which they then collect so that they can be mixed with sperm. However, in natural IVF, the specialist aims to remove the one egg that would be ovulating naturally in that cycle, usually without the use of any fertility drugs. Then, as with conventional IVF, your egg is introduced to the sperm in a petri dish, and any resulting embryo is implanted in your uterus.

Although success rates for natural IVF can be lower than conventional IVF, I do recommend trying this approach first because it's healthier for you and will cost you less money (drugs make up a large part of the cost of conventional IVF). You should especially consider it if you find it hard to tolerate medication (for example, if medication gives you a number of unpleasant side-effects). Sometimes, your doctor will still ask you to take low-dose fertility drugs (called "mild IVF") to stimulate the release of more than one egg. However, the dosages are so low that there's little or no risk of ovarian hyperstimulation syndrome (see box, p.176).

Gamete intra-fallopian transfer (GIFT)

The difference between GIFT and IVF is that in GIFT fertilization takes place in your body rather than in a dish. Your eggs and the sperm are mixed together in

---

ASSISTED HATCHING (AH)

If you're to undergo IVF or ICSI (see p.186) treatment, you may be asked to consider AH, too. During this procedure, an embryologist makes a hole in the shell of the embryo to give it a better chance of hatching and implanting into your uterus lining. Normally, enzymes in the Fallopian tube would have started to soften this shell, but of course this part of the process is missed out during assisted conception. AH seems to improve the success rate for younger women, but not for women over the age of 35.

REFLEXOLOGY TO BOOST FERTILITY

Reflexology can encourage a boost in fertility because it helps reduce stress levels and improve hormone balance, both of which have a significant impact on your fertility. If you can go to see a reflexology practitioner, he or she can work on your specific fertility problem, but in the meantime the following reflexology massage is a good treatment to try at home, up to three times a week if you have the time.

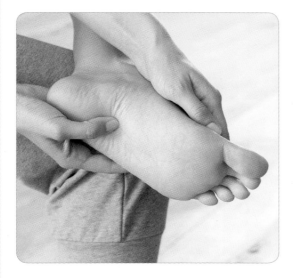 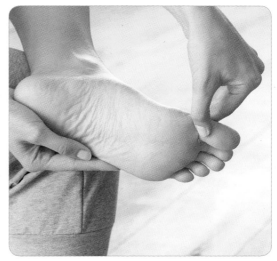

1 Fill a clean bowl with warm water and soak your bare feet in it for 10 minutes. Then gently dab them dry. Place 3 drops of a relaxing massage oil, such as lavender (15 drops of lavender in 6 tsp. of sweet almond), or dab a little of your usual moisturizing cream on each of your palms.

2 (above left) Sitting up, rest your left foot on your right knee. Use your right hand to press and push the sole, particularly around the heel, which in reflexology refers to the reproductive organs. Do this for 2–3 minutes.

3 (above right) Press and push the underside of your left big toe, using firm pressure, but not so as to cause pain. This area corresponds to your pituitary gland, which is the gland responsible for regulating your reproductive hormones. Do this for a further 2–3 minutes.

4 When you've finished massaging your left foot, repeat steps 3 and 4 on your right foot (placed up on your left knee).

the petri dish as in IVF. However, instead of arranging for fertilization to happen outside your body, and then putting the embryo (fertilized egg) back into you, a fertility doctor puts the egg-and-sperm mixture into your Fallopian tubes. In this way, fertilization occurs exactly where it would in natural conception. The drawback, of course, compared with IVF, is that if the treatment isn't successful, no one can know if fertilization didn't ever occur, or if it did but something else went wrong. Because GIFT involves the Fallopian tubes, it is suitable only for women whose tubes are healthy.

Intracytoplasmic sperm injection (ICSI)

If your partner has a problem with his sperm—for example, if he has a low sperm count or a high number of abnormal sperm—treatments such as IVF can be impossible, making ICSI the recommended alternative. Receiving ICSI treatment involves collecting your eggs in the same way as they'd be collected for IVF (see illustration, p.177), but then a single sperm is injected directly into one egg to fertilize it. Fertility doctors then implant the embryo into your uterus, just as with IVF.

IN 1997, doctors reported the first birth resulting from ICSI treatment and frozen eggs.

Although, at 25 to 30 percent, the success rate for ICSI is slightly higher than IVF, I do have one particular concern about it. Because an embryologist decides which individual sperm to inject into the egg, you lose the element of "survival of the fittest"—not necessarily the healthiest or strongest sperm makes its way through the egg wall. Some researchers believe ICSI-treatment babies may be more likely to have problems with their chromosomes or have an inherited genetic problem. Taking all the concerns about natural selection into consideration, I think it's important that if your partner has severely abnormal sperm, he should undergo some genetic testing before you consider any course of ICSI treatment. This will help prevent him from passing on the same infertility problems to a boy baby.

If your partner has no sperm in his semen sample, you may still be able to undergo ICSI treatment through a process of "sperm aspiration," in which a specialist tries to obtain sperm directly from the testes.

IMPROVING THE ODDS OF YOUR IVF OR ICSI TREATMENT WORKING

Undoubtedly, much of the success of any IVF or ICSI treatment you undergo will be determined by the quantity and quality of your eggs and your partner's sperm—and so there are many things you can do to help improve your odds of getting and staying pregnant. First and foremost, make sure you follow my preconception care guidelines on pages 168–173, beginning before your treatment starts and continuing throughout your treatment and after implantation. In a nutshell, throughout this time be sure to eat a healthy, balanced diet and to take your vitamins (including folic acid), minerals, and omega-3 oil supplements.

After implantation, don't do anything too strenuous, watch your stress levels, get gentle exercise (swimming and walking are good choices), and, just as you did before implantation, avoid alcohol, caffeine, and cigarette smoke, and try to get lots of fresh, unpolluted air. Make sure you drink plenty of water and get plenty of rest. Even if things don't work out with your treatment this time, you'll know that your body and reproductive system are as healthy as they possibly can be for a better chance of success next time, should you and your partner decide to try again.

You can also use complementary therapies, such as acupuncture, reflexology (see box, p.185), hypnotherapy, homeopathy, and relaxation techniques alongside your fertility treatments to maximize your chances of success. However, do make sure that you work with a qualified practitioner at all times, and discuss your choices with your fertility doctor.

EGG FREEZING

Doctors have been able successfully to freeze and thaw a man's sperm for the past 50 or so years; since 1983, we have even been able to freeze and thaw human embryos. Egg—or oocyte—freezing, however, has been more difficult for two reasons. First of all, eggs are larger cells with outer layers that are fairly water resistant. When water gets trapped inside the egg, ice crystals form during the freezing process and cause damage. Second, research on the eggs of animals has shown that freezing eggs can damage the control mechanism for genes or chromosomes, increasing the risk of birth defects. However, following the development of ICSI (see opposite), things began to look up. It seemed that, in early trials, sperm found it hard to penetrate the thawed egg, but using ICSI, the sperm could be injected directly into the egg, so the needle did the work. Successful live births ensued, but despite this the process was still regarded with caution.

All this changed in 2007 when perhaps the most exhaustive study yet of children born after the freezing procedure found that they appeared to be as healthy as those conceived through intercourse or by IVF. Today, fertility experts believe that research into a method known as vitrification may well lift the last remaining barriers to routine egg freezing. This may preserve a woman's fertility so that she can delay child-bearing or go on to have children following treatment for cancer that has made her infertile. Vitrification involves flash-freezing eggs after special preparation. Up to 95 percent of vitrified eggs survive the thawing process, compared with 50 to 60 percent of those preserved by older slow-freezing methods. Furthermore, when researchers

assessed the outcomes of 200 children born from vitrified eggs, they found that the rate of birth defects was 2.5 percent, which is comparable to natural pregnancies and IVF.

EGG FREEZING IN PRACTICE

If you want to freeze your eggs, regardless of whether it's because of illness or because you want to plan to have children after the age of 35, you should follow my three-month pre-conception plan on pages 168–173, so that your eggs are of the best possible quality before they're harvested and frozen.

Furthermore, I want to stress that egg freezing is still in its infancy and holds no guarantees for successful pregnancy. If you use your eggs when you're older, you'll have a higher risk of miscarriage purely as a result of your age. If the pregnancy is successful, you may have an increased risk of a congenitally abnormal baby, again because of your age.

I'm fully supportive of the egg-freezing procedure for women who've undergone chemotherapy or other treatments that have caused infertility. However, I would not feel comfortable advising any of my patients to freeze their eggs for the future purely because they want to delay pregnancy as a lifestyle choice. As with other fertility treatments, you may still need to take fertility drugs, which themselves carry medical risks (see p.181). Being able to freeze eggs successfully is a wonderful step forward in the science of fertility treatment. However, for me it is an option for those who may never have children without it, rather than for those who choose to have children later than nature intended.

Fertility and aging

I've been running my clinics for 25 years, and over that time I've seen one undeniable trend: women are waiting longer to get pregnant, making age-related infertility an increasing concern.

WHY AGE MATTERS

You were born with your life supply of eggs already in place—usually about two million of them. However, from the moment you were born these eggs began to die, and by the age of 45 you'll have only about 10,000 of them left. Although this sounds like a lot, not all of them will be of a quality that can make a healthy baby. The older the woman, the older her eggs—and older eggs simply aren't as viable as younger ones. This is because older eggs have a greater risk of chromosomal defects that can either prevent fertilization or, if it does occur, increase the risk of a miscarriage.

In general, fertility declines dramatically after age 35: Your periods may still be regular, but you may not ovulate every month. But don't despair, because, although you can't reverse the aging process in your ovaries, uterus, or anywhere else in your body, there are plenty of things you can do to slow it down. With regard to your eggs, this means improving their quality, even if you can't improve their quantity. Stress, diet, smoking, and alcohol all speed up the aging process, so it's time to cut them out. Regulating your hormones by making adjustments to your diet and lifestyle can also optimize your chances of conceiving for your age.

TESTING FOR OVARIAN RESERVE

Every woman is unique, and although the average age for a decline in fertility is 35, you may be different. One way to assess how much time you have left on your biological clock is to test your "ovarian reserve"—how many eggs you have left in store. The following are the main ways in which your doctor can do this. Remember, though, the tests can reveal only how many eggs you have left—not how good they are (you still need to follow my guidelines to improve your egg quality).

Ultrasound testing Performed during the first half of your cycle, an ultrasound scan examines the size of your ovaries and the number of measurable small (antral) follicles that contain developing eggs.

AMH blood testing This test does not have to be done at a certain time in your cycle, nor does it require a visit to a hospital, only to your doctor. The test measures the levels of a hormone called anti-mullerian hormone (AMH) in your blood. Your ovaries produce AMH each month to encourage eggs to mature and it's also vital for the production of estrogen. The levels of AMH in your body can give a good indication of how well your ovaries are functioning, which in turn can give an indication of both the quantity and quality of your egg supply. In general, the lower the levels of AMH, the lower your fertility level is likely to be.

FSH blood testing The pituitary gland releases follicle-stimulating hormone (FSH) every month to stimulate a group of follicles to grow on the surface of an ovary. At the beginning of a normal cycle, your level of FSH should be low. If a blood test taken on the second or third day of your cycle reveals that it's high, your pituitary gland is probably pumping out extra hormones because the ovaries are not responding to normal levels. The fewer eggs you have, the more FSH the pituitary has to release to stimulate those eggs.

If the tests reveal your egg reserve is low, you need especially to concentrate on improving the quality of the eggs you do have in order to have the best possible chance of conceiving.

YOUR DIET

If you want to conceive, pack your diet with fruits and vegetables. These foods supply you with antioxidants, which protect against the effects of free radicals. These chemically unstable atoms can damage the body's cells and have been linked to a number of health problems, including premature aging. Vitamins A, C, and E, plus the minerals selenium and zinc, are all antioxidants and are contained in brightly colored fruits and vegetables, such as carrots, pumpkins, and cantaloupe, and also in nuts, seeds, and oily fish. If your mother told you to "eat your greens," now it's time to "eat a rainbow" because variety is key.

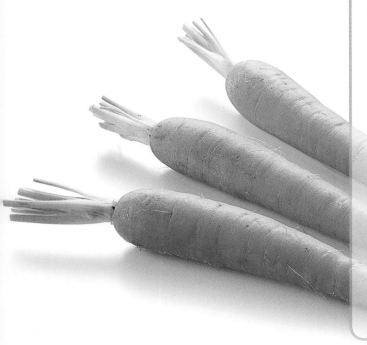

YOUR ANTI-AGING FERTILITY MENU

Here are some ideas for healthy but delicious meals that are packed with anti-aging nutrients.

BREAKFAST Choose organic oatmeal, cooked with water instead of milk and topped with ground nuts, seeds, and colorful berries, such as blueberries and raspberries. Or have a poached egg on toasted wholegrain bread with grilled tomatoes. Or have an organic, plain yogurt with active cultures with chopped up pieces of fruit and sprinkled with nuts and seeds.

LUNCH Make a colorful soup, such as carrot, red pepper, or tomato, and add in a good vegetable protein, such as lentils. If you have a sandwich, choose wholegrain bread and have a good amount of salad ingredient, such as tomato, cucumber, or lettuce, with the filling.

DINNER Steam, roast, or stir fry (in olive oil) heaps of vegetables with your supper and also use plenty of herbs, spices, and flavorings, such as garlic, lemongrass, ginger, tamari, lemon, miso, turmeric, and cinnamon. Tofu and stir-fry vegetables, seasoned with garlic, ginger, and tamari is a great dinner choice. Or try a piece of grilled salmon served with corn on the cob, broccoli, and roasted sweet potatoes.

SNACKS Have a morning and afternoon snack of nuts, seeds, dried fruits, and different-colored fresh fruits.

SUPPLEMENTS

It's important to take the food supplements (or a combined fertility supplement; see p.320) mentioned in my section on pre-conception care (see pp.169–70), but the priority here is to make sure that you have good levels of the antioxidant vitamins and minerals. So along with your fertility supplement, take:

■ ANTIOXIDANTS Every day take 1,000mg (500mg, twice daily) vitamin C with bioflavonoids (as magnesium ascorbate); 600iu vitamin E; 15mg zinc; and 100μg selenium. (Your fertility supplement can count towards these this.)

■ OMEGA-3 FATTY ACIDS (1,000mg fish oil containing at least 700mg EPA and 500mg DHA, daily) These good fats are crucial for your general health and keeping your cells in top condition. (Take flax seed oil if you're vegetarian.)

HERBS

Herbalists have a host of remedies they believe will slow down the aging process and boost fertility. The following are my particular favorites.

■ AGNUS CASTUS (*Vitex agnus castus*) This wonderful herb has a balancing effect on the ovarian hormones because it stimulates the normal functioning of the pituitary gland, which in turn helps normalize levels of FSH and LH. Agnus castus may encourage ovulation and help you get back to having a regular menstrual cycle. Because it is an adaptogenic herb, agnus castus has a balancing effect generally, so if you suffer from low levels of one hormone or an excess of a different one, taking agnus castus can assist your body in achieving normal

levels. Take 1 tsp. tincture in a little water, or 200–300mg in capsule form, twice daily.

■ SIBERIAN GINSENG (*Eleutherococcus senticosus*) This adaptogenic herb has a beneficial effect on your adrenal glands and can help you cope better when under stress. It's important to do whatever you can to cushion the negative effects of stress on your hormonal balance. Take 1 tsp. tincture in a little water, or 250–300mg in capsule form, twice daily.

SELF-HELP

Alcohol Drinking alcohol can delay conception—and if you're over the age of 35, time is of the essence. Research shows that women drinking five units or fewer a week are twice as likely to conceive within six months as women drinking ten units or more.

Stress The stress hormones can cause the menstrual cycle to become irregular and even to stop, and high levels of anxiety may cause your ovaries to release eggs that are not yet mature, wasting your precious store. Try to spend at least 30 minutes each day practicing a relaxation routine, such as the meditation on page 51 or the visualization on page 61. If dedicated relaxation isn't for you, try to make sure that each day has 30 minutes of "me" time in it. Turn off your phones, the TV, and the radio. Use the time to engage in something you enjoy—whether that's painting, reading, or listening to music. Lose yourself in it completely.

Smoking Quit. Cigarette smoke contains substances called polycyclic aromatic hydrocarbons, which are toxic and can make your eggs die at a faster rate than normal, hastening your time to menopause.

Keep fit in the sun All types of exercise are anti-aging except when they are performed to the extreme. However, there's now a large amount of evidence to show that getting outside while you exercise and exposing your skin to the sun for 15 minutes at a time (without sunscreen, but not between 11 am and 3 pm) actually has an anti-aging effect. This might seem contrary to popular wisdom, but as with anything in nature, it's a question of balance. Vitamin D is manufactured through the skin when it is exposed to the sun. Having good levels of this vitamin in the body can slow down the body clock. In addition, vitamin D is thought to play an important role in controlling the immune system, so that it allows you to get pregnant and then goes into override to prevent your body rejecting the embryo (causing a miscarriage).

MALE FERTILITY AND AGE

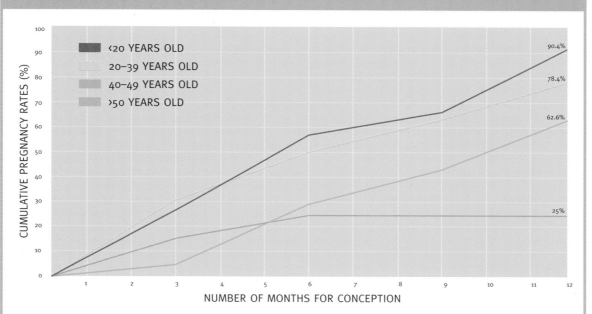

Cumulative Pregnancy Rates (%) vs Number of Months for Conception

- <20 YEARS OLD
- 20–39 YEARS OLD
- 40–49 YEARS OLD
- >50 YEARS OLD

90.4%
78.4%
62.6%
25%

Although most people talk about women's fertility declining with age, men also have a biological clock that starts to slow down around the age of 40. Research shows that in men over the age of 40, the quality and quantity of sperm decline, and there is a higher chance of DNA damage, which increases the risk of his partner suffering a miscarriage or of the baby having birth defects. The rate of declining fertility is demonstrated clearly in this graph, which shows the effects of a man's age on pregnancy rates during the first year of trying to conceive. Pregnancy rates decrease as the man's age increases. What's striking is that the research shows that the effect of decreasing fertility is independent of the woman's age. So, for a man over the age of 50, there's only a 25 percent chance of conceiving in the first year, compared with a 78.4 percent chance for a man aged between 20 and 39.

By making positive changes to his diet and lifestyle, your partner can reduce a high level of sperm DNA damage. Ask your partner to follow my pre-conception care guidelines (see pp.168–73). It's particularly important for him to eliminate smoking and alcohol, as well as to keep baths warm but not hot and to avoid saunas. He should steer clear of additives, preservatives, and artificial sweeteners in food, especially if he is over 35. Instead, he should eat as healthily as possible (see pp.24–9), with plenty of organic fruit and vegetables that are rich in antioxidants. Another important factor in DNA damage is body weight. We know that when body mass index (BMI) is over 25 (see p.297), the incidence of sperm DNA "fragmentation" rises. This is even more of a problem when the BMI is greater than 30. If necessary, encourage your partner to exercise regularly to lose weight.

PREGNANCY, BIRTH, AND BREASTFEEDING

I love to see women bloom as their pregnancies progress, not least because I know that, underneath the glowing exteriors, a mass of intricate work is keeping both mother and baby in prime condition.

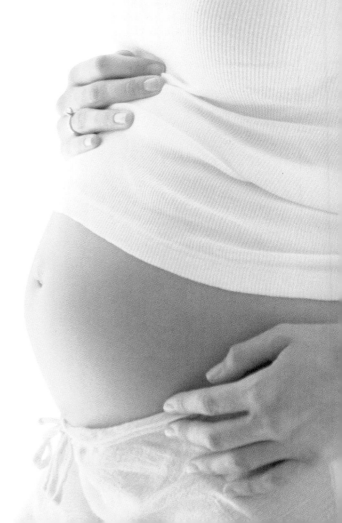

If you're pregnant, your hormones are surging, your muscles and ligaments are stretching, your heart is working overtime, and your body is storing up lots of fluid and fat reserves. Despite all this, for most of your pregnancy, if you're like the majority of women, you'll feel completely healthy. Even so, there's that bit at the beginning (with the morning sickness and ligament pain) and towards the end (with the backache and labor pain) when the incredible changes taking place inside your body can make you feel pretty terrible.

I've found that pregnancy is often the first time many women turn to natural medicine—because, rightly, conventional doctors are reluctant to recommend drugs during pregnancy, and, for the same reasons, many women don't want to take drugs while they're pregnant in case the medication crosses the placenta and is absorbed by the baby. In this section, I'll explore some of the most common, but nonetheless important problems you're likely to encounter as you carry your baby during pregnancy and give birth to him or her, and some of the uncommon problems. I'll give you advice on how nutritional and natural medicine can help you through them—from relieving morning sickness to easing labor pain. However, if you have any concerns during your pregnancy, don't rely upon any book alone. It's really important to see your doctor *before* embarking upon any form of remedial medicine—natural or otherwise—so that you can rule out any serious problems for you and your baby.

Being pregnant, staying healthy

Carrying the life of another human being inside you is both amazing and joyful. Now, more than at any other time in your life, you'll probably want to know which foods and lifestyle choices are best for you.

You'll need to know what foods to avoid, as well as what to eat and what supplements you should try to take. Other aspects of health are important, too—how do you stay fit, but safe, during pregnancy, for example? The following pages provide your one-stop-shop to a natural, healthy pregnancy for you and your baby.

THE IMPORTANCE OF DIET

During the nine months of your pregnancy, you literally "make" your baby—almost from scratch. For this reason, I can't emphasize enough how important it is for you to eat healthy, nutritious food.

To some extent your baby is protected in your uterus—we know that if there isn't enough good food going into your system, your baby will get first call on your reserves, and you'll go without. However, that's not to underplay the effects of what you decide to eat or not to eat on your unborn baby's health. Your developing baby is highly sensitive to your nutritional status; and poor intake of essential nutrients can alter the rate of growth of your baby's organs, and influence their structure and long-term function. The overall result is to increase the risk of health problems for the baby after he or she is born and even into adulthood.

For the nine months of pregnancy—and longer if you breastfeed—your baby is totally dependent on you for all the nutrients it needs. It's important to eat well from the moment you find out you're pregnant. The responsibility is great but not daunting if you follow my guidelines. And if you've already been following my pre-conception care guidelines on pages 168–73,

you probably won't need to change much to cover the extra nutritional demands of pregnancy. You'll just need to listen to your body and follow its lead.

YOUR PREGNANCY DIET

The amount of food you need to eat doesn't have to increase that much during pregnancy. However, to support your growing baby, the need for essential nutrients increases dramatically. You'll require a good supply of B-vitamins, vitamin D, vitamin E, magnesium, selenium, and zinc. In particular, try to improve your intake of the following foods and supplements:

Protein Your body demands more protein when you're pregnant to cope with the growth of your baby—make sure that you have some protein (vegetable or animal) with every meal. For example, if you're having oatmeal for breakfast, sprinkle some ground seeds on top. Healthy sources of protein include legumes, fish, dairy, nuts, seeds, peas, beans, whole grains, and some vegetables (such as broccoli and spinach).

Essential fats Make sure you get enough essential fats from oily fish, nuts, and seeds. These are crucial for brain, eye, and central-nervous-system development in a growing baby, especially in the last trimester (three months) of pregnancy. You may feel a bit confused about oily fish because, on the one hand, we know it's important for you and the baby and, on the other hand, government guidelines recommend no more than two portions of oily fish a week during pregnancy because of the high levels of toxic mercury found in these fish. To optimize your levels of essential fats from fish, I recommend you avoid shark, swordfish, and marlin, and limit tuna to either two fresh tuna steaks a week or four medium cans of tuna. The other oily fish—sardines, salmon (buy wild or organic, not farmed), herring, mackerel, and anchovies are fine. Fish-oil supplements are also fine as long as you know they're from reputable sources, which will have been screened for contaminants. They should contain good levels of both EPA and DHA—in my clinics I use a supplement that contains 700mg EPA and 500mg DHA in just two capsules, taken daily. Do not use cod-liver or any fish-liver oil supplements during pregnancy: They contain high levels of vitamin A, which can be toxic to your baby.

Iron During pregnancy, your blood undergoes a large increase in volume, meaning that you need extra iron to make the hemoglobin for the increased number of red blood cells. Good food sources of iron include eggs, leafy dark-green vegetables, seaweed, apricots, lentils, millet, and whole grains. Avoid liver because it contains high levels of vitamin A (see left). To help your body to absorb the iron in your food better, don't drink black tea fewer than 30 minutes before or after a meal: the tannin in the tea blocks your body's uptake of iron (and other minerals, such as calcium).

Your doctor or midwife will test you for anemia (low levels of iron in your blood) during your pregnancy and advise you to take iron supplements only if you need to. If you do need to supplement, take organic irons, such as iron citrate, or chelated irons, which are combined with an amino acid to make them easier for your body to absorb. Also, always take iron with a vitamin-C supplement and on an empty stomach, both of which also improve absorption.

Calcium Your growing baby needs calcium to build strong bones and teeth. Nature is clever and research shows that during pregnancy, your body increases the amount of calcium you're able to absorb from your food (and it doesn't steal it from your own bones as we once thought). Good food sources include organic dairy

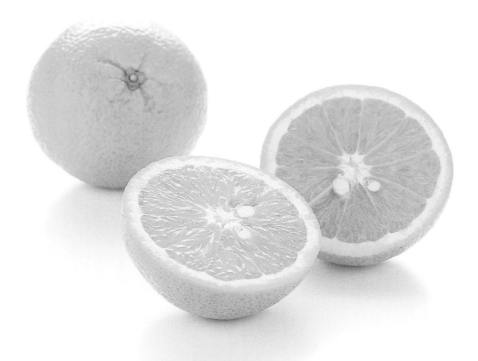

products, leafy green vegetables, sesame seeds, and fish where you eat the bones (such as canned salmon). Avoid spinach and rhubarb, which contain oxalic acid that blocks your body's ability to absorb calcium.

Folic acid This essential pregnancy nutrient is actually a B-vitamin (B9), and it helps prevent the risk of neural tube defects in your baby. You can meet your folic-acid requirement by taking a good prenatal supplement containing 400μg and eating at least one dark green vegetable, such as broccoli, each day. You should also eat two or three servings of fruit (strawberries and bananas are good sources) daily. Try not to overcook your food, as cooking destroys the folic-acid content.

Vitamin C Your baby needs vitamin C for healthy bones and teeth. Good food sources include citrus fruits, berries, broccoli, cauliflower, and peppers. In addition, I recommend a vitamin C supplement, on top of any prenatal supplement you're taking (see box, right). Take 500mg vitamin C with bioflavonoids (as magnesium ascorbate, not ascorbic acid), twice a day.

An organic pregnancy

If you're already eating a healthy, varied diet rich in fruits, vegetables, whole grains, nuts, seeds, beans, legumes, eggs, and oily fish, you're probably making good headway to getting as many essential nutrients as possible from your food, especially if you buy organic.

When you take in chemicals, your baby does, too. Organic food is a better choice when you're pregnant because it will not have been sprayed with pesticides, herbicides, or other toxic substances. If you're on a limited budget, choose organic for foods that are small in size—the smaller the food, the more pesticides it can absorb. Choose organic grain foods (such as oats and wholegrain bread) and buy non-organic bananas, for example. Buy organic carrots and potatoes because you need only to scrub, rather than peel, them, and most of the valuable nutrients are concentrated just under the skin. You could make the decision not to buy organic

onions, as you have to peel those anyway. The kind of society we live in means that we can't avoid exposure to all chemicals, so just do whatever you can with the resources and choices you have, without allowing the process to make you anxious.

How much should you eat?

Pregnancy is a time of extremes: You may never have been so excited or so tired, and you may never have felt

---

RECOMMENDED SUPPLEMENTS

During your pregnancy, take a supplement that contains the following nutrients at levels as close as possible to those in this list. If you can't find a good prenatal supplement locally, you can order one online (see p.320).

Vitamin B1: 10mg

Vitamin B2: 10mg

Vitamin B3: 10mg

Vitamin B5: 10mg

Vitamin B6 (as pyridoxal-5-phosphate): 10mg

Vitamin B12: 50μg

Vitamin C with bioflavonoids: 150mg

Vitamin E: 200iu

Vitamin D3 (cholecalciferol): 5μg

Beta-carotene: 833.3μg

Folic acid: 400μg

Calcium (as citrate): 40mg

Chromium (from saccharomyces): 20μg

Iron (as citrate): 5mg

Magnesium (as citrate): 28mg

Manganese (as citrate): 2mg

Selenium (as sodium selenite): 100μg

Zinc (as citrate): 7.5mg

so hungry. But you may also be worried about gaining weight or you may have started your pregnancy with excess weight already. This is not the time to think about reducing calories or restricting food groups—to do so would be to deprive you and your baby of valuable vitamins and minerals. Also, as you lose weight, toxins that your body stores in your fat are released and passed into your baby before your body excretes them.

If you eat a healthy diet and keep your blood sugar in balance (by eating good food, little and often; see below), you'll lose any excess weight and end up at the weight you should be. During your pregnancy, you should aim to gain not more than 33lb., and not less than 11lb.

You'll be more sensitive to blood-sugar changes during pregnancy, so avoid refined sugar in all its guises. Refined sugar is of no nutritional value, providing only empty calories that make you gain weight, and will send your blood-sugar levels yo-yoing. Take care with fruit juices, too. Although a glass of orange juice may contain eight oranges, it lacks the fiber of the oranges themselves and so can have an adverse effect on your blood-sugar balance (fiber moderates how your body responds to the fruit sugar). Choose smoothies or dilute the juice with water instead.

Another easy tip that helps you know how much to eat is to take your time and chew well. It takes your brain 20 minutes to register that you're full, so if you eat quickly you can consume a lot before your brain says you've had enough.

SUPPLEMENTS

Although it's best to get nutrients to your baby through the food you eat, it's all-too easy to become deficient,

FOODS TO AVOID DURING PREGNANCY

"Unhealthy" foods, such as fast foods, deep-fried food, foods containing hydrogenated (trans) fats, and processed meats (sausages, hamburgers, and so on) are all off the menu while you're pregnant.

Avoid all undercooked meat, poultry, and fish, which can cause food poisoning, as can raw eggs. These can carry salmonella, which won't directly harm your baby, but will cause you to have diarrhea and vomiting and make you feel extremely unwell.

Food-borne illnesses are also rife in meat pâtés, ready-to-eat salads, and unpasteurized soft or blue cheese, such as brie or Stilton. All these foods can contain listeria, which if passed to your unborn baby can cause a miscarriage. Cottage cheese and hard cheeses, however, are fine.

Candy, chocolates, processed foods, and carbonated soft drinks are full of refined sugar and give you no nutritional value (see above), so avoid them. Caffeine can increase the risk of miscarriage, so limit your intake to only one cup of coffee or tea a day; and alcohol can harm your baby's development, so you should abstain completely from drinking it during pregnancy.

However, just because you're pregnant doesn't mean that you have to become a food saint. If about 90 percent of your diet is healthy, you can afford to treat yourself to goodies such as ice cream and chocolate once in a while. But choose the best-quality foods available, so they're not full of artificial sweeteners, preservatives, colorings, and so on. A balanced, healthy diet contains a wide variety of foods—just don't go overboard. Enjoy a little of everything in moderation.

Opposite: Chamomile tea

especially in folic acid and the other B-vitamins, vitamin C, calcium, and iron—that's why it's really useful to take a good prenatal supplement throughout pregnancy (see box, p.195). Whichever prenatal supplement you choose, it's most important to ensure that it doesn't contain more than 2,500iu (daily) of vitamin A, which can cause toxicity in an unborn baby. (However, beta-carotene, which the body uses to convert to vitamin A, is fine.) Remember, though, a prenatal supplement is not a substitute for a healthy diet.

HERBS

Herbs can help with many uncomfortable symptoms of pregnancy. You may want to try ginger tea for morning sickness, or chamomile tea for stress. However, as with essential oils, herbs are potent substances, and there are several that are not safe to take during pregnancy (dong quai and goldenseal among them). Visit a registered herbalist for advice and follow his or her guidance carefully.

OTHER NATURAL TREATMENTS

During your pregnancy, you'll probably find your doctor reluctant to prescribe you with conventional medicines for fear of harming your unborn baby (talk to him or her about any prescription medications you take regularly as soon as you know you're pregnant). For this reason, complementary therapy has a firm place in the well-being of every pregnant woman.

As long as you work with a qualified practitioner, acupuncture and acupressure, hypnotherapy, homeopathy, meditation, yoga, and reflexology have all proven useful in the relief of adverse pregnancy symptoms, such as tiredness, muscle aches and pains, and morning sickness. You may also like to try the following (with the guidance of a practitioner in each field).

Aromatherapy and massage An aromatherapy massage can relax tired muscles, soothe aching legs, or rub away stretch marks (see box, p.198) during pregnancy. Simply inhaling the aroma of some oils can help

relieve anxiety about the birth or relax you during labor. However, always practice aromatherapy under a qualified practitioner's guidance, as several essential oils are contraindicated during pregnancy, and it's important that your treatment not only avoids these but is tailored to you. Oils to avoid during pregnancy are: basil, bay, clary sage, comfrey, fennel, hyssop, juniper, marjoram, melissa, myrrh, rosemary, thyme, and sage.

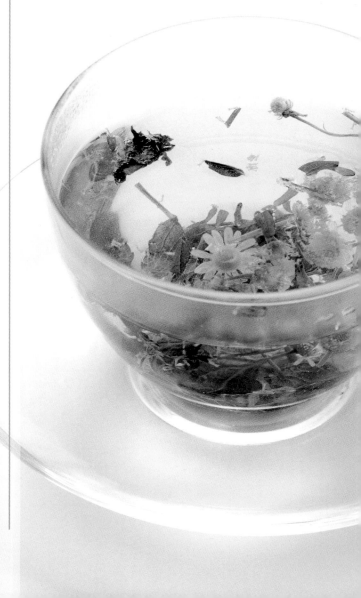

EXERCISE

In the past—when having a baby was considered an illness—you weren't supposed to exercise if you were pregnant. Now, experts encourage expectant mothers to keep active because it does you and your baby good. The only way you might put your baby in danger is if the exercise is exhausting, strenuous, or violent, such as climbing a mountain, boxing, or running a marathon (stomach crunches are out, too). However, moderate exercise, such as 30 minutes of brisk walking or swimming a day, can prevent the problems of excessive weight gain, poor posture, back pain, and poor body image. If you have low points during your pregnancy, exercise will also help lift your mood.

If you achieved a certain level of fitness before pregnancy, you should be able to maintain this. However, do consult your doctor before you begin any exercise program. Try to find a yoga class designed specially for pregnant women. The gentle stretches and postures of yoga can not only help while you're pregnant, but can actually make the labor and birth easier, too.

You may feel that being pregnant is enough of a workout and that instead of exercising you would prefer to put your feet up. While that's understandable, evidence concludes that if you do exercise regularly, you'll manage your weight and strengthen your body for the demands of pregnancy, childbirth, and postpartum recovery. Think of the nine months of your pregnancy as a training period: you're in training to become a fit parent, ready to welcome your baby with vigour when he or she is born, and prepared to withstand the demands of taking care of a new life.

ANTI-STRETCH-MARK MASSAGE

The best way to prevent stretch marks during pregnancy is to eat healthily, drink a lot of water, and moisturize your skin morning and night. Regular massage may also be of benefit because massaging oil or cream into high-risk areas can help keep your circulation working properly and stretch marks at bay. Try the following anti-stretch mark massage as often as you can throughout your pregnancy.

1 Sit in a comfortable position on a chair or on the floor. (If you're more than four months pregnant, lying down isn't recommended.) Place a good amount of vitamin-E oil or cream or cocoa butter into the palm of one hand and rub your hands together.

2 Using light, smooth strokes, begin at the top of your abdomen, one hand over the other, as you make gentle movements in a clockwise motion (to your left first) around your bump.

3 Add some more oil or cream if you need to, then move on to massaging your thighs, one at a time. Rub the tops of the thighs firmly, but without causing discomfort, gently squeezing your flesh between the fingers and thumb of each hand.

4 Finally, gently massage each breast (stop if it feels uncomfortable or sore), using smooth, gentle strokes over and around the whole breast area.

Prenatal depression

You've probably heard all about the postpartum "baby blues" and postpartum depression, but you may not have heard about a surprisingly common condition called prenatal depression.

Pregnancy, particularly if it's planned or longed-for, is meant to be a time of great joy. However, it's now thought that more women are likely to feel depressed during the pregnancy than after. A study in the *British Medical Journal* showed that almost three in 20 women suffered depressive disorders during pregnancy, with the worse time being around 32 weeks. Happily, in the great majority of cases, the depression seems to lift as soon as the baby is born, and it doesn't appear that those women who suffer prenatal depression will suffer postpartum depression, too.

SYMPTOMS

Low mood and depression are different things. Pregnancy is a traumatic time—your hormones fluctuate wildly, your organs are squashed, and, generally, your whole body, physically and mentally, is put under strain. With all this to deal with, it's no wonder that a woman experiences massive dips in mood at times during her pregnancy—but is this depression?

The answer is no. Mood swings, even short periods of sadness, are different from depression, which is characterized by a chronic, ongoing dark mood. The signs of prenatal depression are as follows. You may be unable to sleep, or you may want to sleep all the time; you may be excessively irritable, angry, and sensitive; you'll probably be prone to bouts of crying; and you may withdraw from your friends and family. You may even have thoughts of harming yourself or the baby; you almost certainly will stop taking care of yourself. The most important thing is to recognize these symptoms and to get help—you have a very real illness, and there is no shame in asking someone (even if, at first, that person is simply a close friend) to guide you.

CAUSES

Some factors appear to predispose women to prenatal depression—although being able to say categorically who'll get this illness and who'll not is impossible. If you think any of the following apply to you, you may be at risk. Watch out for the symptoms and talk to someone as soon as you can if you think depression is setting in—but don't become paranoid.

Heredity Many forms of depression have a heredity factor—that is, you're more likely to suffer from some form of depression if a parent, grandparent, or even aunt or uncle suffered from a form of it; and you're more likely to suffer from prenatal depression if you have suffered another form of depression in the past.

Additional anxiety and stress Pregnancy, as joyful as it should be, can also be a time of great physical and mental stress. If you also have other stresses in your life—a difficult or new job, a bereavement, a separation or other relationship problems—life can simply become too much and depression can set in. The stress of abusive relationships, past or present, is also a trigger. When so much about your own body is out of your control, having been emotionally, physically, sexually, or verbally abused can make becoming a parent a traumatic rather than a joyful experience.

Pregnancy itself Being pregnant for the first time is a catalogue of "unknowns." All sorts of changes take place in your body that have never happened before, and the weight of the responsibility for nurturing your unborn baby and then caring for a new life can be overwhelming. Equally, many second-time mothers can become depressed—how will she cope with two? How will the first know that he or she is loved just as much as before? And how will the second ever measure up to the first? The less pleasant aspects of pregnancy—severe morning sickness, for example—are also triggers for prenatal depression. Finally, if you've had frequent miscarriages in the past, or if you've lost a child, being pregnant now can bring on all-consuming anxiety that leads to depression.

This all sounds very gloomy, but remember that for the majority of women pregnancy is a happy time—but often only with support from others.

CONVENTIONAL TREATMENTS

Be open with your doctor and talk through your feelings. It's unlikely any doctor will prescribe you with antidepressants, which are not recommended for use during pregnancy. The only exception may be if the doctor believes you're suicidal.

Counseling is the most important help anyone can offer you—and if your doctor doesn't suggest it, I urge you to find a counselor yourself.

YOUR DIET

What you eat can have an enormous impact on your brain chemistry. Although changes in your diet—perhaps feeling that you don't want to eat, or bingeing on junk foods—are a common symptom of prenatal depression, try to keep to good eating habits. Ask someone else to cook for you, if need be.

Balancing your blood sugar is essential, so eat little and often (aim for six small meals a day) and eliminate added sugar (such as in cakes, cookies, and many juice drinks) and stimulants (such as caffeine). Try to combine foods in the right way, too.

Many antidepressants, such as Prozac (fluoxetine), are called selective serotonin reuptake inhibitors (SSRIs) because they optimize the use of serotonin, one of the neurotransmitters involved in controlling mood. Amazingly, starchy carbohydrates help increase serotonin levels—one study showed that making your evening meal carbohydrate-rich and protein-poor can reduce symptoms of depression and fatigue.

But why? In order to manufacture serotonin, your brain needs additional help in the form of tryptophan. This amino acid occurs naturally in dairy products, fish, bananas, dried dates, soy, and almonds, but these and other forms of protein also contain other amino acids. When you eat protein, your body breaks it down into its constituent amino acids, and these enter your bloodstream. When they get to your brain, they meet your blood-brain barrier, which lets only some of the amino acids through. Because there are always fewer tryptophan molecules than the other amino acids, the others get through, leaving the tryptophan behind. However, all this changes if a meal contains starchy carbohydrates as well. Carbohydrates help the body release insulin, which makes use of the other amino acids before they get to the blood-brain barrier, leaving the tryptophan to dominate So make sure you always combine a protein with a carbohydrate. For example, if you're having fish and vegetables, have potatoes, brown rice, or wholegrain pasta with it, too.

When we feel depressed we tend to want to eat bread, cakes, sweets, and sugary foods, all of which are starchy carbohydrates. In a sense, the body is trying to prescribe its own medication. But remember that much of the quick-fix food we crave combines sugar and refined carbohydrates, which will give you a quick high followed by a crash. Try to train yourself to resist temptation and go for good-quality starchy carbohydrates, such as brown rice, wholegrain bread, and so on.

SUPPLEMENTS

Deficiencies in certain nutrients can contribute to depression, so it's vital that you take your prenatal supplement. Also include more zinc, low levels of which can affect your mood. Take at least 30mg daily altogether. Finally, take a good omega-3 fish-oil supplement (1,000mg containing at least 700mg EPA and 500mg DHA, daily). Good levels of these oils are known to help relieve depression and low mood.

HERBS

Although several herbs, such as St John's wort, are well known to treat depression, I strongly advise against self-prescription of any herb during pregnancy. However, do visit a qualified herbal practitioner, who will be able to advise you on what's safe.

OTHER NATURAL TREATMENTS

Homeopathy You have nothing to lose and everything to gain by using homeopathy if you suffer from prenatal depression. It's important to get help from a professional homeopath, but the following are some useful remedies to try at home. Take the remedy that is most appropriate for your symptoms in a 30c potency, three times a day between meals.
• Lycopodium can help when your depression is accompanied by a bad temper
• Pulsatilla can help when you feel tearful and sad but you can find no obvious reason
• Sepia can help if you feel irritable, weepy, and emotionally flat

Aromatherapy Essential oils can be extremely useful for lifting mood during pregnancy. However, use them only once you're in your second trimester (or week 24 in the case of lavender essential oil). Use 2 or 3 drops of each of the following oils in your bath water, or use a total of 15 drops in 6 tsp. carrier oil (such as sweet almond oil) for a massage.
• To reduce depression and irritability: bergamot and Roman or German chamomile
• To ease depression and anxiety: jasmine
• To encourage sleep: lavender
• To lift mood: rose

SELF-HELP

Do some exercise You may not feel like exercising at all, but the effort will be well worth it. Exercise releases endorphins, brain chemicals that help you feel happier. It can also improve your self-esteem, which is important if your confidence has taken a dip since becoming pregnant. Swimming, yoga, and walking are good forms of exercise for pregnant women. Try to take at least 30 minutes of exercise a day.

Keep a journal Noting down your feelings and thoughts each day can provide a release for some of the confusion that often goes with depression. Also, each day make a note of the things that are good in your life and the positive things that have happened that day.

Use visualization Sitting or lying down in a quiet room, without any distractions, and imagining yourself somewhere beautiful, such as a pretty garden or a beach somewhere warm, can be highly effective if you practice it every day for around ten to 15 minutes (the longer the better). Try to capture all the sights, sounds, and smells of the place you visit in your mind's eye.

MUSIC THERAPY

Any music that has happy connotations for you can lift your mood. Choose a piece of music and listen to it quietly, imagining all your anxiety flowing out through your fingers and toes. Focus on the wonderful life growing inside you. Transmit feelings of positivity to your baby—and imagine the baby doing the same back to you. Put your piece of music on an MP3 player and carry it with you. Listen to it when you feel sad. Before long, the music should provide a trigger to quickly lift your spirits.

Morning sickness

If you suffer from motion sickness, you'll know that horrible, queasy feeling that doesn't go away until you stop moving. Morning sickness is just like that—but there's no opportunity to stop!

In the first three months of pregnancy, more than 80 percent of expectant mothers will suffer some level of morning sickness—which, despite its name, doesn't occur only in the morning.

Thought to be caused by chemical by-products or increased hormonal activity building up and creating toxins in your body, morning sickness is associated with a range of symptoms including cramps, heartburn, cravings, intense hunger, a metallic taste in your mouth, and feelings of weakness and tiredness. Vomiting, which can occur without warning, temporarily relieves the heaviness of the nausea, but can leave you feeling exhausted, provoke nosebleeds, and make your head ache. Unfortunately, this is all just a part of being pregnant, and your doctor won't be able to prescribe you anything to relieve the symptoms, which are usually confined to the first trimester of pregnancy.

Although morning sickness can be an awful experience, I'd like to offer you some comfort in that a study by the National Institute of Child Health and Human Development in the USA found that women who vomit during pregnancy are more likely to carry all the way to term and deliver healthy babies. Horrible as it is, morning sickness can be a good sign.

MORNING SICKNESS AND WEIGHT GAIN

I see many women who are anxious that their morning sickness is preventing them from gaining weight, which also makes them concerned about the nourishment of their baby. However, in the great majority of cases, your clever body will meet the needs of your baby before your own, even if you're vomiting a lot. In addition, your symptoms will typically disappear in the early part of the second trimester when your placenta is fully formed, and you'll still have plenty of time to gain weight. However, if at any time you lose more than five percent of your pre-pregnancy weight, it's important that you consult your doctor.

YOUR DIET

Even though morning sickness can make a woman wonder if she'll ever enjoy eating food again, I have seen that it can have some positive effects on the

HYPEREMESIS

For most women, the symptoms of morning sickness are mild to moderate. However, for some, morning sickness occurs in its most severe form, known as hyperemesis. If you suffer from this condition, you may vomit so much that you can't keep any food or drink down, and you may have to be hospitalized and fed fluids intravenously. The condition can be dangerous for you and your baby, so if you're vomiting so much that you can't eat or drink, it's essential that you consult your doctor immediately.

Opposite: Almonds

women who visit my clinic. Fear of it striking again can make a woman more thoughtful and careful about her food choices, especially if they were poor before her pregnancy. Morning sickness can give her the incentive she needs to change her diet and make a fresh start with her nutritional choices.

In general, try to steer clear of fried and spicy foods, avoid caffeine, and don't brush your teeth straight after a meal as this can make you gag. Keep your food choices simple. It also helps to avoid doing the cooking yourself and to keep away from bad smells, wear loose clothing, and keep car, coach, or plane journeys to a minimum. All of these things can make your symptoms worse. Very hot or cold food can also irritate your stomach. If you're being or feeling so sick that you're finding it hard to take your prenatal supplements, try taking them at the time of day when you feel least queasy and always take them with food. Furthermore, try the following tips for helping to ease away the feelings of pregnancy nausea.

Eat little and often You may be able to ease your symptoms by keeping your blood-sugar levels balanced. Eat snacks that combine complex carbohydrates with a little protein and don't go for more than three hours without eating. Good snack choices include organic hummus on a wholegrain toast or rye crackers, or well-cooked scrambled egg on wholegrain toast. Try eating just a plain, dry wholegrain cracker first thing in the morning, and carry some in your handbag so that you can eat one when nausea strikes.

Try apple cider vinegar First thing in the morning have a cup of warm water and add to it 2 tsp. apple cider vinegar. Apple cider vinegar is pH neutral, so it can help settle stomach acid, which can cause nausea.

Eat almonds Soak ten almonds (unroasted) overnight, and the next morning peel off the skins and eat them. They're a good source of protein and calcium, both of which can settle your stomach.

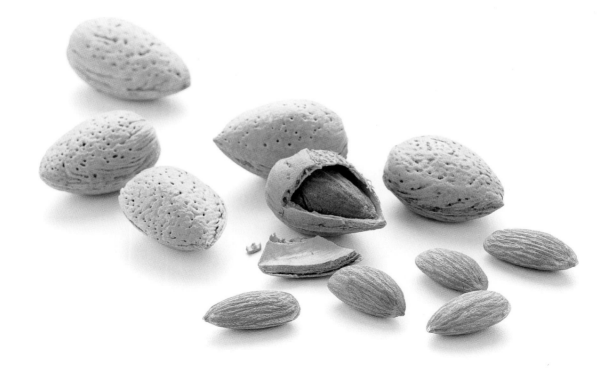

Drink water Although drinking water in itself won't settle your nausea, doing so is essential to compensate for the fluids you lose during any vomiting (not all women vomit, however). A drink that may be helpful to keep by your side is 2 cups mineral water with the juice of half a lemon and a pinch of salt added. The lemon juice makes the water more alkaline, and this seems to settle the stomach.

SUPPLEMENTS

■ VITAMIN B6 (25mg, daily) Some experts believe that morning sickness is caused by high levels of estrogen in the system. Estrogen can build up when the liver isn't efficiently flushing away the excess. Vitamin B6 can help clear away excess toxins by optimizing liver function.

HERBS

■ GINGER A tried-and-tested home remedy for nausea, ginger can be extremely effective for morning sickness. Ginger supplements have been proven to ease nausea by helping food to pass more rapidly through the digestive system, as well as reducing the stimulation to the part of the brain that prompts a burst of nausea or vomiting. There are many different ways to take ginger, although liquid form is the most effective. So, to make a fresh ginger decoction, take a piece of fresh gingerroot, peel it and grate it to give 1 tsp. In a pan, bring 1 cup water to a simmer, add the grated ginger and simmer for ten minutes. Strain the liquid into a cup and drink. If you need it sweetened, drink it with a splash of real maple syrup (not maple-flavored syrup) or honey. Alternatively, you can take ginger in capsule form (1g daily, taken in two or three doses, depending on the amount in each capsule).

OTHER NATURAL TREATMENTS

Homeopathy Although it's always best to have an individual consultation with a registered homeopath, the following are remedies you can try yourself at home. Take the most appropriate in a 30c potency, four times a day for three days. If you have no improvement, try another, or see a qualified practitioner.
• Arsenicum is best if you have a sense of constant nausea, some vomiting and if you feel exhausted or faint
• Ipecac for morning sickness that isn't relieved by either vomiting or eating
• Nux vomica if you feel nauseous but better if you actually vomit
• Sepia if you feel constantly nauseous, but a little better if you eat little and often

Acupressure One study showed a 60-percent improvement in morning sickness in women who used acupressure. The acupressure point for nausea is at the base of your wrist, about 2in. from the crease of

---

CRAVINGS

It's important to listen to your body when you're pregnant because it can tell you what it needs or doesn't want. For example, you may well find that you instinctively go off certain foods and drinks, such as coffee, and simply can't even stand the smell of them. You may also find that you get powerful cravings for a specific kind of food.

Sometimes cravings can be a sign of nutritional deficiency and give you a clue about the kind of food your body needs. Ice-cream cravings, for example, may indicate a need for fat, protein, or calcium. Whatever food you crave, stick to a healthy diet and always aim for the healthiest option. So, if you crave sweets, try adding more protein to your diet to help balance your blood sugar, which will stop the sweet cravings; or choose healthier sweet options, such as raisins.

your wrist on the inside of your arm. (Or, find the point by placing your index finger and middle finger horizontally across your wrist from the base of your palm.) Press on the point for several seconds each time you feel nausea coming on. Alternatively, you can buy acupressure bands to do this job for you—they are the same as the bands used to relieve motion sickness. If you want a tailored treatment, see an acupuncturist. One session twice a week for three or four weeks may ease your symptoms, but if the thought of needles makes you feel even more unwell, try homeopathy.

Aromatherapy Try putting a few drops each of rosewood and lavender essential oils onto a tissue or handkerchief and inhale during the day.

SELF-HELP

You can help yourself by getting as much rest as possible (nausea could be your body's way of telling you that you're overdoing it); and, if at all possible, taking your time getting up in the morning and separating your food from your drinks (drink little and often throughout the day and away from your mealtimes). In addition, try the following tips.

Go for a walk Going for a walk and getting fresh air can not only relieve stress, it can also help take your mind off your nausea. It's better if you can find a green space to walk in rather than the street because it means you can breathe deeply away from any traffic fumes.

Take it easy There's a link between morning sickness and fatigue and stress, so try to relax and unwind as much as you can. Use the tips on pages 309–11 for some ideas. Try to practice relaxation every day.

Try lemon therapy Lemon juice can help relieve nausea—even by just inhaling its fragrance. Cut a lemon in half and rub the juice on your hands, then hold them to your face and take a deep breath whenever you feel nauseous. Alternatively, add the lemon juice to hot or cold water and drink.

PREGNANCY CONSTIPATION

The muscular wall of a healthy bowel contracts to push a stool along until it can be expelled from the body. One of the reasons for constipation is a breakdown in this mechanism, meaning that the stool becomes stuck and hardens in the bowel. Unfortunately, the hormones your body produces during pregnancy can do just this, making your bowel work less efficiently. The pressure from your growing uterus on the bowel wall can also hamper its usual muscular squeezing action. Although it seems only a minor complaint, constipation can lead to hemorrhoids (piles), as a result of straining to pass a stool.

Avoid using laxatives, which can make your bowels lazy. Try simple dietary changes, such as drinking more fluids—plain water and herbal teas are both good choices. Also, eat plenty of good-quality fiber from fruits and vegetables (leave the skins on if you can) and whole grains. Avoid psyllium and bran, though, which can cause bloating and flatulence. Try soaking 1 tbsp. whole organic flax seeds overnight in water, then swallow the whole lot before breakfast the following morning. Finally, don't hold on to a movement when you feel the need to go, and try to walk for up to 30 minutes a day, as exercise can help keep your bowels regular.

Back pain

The weight of an unborn baby and the softening of ligaments during pregnancy mean that between half and three-quarters of expectant mothers experience some form of back pain during their pregnancy.

Fortunately, there are many things you can do to prevent back pain, or, if you do experience it, to alleviate the pain and prevent it from turning into a long-term problem after your baby is born.

CAUSES

All the reasons that cause back pain when you aren't pregnant apply just as much—if not more—during pregnancy. Poor posture, bad lifting technique, weak or tight muscles, and injury can all put your ligaments, muscles, discs, and joints under stress or strain. If you're pregnant and you've been on your feet for a long time, you may find that your back pain gets worse. It can also worsen towards the end of the day because your back muscles become tired and your ligaments stretch slightly from the weight of your body. The additional weight of the growing baby makes the strain—and the pain—worse. However, there are also issues specifically related to pregnancy that can contribute to back pain.

Pregnancy-specific causes

Changes in your hormone levels can cause your muscles and ligaments to become more relaxed, especially during the last few months of pregnancy, as your body prepares itself for labor. The weight of the growing baby may lead to a curvature of your lower spine, causing your ligaments and muscles to feel strained. The growing baby also forces your organs to move up and

A GROWING BABY shifts your balance, straining your spine.

back, which in turn can cause your rib cage to expand, resulting in pressure on the muscles that connect your ribs. Finally, your center of gravity slowly shifts, again to accommodate the weight of the baby, which in itself can result in back pain. To correct this, try to consciously stand with a firm base, keeping your feet shoulder-width apart.

Other common causes of back pain during pregnancy include pelvic girdle pain (PGP) and sciatica. PGP results from the softening effect of the ligaments and leads to instability in the pelvis, which in turn creates pain and inflammation. (If you have pain that's located at the front of your body, this can be the result of a condition known as symphysis pubis dysfunction (SPD), where the softening effect on the ligaments is targeting the usually stiff joint (symphysis pubis) that connects the two halves of your pelvis. The softening effect can then produce pain and inflammation at the front of the body.)

The sciatic nerve is the longest nerve in the body, running the length of your spine and down each leg. Sciatica, which is the name given to describe the pain you feel (the symptom), occurs when something compresses or causes inflammation in the sciatic nerve as it leaves the spine. In the case of pregnancy, the compression comes from your expanding uterus. This can sometimes impair nerve function, causing tingling in your legs and pain down the back of your leg. The problem can be ongoing, even after your pregnancy is over.

WHEN BACK PAIN IS CAUSE FOR CONCERN

Most pregnancy-associated back pain will subside when your body readjusts after the delivery of your baby. However, there are several kinds of backache during pregnancy that need treatment, so never ignore anything that you think seems unusual or suspicious. A dull, low backache may be a sign of pre-term labor, while severe back pain or back pain accompanied by vaginal bleeding or discharge needs to be checked out by your doctor. As a rule of thumb, if you're concerned about your back pain, contact your doctor right away.

CONVENTIONAL TREATMENTS

Although back pain can be debilitating, always check with your doctor before taking any kind of painkilling medication while you're pregnant. In my opinion, unless your pain is excruciating and prevents you from functioning properly, you should avoid any kind of drug during pregnancy and instead try the natural approaches I've suggested below.

NATURAL TREATMENTS

Osteopathy Gentle osteopathic manipulations can help support all your muscles and ligaments, in turn assisting your body to support the weight of your unborn baby. As a result, the baby should not put quite so much strain on your back.

Acupuncture A useful treatment for back pain, acupuncture can help reduce inflammation and swelling, as well as helping to relax your muscles. An acupuncturist will often place the acupuncture needles at the site of the pain and then add several more needles along the meridian (see p.47) that is connected to the pain site.

Massage During pregnancy, massage can help relax the muscles in your back and generally ease away any tension that you're holding throughout your body. I firmly recommend that you see a qualified, registered practitioner during pregnancy, so that you can have a massage that's suited to your needs.

SELF-HELP

My simple self-care strategies and natural therapies can help you ease, treat, or even prevent the discomfort of generalized back pain during pregnancy. However, if you think that you have PGP, SPD, or sciatica (see opposite), or if you have general backache and the self-help measures below do not prove successful, it's important to see your doctor, who may refer you to a physiotherapist for treatment.

Practice good posture It's amazing how many women can resolve their back issues simply by practicing good posture. To stand comfortably and correctly, keep your feet slightly apart and your legs straight with your hands by your sides or behind you. Pull yourself up straight and tuck your buttocks slightly under because this helps you roll your shoulders back and open your upper chest so that breathing is easier. To walk with your spine and head erect, look straight ahead. Wear flat, comfortable shoes, carry your bag diagonally across your body or distribute your weight between bags, so your hands, arms, and shoulders are balanced. Roll your shoulders back and down towards your waist, without tilting your spine.

Sit and stand with care Try not to stay in one position for too long, especially standing. If you must stand, use the posture given above, or stand with one foot resting on a low stool. When you're sitting, keep your feet flat on the floor and slightly apart and position your chair so your knees are higher than your hips, or use a wedge cushion to help push your spine into the correct posture. If you sit at a desk, make sure it's at the correct height for you to work without slumping.

Sleep on your side and get out of bed carefully Sleep on your left side with your knees bent. It may also help to place a pillow between your knees and another under your abdomen. Some women find relief with a full-length pillow. When you get out of bed, stretch the length of your body, bend your knees, and roll on to the side you get up from. Stay there a few moments, then slowly come up to a sitting position with your legs over the side of the bed. Place your feet firmly on the floor and gently push downward on your hands to lift yourself up.

Learn to lift properly If you need to lift something small, squat down, bending at your knees, hold the object close to your body, and raise yourself by straightening your knees. Don't bend at your waist or lift with your back, and try not to twist. Avoid sudden reaching movements or stretching your arms over your head. Ask someone else to lift heavy objects for you.

Keep fit Regular, gentle, pregnancy-appropriate exercise will help keep your back strong and may even relieve back pain. Walking is excellent exercise for your back, as long as you follow my guidelines on good posture (see p.207); while research shows that swimming, and in particular aquanatal classes, can reduce back pain during pregnancy. However, if you're swimming, practice only those strokes in which you dip your head into the water as you swim (for example, breast stroke or front crawl) because holding your neck up puts more strain on your back. Pelvic floor exercises (see box, p.127) will help support your back muscles, and the yoga Cat stretch (see box, p.123), which is perfectly safe to practice during pregnancy, may also offer relief for lower back pain.

Think hot and cold Apply heat to your back by soaking in a warm bath or using a hot water bottle or heating pad. Some women find relief by alternating heat with ice packs. A warm jet of water directed at your back from a shower head can also bring relief.

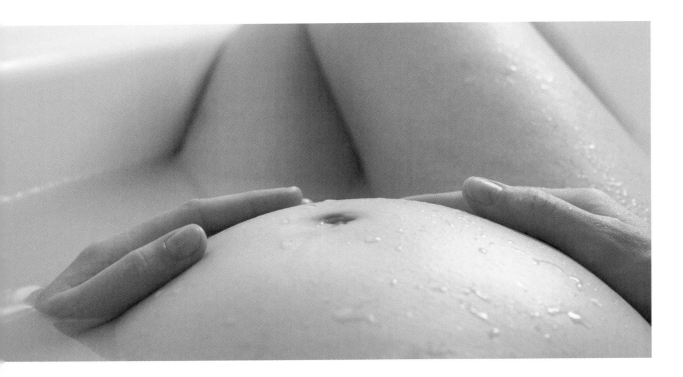

Gestational diabetes

It's estimated that pregnancy—or gestational—diabetes affects between two and three percent of pregnant women. Although the condition can cause concern, it's perfectly treatable.

Diabetes is a condition in which your blood-sugar level is high because your body doesn't produce enough insulin (the blood's sugar-regulating hormone), or the insulin you do produce isn't working properly.

SYMPTOMS

Increased thirst, a frequent need to urinate, and feelings of fatigue are all signs of gestational diabetes. But, these are also all symptoms of a normal pregnancy. For this reason, diabetes can be overlooked, so your routine screening blood and urine tests (usually given by your doctor or midwife) are absolutely crucial.

CAUSES

During pregnancy, various hormones typically block the usual action of insulin to make sure your baby gets enough glucose for its own development. To compensate, your body produces more insulin. Gestational diabetes develops when your body can't compensate properly. As a result your blood-sugar levels rise, and this can lead to problems for both you and your baby.

No one knows why some women develop gestational diabetes and others don't, but you're more at risk if the condition runs in your family. Your risk also increases if you have had a stillbirth or given birth to a large baby (weighing more than 9lb. 14oz.), if you're overweight or obese, or if you have PCOS (see pp.83–7).

DIAGNOSIS

Gestational diabetes usually begins in the second half of pregnancy, between 20 and 24 weeks. Your doctor or

BLOOD-SUGAR BALANCE

This graph shows what happens when blood-sugar levels are out of control—fluctuating on a roller coaster of highs and lows (light gray line)—and what you should be aiming for (dark gray line), where levels slowly rise and fall over the course of a day. If you have gestational diabetes, your blood-sugar levels are high all the time (hyperglycemia), as in the orange line. By eliminating foods and drinks that cause blood-sugar levels to rise (such as sugary and refined foods, as well as caffeine), you can bring your blood-sugar levels down naturally.

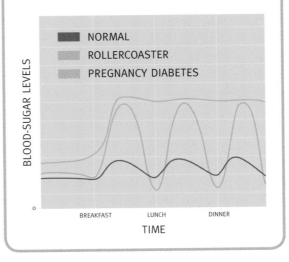

NORMAL
ROLLERCOASTER
PREGNANCY DIABETES

BLOOD-SUGAR LEVELS

0

BREAKFAST   LUNCH   DINNER

TIME

midwife will give you regular blood or urine tests throughout your pregnancy that will pick up the condition, and a glucose tolerance test will confirm it. If the tests are positive, rest assured that the condition will usually go away after your baby is born; if it doesn't, the chances are you were already at a high risk of developing non-gestational diabetes.

RISKS

The biggest risk is that gestational diabetes is a symptom of a condition called preeclampsia (see pp.212–15). Preeclampsia causes high blood pressure, too much amniotic fluid, and premature labor and can also cause your baby to grow larger, which can make delivery difficult. As a result, women with gestational diabetes are more likely to have a Caesarean delivery than women who don't. After the birth, you may be at a greater risk of developing type II diabetes.

Your newborn baby may also have low blood sugar (hypoglycemia) because after birth he or she may continue to make extra insulin. Fortunately, in many cases normal feeding with breast milk or formula is enough to balance a baby's blood-sugar levels, but in some cases your doctor may recommend that your baby be given a sugar (dextrose) solution through a drip. Very rarely, if doctors can't bring your baby's blood-sugar levels under control, there's a slightly increased risk of infant death. Your baby is more likely to develop jaundice (yellowing of the skin and whites of the eyes). This usually isn't serious, and will fade without the need for medical treatment. Gestational diabetes can increase the risk of your baby being born with congenital problems, such as a heart defect or respiratory distress syndrome, and your child may be more prone to obesity and diabetes in later life—but the risks are very small.

CONVENTIONAL TREATMENTS

If you're diagnosed with gestational diabetes, your doctor may refer you to a clinic with doctors and nurses who specialize in the condition. You'll be told how often you'll need to have tests to measure your blood-sugar levels and the kinds of blood-sugar results you need to be aiming for. This is one area where natural medicine and conventional medicine are in complete agreement, and you'll be given a carefully planned diet and exercise program. Your meal plan will focus on controlling your blood sugar and ensuring that you get the right balance of protein and carbohydrates. It's well known that regular, moderate exercise can help balance blood-sugar levels, so you will be urged to do at least 30 minutes of activity that gets you slightly breathless each day.

If diet and lifestyle changes don't settle your blood sugar, then you may need daily injections of insulin, and your doctor or specialist midwife will teach you how to do this. You'll also be taught to recognize the symptoms of low blood sugar (hypoglycemia), such as paleness, shaking, hunger, and sweating. You'll be given advice on what to do if you have these symptoms, such as keeping a sugary soft drink handy. In rare cases, low blood sugar can cause you to faint, and you'll need an injection of glucagon, which causes the liver to release glucose into the blood to restore your body's glucose levels. It's a good idea to make sure your family and friends know what to do if you faint, and even to carry a note about your condition—and what to do in an emergency—in your handbag.

When your baby is born, your doctor or midwife will monitor both your and your baby's blood-sugar levels.

YOUR DIET

Everything you eat and drink affects your blood-sugar levels, and I have seen women with a history of gestational diabetes avoid the condition in subsequent pregnancies simply by getting their nutrition right. The same goes for women referred to me with borderline blood-test results.

Your daily diet won't actually be that different from a usual healthy pregnancy diet (see pp.193–7), but you will need to stick to it rigidly. In general, you'll need to drink lots of water (at least eight glasses a day) and eat three regular meals and three regular snacks a day. It's

A "PERFECT DIET" DAY

The following is an ideal menu plan for a woman with gestational diabetes.

BREAKFAST Organic oatmeal made with water rather than milk (instant oatmeal doesn't count) and topped with ground mixed seeds; or scrambled egg on wholegrain or rye toast.

MID-MORNING SNACK Piece of fruit with a handful of nuts and seeds.

LUNCH Grilled sardines on wholegrain or rye toast; or hummus and vegetables in wholegrain pitta bread.

MID-AFTERNOON SNACK Rice cakes with cashew-nut butter and pure fruit jam (no added sugar).

DINNER Quinoa and roasted vegetables; or lentil and vegetable curry with brown Basmati rice.

important to space your meals over the course of the day and to mix good wholegrain carbohydrates with healthy protein at every meal, and snack to keep your blood-sugar levels steady. You'll need to avoid sugar and sweet foods, but also refined carbohydrates, such as white bread, cakes, candy, and processed foods, because your body converts them into sugar too quickly. Eat fresh, natural, unrefined foods—such as whole grains, nuts, seeds, legumes, and vegetables—that release their glucose steadily. Finally, avoid undiluted fruit juices because the sugar in undiluted fruit juice will hit your bloodstream too quickly, causing a sharp rise in blood-sugar levels.

SUPPLEMENTS

Make sure you're taking a good prenatal supplement (see p.320), as well as the following.

■ VITAMIN C with bioflavonoids (500mg, twice daily, as magnesium ascorbate) Vitamin C is connected to glucose metabolism and can help regulate blood sugar and prevent diabetes. This dosage is a total daily dosage, so account for your prenatal supplement, too.

■ CHROMIUM (200µg daily, including the amount already in your prenatal supplement). If you've been given some time to sort out your gestational diabetes with a nutritional approach (that is, if your condition does not need urgent treatment), boost the chromium in your supplementation. It helps improve insulin's ability to move glucose into the cells, so it helps lower blood-sugar levels. Don't take extra chromium if you have been given diabetic medication.

■ OMEGA-3 FATTY ACIDS (1,000mg fish oil containing at least 700mg EPA and 500mg DHA, daily) Fish oils are important against gestational diabetes, because they help keep your cells soft, so that the insulin receptors on the surface of your cells are more able to use insulin effectively. (Use flax seed oil if you're vegetarian.)

HERBS

A number of herbal remedies may help stabilize glucose levels in your blood, and these include cinnamon and fenugreek. However, because some herbs can have a rapid effect on blood-sugar levels and because their effects vary from person to person, it's important to talk to a qualified herbalist and to let your doctor known what you're doing, rather than self-prescribing.

OTHER NATURAL TREATMENTS

Acupressure and acupuncture The World Health Organization endorses the use of acupuncture for help with diabetes. In Chinese medical terms, diabetes is thought of as a deficiency in yang energy in the body. An acupuncturist may use up to a dozen acupuncture points in one treatment session.

Preeclampsia

Characterized by high blood pressure and protein in the urine, preeclampsia is a condition that, if allowed to develop into full-blown eclampsia, can have serious implications for you and your baby.

Preeclampsia occurs in about one in 14 pregnancies and usually some time after the 20th week. Its severity varies, but the more severe the condition becomes, the greater the risk of complications.

SYMPTOMS
The condition is especially characterized by high blood pressure. When your blood pressure becomes too high, the amount of blood your body delivers to the developing fetus falls and an undernourished fetus can fail to grow normally. As a result, your baby may be unusually small—a condition known as intra-uterine growth retardation (IUGR). Normal blood pressure in a healthy (pregnant or otherwise) woman is around (or ideally just below) a reading of 120/80mmHg. The upper number is your systolic blood pressure, the most pressure your blood is under during a heartbeat, when your heart is pumping hardest; the lower number is your diastolic blood pressure, the least pressure your blood is under when your heart is at rest, during a heartbeat. The blood-pressure reading is taken in millimetres of mercury (mmHg).

Preeclampsia is classed as mild or severe. In mild preeclampsia, your blood pressure reading will probably be around 140/100mmHg and accompanied by slight swelling in your hands and feet, but no detectable protein in your urine. In severe preeclampsia, your blood pressure can rise much higher, to around 160/110mmHg, and your urine sample will show traces of protein because your kidneys are struggling to function properly. These symptoms, as well those given

opposite, indicate that your preeclampsia is severe and you need urgent medical treatment.

Other symptoms include edema (fluid build up in the tissues) and protein in the urine alone. Your regular prenatal health checks with your doctor or midwife will pick up these signs as soon as they become apparent, which is why the checks are so important.

Occasionally preeclampsia develops very quickly, so don't hesitate to call your doctor or midwife if you have any of the following symptoms in the second half of your pregnancy (or in the first few days after you've had your baby, as preeclampsia is still a risk up to four weeks after the birth): rapid weight gain or sudden swelling in your ankles or face; blurred vision; decreased urine output; headaches; confusion or anxiety; shortness of breath on exertion; nausea or vomiting; and pain in the top of your abdomen.

CAUSES
No one really knows what causes preeclampsia, although some believe it may be a malfunction in the placenta. You're at greater risk of the condition if you fall into any of the following categories. If this is your first pregnancy; if you're carrying multiple babies (such as twins or triplets); if you have pre-existing high blood pressure (hypertension), diabetes mellitus, kidney disease, connective tissue disease or vascular disease; if you're under 25 or over 35; if you're overweight or obese; or if you or members of your family have had preeclampsia or eclampsia. However, please rest assured that stress, worry, and working during

pregnancy will not cause preeclampsia and there's no reason not to live a normal life while you're pregnant.

RISKS

Around one in five women with severe preeclampsia develop hemolysis, elevated liver enzymes and low platelets (HELLP) syndrome. This basically means that blood cells start to break down and your liver stops functioning effectively, which in turn increases your risk of serious bleeding.

However, most serious of all is when preeclampsia deteriorates into a life-threatening condition called eclampsia. About one in a hundred women with preeclampsia develops eclampsia, which is associated with convulsive seizures and coma (in the mother). It's estimated that approximately 150 women and 1,200 babies in the USA and approximately ten women and several hundred babies in the UK die each year from the complications of severe preeclampsia. The main aim of any treatment program for a woman with preeclampsia, therefore, is to prevent eclampsia. Happily, we are able to diagnose and manage preeclampsia so effectively that eclampsia is now a rare condition.

CONVENTIONAL TREATMENTS

If you've been diagnosed with mild preeclampsia, you may need only regular checks with your doctor or midwife, as long as the condition remains mild. You should have as much bed rest as possible, lying either on your left-hand side, because this improves the flow of blood to the placenta, or sitting well propped up. A midwife will probably visit you on a daily basis to check your blood pressure and, if it worsens significantly, you're likely to be admitted to hospital. When you're in the hospital, the doctors will use scans to monitor your baby's growth. A CTG (cardiotochograph) is attached to your bump via a pad to check his or her heart rate.

The most effective cure for preeclampsia is to deliver the baby. This is because, after birth, your blood pressure and any other symptoms you've experienced will usually soon settle. For this reason, your doctor may decide to induce your delivery early (or to deliver your baby by Caesarean section). The risk to the baby is small if he or she is born just a few weeks early, but you may need to make a difficult decision if you develop severe preeclampsia early in your pregnancy. Both you and your partner, as well as your doctor, will need to take into account the severity of your condition and the risk to you of complications. You'll also need to consider the relative risks to the baby if you continue with the pregnancy (remember that a preeclampsia baby often doesn't grow well), rather than delivering the baby prematurely.

Medicines A large research study published in 2002 found that giving mothers with preeclampsia magnesium sulphate roughly halves their risk of developing full-blown eclampsia (and also reduces their risk of seizures, a symptom of severe preeclampsia). The medication is administered for about 24 to 48 hours by drip and is used especially in women with severe preeclampsia, where there is a great risk that it will progress to the more dangerous condition. If your preeclampsia is not severe, you may be given medication to normalize your blood pressure.

YOUR DIET

A healthy, balanced diet with sensible pregnancy weight gain can help control high blood pressure. Follow my guidelines for eating healthily during pregnancy on pages 193–7 and, in addition, ensure that you maintain an adequate salt intake (within overall healthy guidelines) because, contrary to advice for non-pregnant women (and for that matter, for men), during pregnancy the sodium in salt helps keep up the flow of fluids in your body, which helps reduce blood pressure and swelling. Drink plenty of fluids, too.

THE WORD eclampsia is from the Greek meaning "bolt from the blue."

SUPPLEMENTS

A study in 2006 showed that pregnant women taking a prenatal supplement were 45 percent less likely to develop preeclampsia than pregnant women taking no supplements at all (the success rate was 71 percent in pregnant women who were not overweight). So, make sure that you take a good-quality prenatal supplement (see p.320) and top up to the following levels.

■ B-VITAMINS (folic acid 0.5–5mg; B6 25–50mg; B12 500μg) These B-vitamins help control levels of homocysteine in your blood, which have been shown to be high in pregnant women who suffer from preeclampsia. Homocysteine results from a natural process in which your body breaks down an essential amino acid called methionine. When your body doesn't detoxify the homocysteine properly, levels become high. This contributes to blood-vessel damage and makes the blood more likely to clot.

■ CALCIUM (700mg, daily) Research shows that calcium supplements may reduce the risk of women developing high blood pressure and preeclampsia during pregnancy. Calcium plays an important part in blood clotting and cell structure, so having good levels of calcium can prevent abnormal blood clotting and high blood pressure in your body.

■ ANTIOXIDANTS (Vitamin C with bioflavonoids—500mg, twice daily, as magnesium ascorbate; vitamin E 400–600iu, daily) Although the cause of preeclampsia is unknown, it's thought that increased oxidative stress and reduced antioxidant defences may play a part.

■ GARLIC (1,000mg aged garlic, daily) This superfood has well-known effects on lowering blood pressure and is completely safe for you to take during pregnancy.

■ OMEGA-3 FATTY ACIDS (1,000mg fish oil containing at least 700mg EPA and 500mg DHA, daily) Having low levels of omega-3 fatty acids has been linked to an increased risk of preeclampsia. One piece of research showed that the incidence of preeclampsia was over seven times more likely in pregnant women who had the lowest levels of omega 3. (Use flax seed oil if you're vegetarian.)

NATURAL TREATMENTS

Homeopathy Preeclampsia can be serious, so see a homeopath for individual treatment (talk to your doctor first). However, the following are useful remedies, taken in a 30c potency four times a day for five days. Use the remedies that are most relevant to you. If you show no signs of improvement after five days using these remedies, you need to see a qualified homeopath and be monitored by your doctor.
• Aurum metallicum if you have high blood pressure, feel stressed, and are craving sweets
• Belladonna for high blood pressure that is accompanied by a flushed, red face, but cold hands and feet
• Nat mur to help reduce fluid retention and swelling

Acupuncture High blood pressure can respond well to acupuncture—a course of treatment can also help to reduce swelling in your hands and feet.

Aromatherapy Use essential oils such as ylang ylang, orange, and sandalwood—all these oils can help lower blood pressure, calm the body, and regulate the heart rhythm. Place 1 or 2 drops of each oil in a bathful of water and relax in it for up to 20 minutes. Alternatively, use up to 15 drops of one or a combination of the oils diluted in 6 tsp. carrier oil, such as sweet almond oil, for a neck and shoulder massage (ask your partner to help).

SELF-HELP

Relax Any kind of relaxation technique, including meditation and gentle yoga, is useful for lowering blood pressure. Any of the meditation exercises in this book can be helpful; and for yoga postures see a yoga instructor who can advise you on safe yoga practice during your pregnancy. I would recommend that you use a relaxation technique at least once a day and twice if you can manage it, for at least 15 minutes each time.

Adjust your sleep position Sleep on your left side, which will take the weight off your large blood vessels.

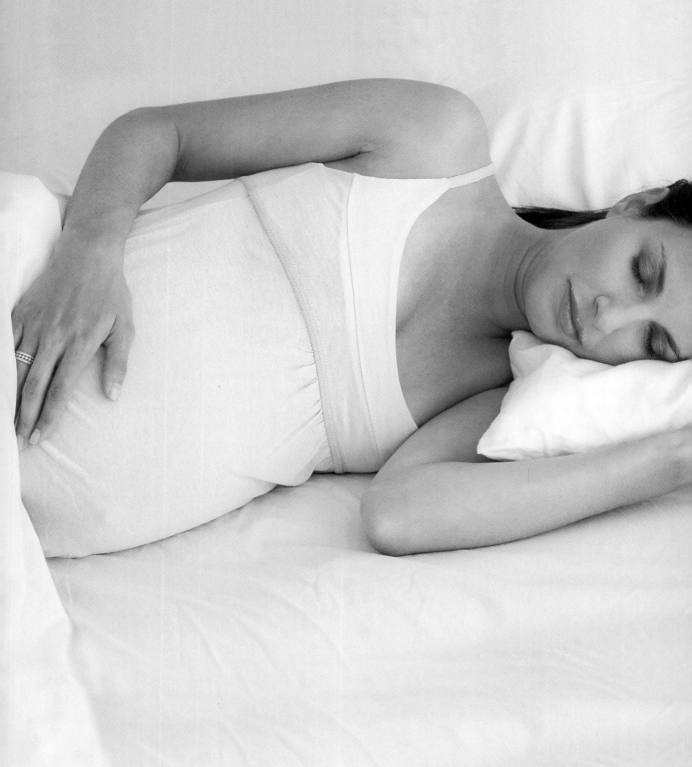

Ways to give birth

Having grown inside you for around 40 weeks, a baby is now ready to be born—a final stage of your pregnancy, and perhaps for some expectant mothers the most daunting stage of all.

Although birth may be nothing like it is in the movies, one thing's for sure: holding your baby in your arms for the first time will make all the effort of labor seem a dim and distant memory.

NATURAL (VAGINAL) BIRTH

The simplest way to get a baby out is also the way nature intended—through the birth canal and out through your vagina. Life doesn't always let things happen the way they should. However, a healthy pregnancy is more likely than not to lead to a healthy, natural delivery, so here are the three main stages of labor.

First stage Changes to the hormone balance in your body make your cervix softer, perhaps producing a "show," when the mucous plug that acted as a seal in your cervix comes away. These hormone changes also start off your contractions. The contractions in this stage are usually "quiet" and irregular at first and can be up to 30 minutes apart. The time it takes to progress through this stage varies from woman to woman, but gradually your contractions will become stronger and more frequent until they're only a couple of minutes apart. Your water may have broken before labor started, or it may break during this first stage. This stage ends when your cervix is fully dilated, which is when it is approximately 4in. in diameter.

Second stage This is the "active" stage of labor, during which your baby is born. As the cervix is fully dilated, the baby's head gets lower. Your contractions become stronger and more frequent and you'll get the feeling that you want to push. If at all possible, it's better to remain upright during this stage of labor because gravity helps open your pelvis, which in turn helps the baby down through the birth canal. The pushing motion moves the baby further down, until the first sign of the baby's head in the vagina, called "crowning," signals that the baby is ready to be born. In a normal delivery, your baby will be born headfirst, followed by the shoulders and then the rest of the body.

Sometimes in the second stage of labor, you might need assistance in order to give birth. Forceps, which look like large tongs, fit round the baby's head and can gently pull the baby out. Or, you may be given a vacuum extraction. In this method, a cup is placed on the baby's head and then the air is sucked out of the cup creating a vacuum that attaches to the head. The midwife can then pull out the baby while you push.

Third stage Once your baby is born, your uterus will start to contract in order to expel the placenta (also known as the afterbirth). Medical staff may actively manage this stage: as the baby's shoulders are born, you may be given an injection of oxytocin and ergometrine to cause your uterus to contact strongly to push out the placenta. However, if your pregnancy has been straightforward, you might like to try delivering your placenta naturally. If you're able to put the baby to your breast, the sucking will stimulate the release of your own oxytocin. The baby's cord is clamped and cut only once the placenta has been delivered.

BREECH POSITIONS

There are three most likely positions for a breech birth.

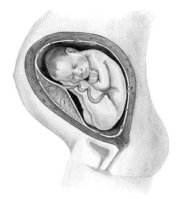

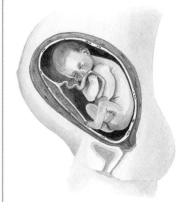

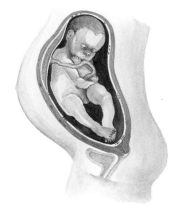

FRANK BREECH

The most common breech position, the frank breech is when the baby's buttocks are lowest and the feet are up by the head, so the buttocks are born first.

COMPLETE BREECH

In this position the baby's feet are tucked under the buttocks and both knees are bent, often with the ankles crossed. The feet and buttocks are both born together.

FOOTLING BREECH

In this position the baby appears to be "standing" on straight legs. Sometimes just one leg will be straight. One or both legs are born before the baby's buttocks.

BREECH BIRTH

In three percent of pregnancies, the baby's buttocks or legs are born first, usually in one of three main positions (see box, above). This is known as a breech birth. However, if your baby is breech, it's likely that your doctor will recommend that you have a Caesarean section (C-section) to avoid any complications. Among these complications, the greatest risk is that the umbilical cord becomes compressed while the baby's head is still inside you, starving the baby of oxygen. Being born legs first can also cause hip dislocation.

Even if your baby is breech at the end of your pregnancy, you can still try to help turn the baby (many babies turn at the last minute of their own accord).

Medical help to turn the baby

A technique called external cephalic version (ECV), can be performed from week 36 and involves gentle massage and manipulation of your abdomen, together with ultrasound scanning to monitor what's happening. This technique is successful for 60 percent of pregnant women with a breech baby, but your doctor won't recommend it if you have had a previous C-section or show signs of having low levels of amniotic fluid.

Natural help to turn the baby

I recommend you try both of the following natural methods to turn your baby—what works for one woman and her baby may not work for another.

Acupuncture Acupuncturists use a technique called moxibustion to turn a breech baby. The acupuncturist burns the herb mugwort and places it on the outer side of your little toe. The treatment is repeated regularly until the baby turns. Find an acupuncturist who has treated pregnant women before.

Exercise The aim of this exercise is to disengage the baby's buttocks from your pelvis so that he or she is free to turn. Kneel down with your knees and legs wide apart and your forearms on the floor in front of you. Rest your head on your forearms and lift your buttocks high into the air. Try to hold this position for about five minutes. Do this exercise twice a day. (If at any time you feel dizzy, uncomfortable, or unwell, stop.)

CAESAREAN SECTION

If doctors believe a vaginal delivery would be a risk to you, your baby, or both of you, he or she will recommend that you have a C-section, where a surgical incision is made through your abdomen and into your uterus to deliver your baby. If you choose to have an elective Caesarean, be aware that it's a major operation, with risks attached.

What happens during surgery?

You'll be asked not to eat or drink anything for up to six hours before surgery. You'll probably be given an epidural, rather than general anaesthetic, so that you can have immediate contact with your baby after birth.

A doctor makes an incision horizontally across your bikini line to get to your uterus, where he or she cuts the amniotic sac, pulls out the baby, and then clamps and cuts the umbilical cord. The doctor delivers the placenta and stitches up the uterus and abdomen.

After surgery

Once you've had your surgery, it's important to rest as much as you can. When you're back at home, you need to take things slowly, and enjoy some pampering and some uninterrupted time with your new baby.

Natural ways to speed your recovery

Diet Make sure you eat healthily, according to my guidelines on pages 24–9. Choose foods that are easy to digest and also warming, such as oatmeal, soups, and so on, so as not to put extra strain on your body.

Supplements Take your prenatal multi-vitamin and mineral supplement (see p.320) as well as vitamin C with bioflavonoids (500mg, twice daily, as magnesium ascorbate) and fish oil (1,000mg, containing at least 700mg EPA and 500mg DHA, daily). The fish oil is good for your general health but is also an anti-inflammatory. Take some extra vitamin E (300–400iu), as this powerful antioxidant will help your skin to repair quicker. As well as taking vitamin E by mouth, each day open one or two of the capsules and pour the oil over your scar. Gently rub in the oil until it's well absorbed. You'll probably be given antibiotics after surgery to prevent infection, so take a probiotic daily to restore the balance of healthy bacteria in your gut. Find one with at least ten billion bacteria per capsule.

Homeopathy After a C-section, homeopathy can help speed recovery healing. Take the following remedies in a 30c potency, three times a day for a week. Visit a registered homeopath for an individualized treatment plan.
• Arnica is recommended after any kind of surgery because it can help control bruising and inflammation and promote healing
• Calendula to improve wound healing
• Hypericum can help offset the effect of the epidural

Aromatherapy Essential oils such as tea tree, lavender, Roman or German chamomile, and thyme can help speed up wound healing and reduce the appearance of scar tissue. Use a few drops of each in your bath. If you can find it, also use the essential oil of *Helichrysum italicum* (sometimes referred to as everlasting essential oil, or immortelle) which has particular healing qualities for the skin.

Labor and labor pain

When your contractions become progressively more frequent and painful, move all the way around your middle, from front to back, and aren't relieved by any change in position, you're probably in labor.

You're about to go through the most natural thing in the world. Call your doctor or midwife for advice on what to do next, and try not to panic. However, what should you do if your labor doesn't start seamlessly, or you're past your due date and don't want to be induced? Sometimes nature needs a little help.

HOW TO GET YOUR LABOR GOING

A daily walk or gentle exercise will encourage your baby to engage, which in turn will help prompt your labor to begin. If you're more than 37 weeks pregnant, drink three cups of raspberry leaf tea a day, which can trigger your uterus to contract. In addition increase your intake of fiber and spicy foods because these foods can stimulate your bowels, which in turn can stimulate labor, although no one is sure why. Making love may also get things going, as semen contains natural prostaglandins, which can help induce labor; an orgasm can help start off contractions.

KEEPING YOUR LABOR GOING

Labor is unpredictable, and what can seem like a run to the finish line can slow down or even stop completely. Try the following to keep things moving along.

Stay upright During the early stages of labor staying upright and moving around as much as possible will encourage the baby's head downward, and walking or moving during a contraction will help ease the pain. Squatting between contractions opens up your pelvis. When you're upright, your uterus is tilted forward and

there isn't any weight bearing down on your blood vessels, so the flow of blood and oxygen around your body is better. Your sacrum is also more mobile, which helps the pelvis joints expand and adjust to the shape of the baby's head as it descends.

Practice yoga During your labor, you could try sitting with the soles of your feet together and your knees flopping outward. This will encourage your pelvic area to open and relax to let the baby out more easily.

Stimulate your nipples Try to get some time alone with your partner and encourage him or her to stroke or massage your nipples. Studies show that nipple stimulation can be more effective than synthetic hormones to induce contractions.

If you're not ready, don't push Pushing against a cervix that isn't fully dilated will delay your labor, so if you aren't ready yet, take lots of deep breaths in and out and try to stay calm.

EASING THE WAY

The following techniques will help you feel more comfortable and relaxed, helping to make your labor an altogether more pleasant experience.

Dim the lights If you can, try to create a cozy, comforting atmosphere in which you're able to feel calm. The more relaxed you are during labor, the easier and quicker your labor will be.

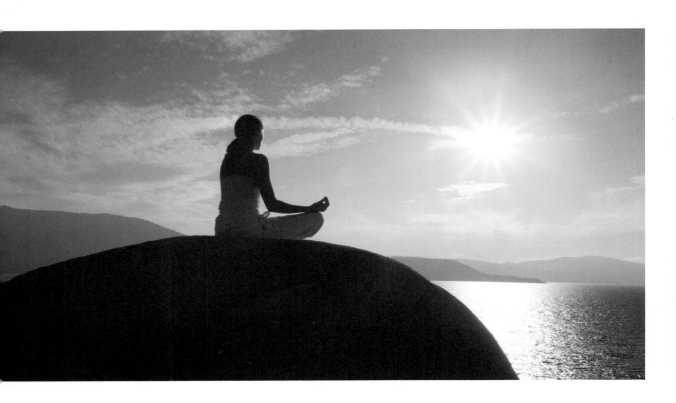

Immerse yourself in water You don't have to opt for a water birth, but getting in a warm bath or even a shower during the early stages of labor will encourage your birth hormones to flow and make you feel relaxed and refreshed, ready for the task ahead.

Sing Try singing or chanting, which amazingly will help relax your pelvic floor, easing the way for the baby to come out. If you want to test this for yourself, try clenching your teeth and relaxing your pelvic floor at the same time; you'll find it virtually impossible. But if you sing (or blow raspberries!), your pelvic floor will relax and open.

Use scent If you're in labor, try putting a few drops of clary sage (*Salvia sclarea*) in a bowl or on a hot cloth and breathe in the scent. Don't use clary sage if you're not in labor, as it can stimulate contractions.

NATURAL PAIN RELIEF

When you go into labor, your body produces natural painkillers called endorphins, which act on your brain to reduce the sensation of pain. Endorphins are also released during exercise. Although they can help you through labor, they are often not enough without additional pain relief, be it medical remedies or self-help or natural therapies. Listed below are the most popular and successful natural pain-relief methods I recommend to my patients. However, keep in mind that your experience of childbirth should be a happy one and if at any point in your labor the pain gets too great or there are complications, there is absolutely no shame in requesting medical assistance or an epidural if you need one.

If you decide to experiment with any of the complementary therapies (acupuncture and so on), be sure to explore them during your pregnancy to see if they're right for you to use during labor. Tell your doctor which complementary therapies you intend to use and be sure to consult a qualified and experienced practitioner in each of them, before you go into labor.

Try deep, slow breathing If you've been to your prenatal classes, you've probably learned a number of breathing techniques to help ease the pain of labor. These really are the most basic and effective ways to deal with the pain. However, if you find that breathing techniques don't help, just focus on your out-breath, making sure you expel all the air from your lungs with each breath. Breathe out slowly and deeply, preferably with your partner who can help keep your breathing steady if you start to panic. Concentrating on breathing out, and letting your in-breath happen naturally, should be enough to help keep you focused on the moment and take your mind off the pain.

Still your mind In the early stages of labor, try to keep yourself busy by singing, listening to music, or even watching a movie. Visualization techniques, such as imagining yourself on a sunny beach or in a beautiful garden, can help you turn off from your pain. You could plan a visualization to a "happy place" in the weeks before your labor, so that you can transport yourself there quickly when the time comes. Remember to use all your senses.

Make a compress A contraction goes all the way around your abdomen and lower back. Try soaking a towel in hot or cold water (your preference). Wring it out and ask your partner to hold it against your back. An ice pack or hot-water bottle is a good option, too.

Have a massage The more relaxed you are, the better the blood and oxygen flow to your muscles and reproductive organs and the less painful your contractions will be. Having your scalp, shoulders, arms, and lower back massaged with firm pressure and downward strokes during labor can be very relaxing. Try combining geranium, clary sage, marjoram, and lavender essential oils to relieve pain (15 drops of essential oil in 6 tsp. carrier).

Hand massage may also be comforting. Hold your hand out and, when you breathe in, ask your partner to apply gentle thumb pressure to the dip in your palm just below the fleshy pad beneath your middle finger and to release that pressure when you breathe out. Massaging around the joint at the base of your thumb on each hand will also help you stay calm. If you don't like being massaged, relaxation and breathing exercises can also help cut down on muscle tension.

Use water power Once your cervix is dilated 2 to 3in., try sitting on a stool under a shower. Water is a fantastic pain-reliever. You may even want to direct the shower jet towards the part of you that hurts the most.

Complementary therapies
Acupuncture and TENS These strategies can trigger your brain to release your body's natural pain-killers, called endorphins. Some hospitals have midwives who are trained in acupuncture. However, the majority of midwives use electrodes called TENS (transcutaneous electrical nerve stimulators) instead to cover key acupuncture points. The TENS machine has electrode pads that are placed on your back to discharge electrical currents, which block the pain. This method works for some, but not all, women. If you intend to use the machine, practice using it during your pregnancy, as it can be fiddly to master. You can usually rent a TENS machine from your hospital or local pharmacy.

Acupressure Ask your birthing partner to place the knuckles of two fingers either side of your spine between the dimples at the bottom of your spine and your buttocks. He or she should press as you breathe in, then hold the press for five seconds. They should release the press as you breathe out. Continue while you're comfortable.

Breastfeeding

Doctors, midwives, and even manufacturers of baby formula agree that breastfeeding is best for both you and your new baby. For this reason, I encourage you to give it a try.

No sooner has the pain of labor subsided and you've been handed your beautiful new baby, than your responsibility as chief provider for this new life kicks in. Almost the first thing any doctor will do once your baby is born and has been checked over, is put him or her to your breast and ask you to start feeding.

The optimal length of time to breastfeed a baby is for six to 12 months. But even if you manage only a few weeks, I urge you to start out by breastfeeding because nature has formulated the best food—and food-delivery system—your baby could ever want.

WHY BREAST IS BEST

It's all very well people telling you (and they will) that breast is best, but what exactly are the reasons?

Complete nutrition Your breast milk contains not only nutrients but also ingredients that can never be replicated in infant formulas, such as antibodies to arm your baby's undeveloped immune system (see right). Breast milk also contains the perfect ratios of certain ingredients (for example, the ratio of iron to protein), whereas in formula milk these ratios are out of balance. Your breasts also have the ability to manufacture milk at a rate that is attuned to your baby's ever-changing needs.

Digestibility Breast milk is perfectly designed for a baby's developing digestive system, and its protein and fat content is more easily handled by the baby's gut than the protein and fat in formula milk. This means

that breastfed babies tend to be less likely to suffer from colic, gas, and vomiting.

Antibodies Colostrum, which is the sticky "pre-milk" that makes up your baby's first feed, is full of antibodies that can protect him or her from infection and disease. Breast milk itself protects your baby from constipation, allergies, and obesity and makes his or her bowel movements sweeter smelling.

Convenience Breast milk is not only completely cost- and bottle-free, it's something you always have with you. In addition, you will deliver it at exactly the right temperature, making it hassle-free, too.

Faster recovery for you As well as providing closeness, which aids the bonding process between mother and baby, breastfeeding will help your uterus shrink back to its pre-pregnancy size more quickly (this shrinking causes the cramping sensation you may feel when your baby breastfeeds) and will help you shed leftover pregnancy weight because you have to burn calories to produce breast milk. In addition, breastfeeding forces you to stop during the day, encouraging you to sit down and rest while you feed the baby.

All this isn't to say that there aren't any advantages to bottle-feeding. Choosing to use a bottle, or having to use one if you're unable to breastfeed, allows you more freedom (perhaps to spend time with the baby's siblings and even for an evening out), makes it easier to

POSITIONS FOR BREASTFEEDING

The four main breastfeeding positions are outlined below. It takes time to feel really comfortable breastfeeding; find a position that works best for you and your baby.

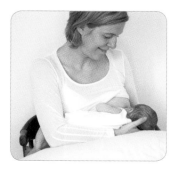

THE CROSS-CRADLE HOLD
Sit up straight in a chair with arm rests and hold your baby across you in the crook of your arm, opposite to the breast you want to feed from—so right arm for left breast and left arm for right breast.

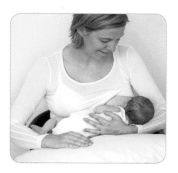

THE CRADLE HOLD
Sit up straight in a chair with arm rests and support your baby with the arm on the same side as the nursing breast. Cradle your baby and rest his or her head in the crook of your elbow.

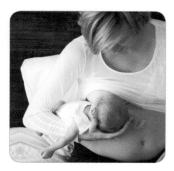

THE FOOTBALL HOLD
Sitting up, hold your baby at your side with your forearm. With your open hand, support the head and face the baby towards your breast. This position is especially good if you're recovering from a C-section (the baby doesn't rest on your abdomen).

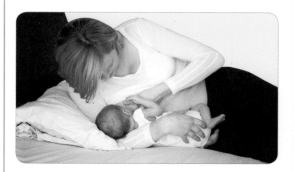

THE LYING DOWN HOLD
Lie on your side and lay your baby next to you, facing towards your breast. Support the baby with the arm and hand of the side you're lying on. With the other hand grasp your breast and place the nipple in your baby's mouth.

monitor your baby's intake of food, and gives the baby's father an opportunity to enjoy the feeding process and bond with his baby, too. Bottle-feeding may also be less stressful in public.

Because of the evidence to promote breastfeeding, choosing not to breastfeed—or not being able to—can cause some women to feel immensely guilty. However, if something isn't right for you—and that includes breastfeeding—then it won't be right for your baby. A bottle given by a relaxed, happy, and loving mother is preferable to a breastfeed given by a mother who is stressed and unhappy.

HOW DO YOU PRODUCE MILK?

Your milk is produced in cells called alveoli in your breasts. It travels down the milk ducts and collects in a sort of reservoir. The hormones prolactin and oxytocin control milk production by causing the milk-producing cells in your breasts to contract, squeezing milk down the ducts and out of your nipple. This is known as the "let-down reflex," and it can be so effective that sometimes your breasts feel as though they are going to burst, and you look forward to feed time as much as your baby.

FIRST STEPS WITH BREASTFEEDING

First, let me debunk some myths. Contrary to popular belief, you can breastfeed if you have small breasts or flat nipples. Breasts and nipples of all shapes and sizes can satisfy a baby, and the size of your breasts has nothing to do with the amount of milk you produce. And contrary to another popular myth, breastfeeding

HOW TO PUMP YOUR MILK

Pumping milk is when you squeeze milk from your breasts by hand or by a pump, store it, and save it in a container so you can feed your baby later. It's a great way to relieve engorged breasts, but it's also good if you need to be away from your baby for a few hours but still want him or her to have the benefits of your breast milk. In addition, your baby's father can feed the baby pumped milk, helping him to feel more involved.

It's possible to pump breast milk by hand, but it's time-consuming, inefficient, and often messy, and many women prefer to use manual or electric breast pumps instead. To use a manual pump, you put a suction cup over your breast and pump milk into a container by using the squeeze mechanism on the pump. With an electric pump, you put the suction cup on your breast, turn the machine on, and let it do the work for you. It typically takes 15 to 40 minutes to pump your milk from both breasts.

As soon as you have pumped your milk, you need to store it correctly in sealed bottles. Remember to put a date on the bottle before storing it in the freezer or fridge. You can store pumped milk in the coldest compartment of a refrigerator for up to a week and for up to four months in a freezer set at 0°F or colder. Freezing does destroy some of the milk's antibodies, but I think that frozen breast milk is still a preferable alternative to using commercial formula. Fresh breast milk will keep in the fridge for only 24 hours.

To thaw and warm the milk, place the bottle in a bowl of warm water. Don't use the microwave because this kills nutrients. Never refreeze any milk that your baby has only partly drunk—just throw it away.

doesn't ruin your breasts or affect their shape or size. Only hereditary factors, age, poor support, and weight gain during pregnancy can make your breasts less firm after childbirth.

Don't expect to have a breast full of milk right away. Babies are not hungry when they're born, and it isn't until the third or fourth day that your milk will start to come in. This doesn't mean your breasts are empty. The first, pre-milk feeds are of colostrum, and each will average less than half a teaspoon. Even so, these tiny feeds give your baby all the nourishment and antibodies he or she needs to keep healthy.

COLOSTRUM is sometimes known as "liquid gold."

When your milk does come in, your baby will be ready for his or her first "proper" feed. Have a glass of water just before you begin and make yourself comfortable. Your baby needs to be facing you so that he or she has to tilt their head back to get your nipple in their mouth, but experiment to find a feeding position that works best for you (see box, p.223).

PROBLEMS WITH BREASTFEEDING

Breastfeeding looks so easy and natural when you see other nursing mothers out and about, yet the first time you put your baby to your breast it may feel anything but. The whole process can be incredibly frustrating— your baby may not latch on properly or may not show any interest in your breast, and you may find breastfeeding painful and uncomfortable. Breastfeeding, like everything else about parenthood, is something you need to learn. Ask your healthcare visitor for advice and support. Try not to get stressed and impatient, and relax as much as possible. Give yourself and your baby time to learn and adjust and, in the majority of cases, soon you will be making breastfeeding look easy and natural, too.

However, on the road to breastfeeding ease, there are several conditions and problems that you, like many women before you, may need to overcome. Here are the most common.

Engorgement Almost every mother experiences engorgement when her milk first "comes in" after the baby is born. It can make your breasts feel hot, swollen, and hard, and it's caused by the increased blood flow to the breasts. Although engorgement can feel very uncomfortable, it's a positive sign that you're producing milk to feed your baby. The condition passes pretty quickly, usually within two to four days, and breastfeeding will help it go away. Once the engorgement passes, your breasts will be softer, although still full of milk. Until then, try the following.

• Reduce the swelling by applying a cold compress to your breasts as often as you need. Use a flannel wrapped around ice cubes or an ice pack.

• Wash your breasts in warm water before a feed.

• Bruise a cabbage leaf and leave it inside your bra against the engorged breast for up to 24 hours. This has an anti-inflammatory effect.

• Nurse frequently—every two to three hours—even if it means waking your baby. This is really important because unrelieved engorgement can cause a permanent drop in your milk production.

• Pump your milk (manually or with a pump) until your areola—the dark area around your nipple— softens, making it easier for your baby to latch on. You may find it easier to manually pump milk in the shower; the warm water by itself may cause enough leakage to soften the areola. Bear in mind that excessive or habitual pumping can lead to overproduction of milk and prolonged engorgement, so avoid pumping unless absolutely necessary.

• Gently massage the breast your baby is sucking on. This encourages milk to flow and will help relieve some of the tightness and discomfort.

• Take echinacea tincture (1 tsp. three times a day in water) to reduce the possibility of infection.

Blocked ducts If you feel feverish and notice tender lumps on your breast, you may be suffering from

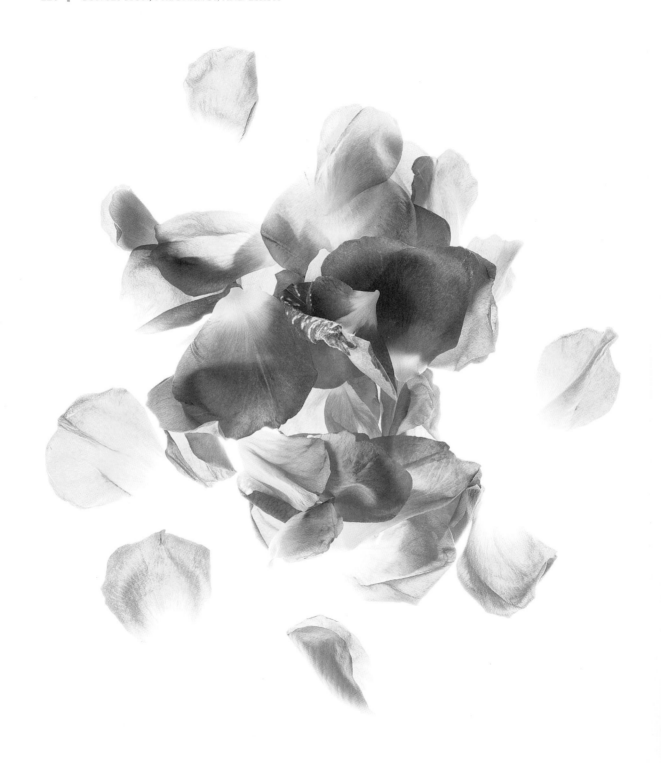

blocked ducts, perhaps caused by a bra that is too tight or by feeding your baby in an awkward position. The tenderness in your breasts can make feeding painful, but don't be tempted to stop feeding altogether because this will actually make things worse. Instead, massage the lump gently in the direction of your nipple to clear away the blockage. You can also apply hot and cold compresses to soothe any pain and inflammation. Offer the tender breast first at feeding time so the baby's strongest sucking, when he or she is hungriest, will help get milk flowing through the ducts again. Other remedies include the following.

• Try a compress made by soaking a breast pad in one drop each of rose, geranium, and lavender essential oils diluted in 2 cups cold water. Apply this as often as you can until you notice some relief.

• Vary your nursing position or try positioning the baby at your breast with his or her chin pointed towards the sore spot. This can direct suction at the plugged duct and can promote healing.

• Try the homeopathic remedies of Aconite, Belladonna, and Bryonia (all at 30c potency, taken three times a day). If these don't work, I advise you to see a registered homeopath who can tailor your treatment.

• If you have an infection, take aged garlic (1,000mg, daily), as well as vitamin C with bioflavonoids (500mg, twice daily, as magnesium ascorbate) and echinacea (1 tsp. tincture, three times daily in water; or 300–400mg capsules, twice daily).

To help prevent recurring plugged ducts, avoid long gaps between feeds and buy a well-fitting nursing bra.

Insufficient milk If your milk supply seems to be insufficient, stress, poor diet, not drinking enough water, or not enough rest on your part may be the culprits, so make sure you eat healthily and take time out to put your feet up more often. Herbs that can stimulate milk supply are called galactagogues, and they can be very helpful. They include fennel (*Foeniculum vulgare*), blessed thistle (*Cnicus benedictus*), fenugreek (*Trigonella foenum-graecum*), and nettle (*Urtica urens*—which can also be used as a homeopathic remedy, see below). Make up a combined tincture of all these herbs by mixing their individual tinctures in equal parts. Take 1 tsp. of the combined tincture in a little water, three times a day. If your milk supply fails completely, try taking 1 tsp. agnus castus (*Vitex agnus castus*) tincture in a little water, three times a day, for up to one month. You could also try the homeopathic remedies of pulsatilla or urtica urens, both in a 30c potency, twice a day.

Sore and cracked nipples Sore nipples are so common in breastfeeding that many new moms think they're normal, but they most certainly are not. It's normal to have an initial pain when your baby first latches on, but it's not normal to have pain throughout an entire feed. The most common cause of sore nipples is incorrect positioning—the baby isn't taking a large enough mouthful of breast tissue. Position your baby so his or her body is turned towards your body, and he or she doesn't have to turn his or her head to grasp your breast. The baby's bottom lip should be turned downward and most of the areola should be inside the baby's mouth. If the pain lasts more than about 15 seconds, break the suction carefully and latch your baby on again. If you still have problems with sore nipples, you can try the following preventative measures.

• Expose your breasts to the air as much as possible.

• After each feed, pump a few drops of milk and smooth them over your nipples and areolae.

• Apply a little soothing marigold (sometimes sold as calendula) or Roman or German chamomile ointment after each feed, but be sure to wash it off before the next feed. Or, use the ointment given in the box on the following page.

PROBLEMS WITH breastfeeding can almost always be overcome—ask for help if you need to.

Opposite: Rose petals (*Rosa* spp)

• Don't just pull your baby off your breast—always break the baby's suction first by placing your finger in the corner of the baby's mouth before removing him or her from your nipple.

• If the pain gets too great, consult a lactation consultant so you can fix what's wrong.

Mastitis About one in ten mothers gets mastitis, an inflammation of the breast, which can lead to infection. It can cause similar symptoms to a blocked duct, but you may feel more tired and sick, almost as if you have come down with the flu. Common, and more serious, signs of mastitis include chills, a headache, a temperature of over 101°F, and exhaustion. These symptoms are not typically caused by infection but by milk entering the small blood vessels in your breast and being treated by your body as a foreign protein.

Infective mastitis may be caused when invading germs from your baby's nose are transmitted to your breast. Some women who have mastitis have had cracked nipples, and the infection may have passed through the crack or fissure in the nipple into the lymphatic system of the breast.

If you suffer from mastitis, don't stop feeding—although mastitis is painful for you, it won't affect your baby, and it's safe for your baby to feed from the affected breast. Follow the guidelines I've given for treating engorgement and blocked ducts (see p.225–7). In addition, try warm cloths on your breasts for several minutes before each feed—this should help your letdown reflex and make feeding more comfortable. Some mothers find that a cold compress or a warm shower works better.

If it helps to massage your breasts, do so gently while your baby is feeding to help the milk to flow from them. Massage that is too vigorous can make mastitis worse by pushing the leaked milk further into the breast tissue. If your baby doesn't empty the inflamed breast during each feed, use a breast pump to empty it; or if it is simply unbearable to breastfeed, try pumping your milk and giving it to your baby in a bottle.

CRACKED-NIPPLE OINTMENT

The following oil or ointment can help create healthy, flexible nipple tissue that is resistant to cracks, tears, and chapping, and it can ease the discomfort of already sore or cracked nipples. Rub the ointment into your nipples after each feed but wash it off again before the next.

Mix one part pure vitamin-E oil to eight parts sweet almond oil in a 50ml bottle and add two drops marigold (*Calendula officinalis*) tincture. Shake the bottle to mix thoroughly. You can make up a thicker ointment by adding a few drops of marigold tincture to some shea butter, if you prefer.

If none of these techniques helps, talk to your doctor or healthcare visitor as soon as possible. If diagnosed early, mastitis is easy and quick to treat, although you may need antibiotics. (Do try my self-help measures first, though.) Once you have mastitis, pay close attention to your condition because if it doesn't start to improve, it can develop into a breast abscess, which will require immediate medical attention (and sometimes surgery) to drain it. If you develop an abscess, breastfeeding on the affected breast must stop temporarily, although to encourage milk production you should continue to pump until healing is complete. In the meantime, your baby can keep feeding from your healthy breast (your body will compensate so that your baby gets enough milk).

If you do need to take antibiotics (you may be able to continue breastfeeding while on them), take a daily probiotic, containing at least ten billion beneficial bacteria per capsule, at the same time. The antibiotics will wipe out all the beneficial bacteria in your gut, and the probiotic will help redress the balance.

Postpartum depression

Postpartum "baby blues" are a normal response to dramatic shifts in hormone levels in your body after you've had a baby. However, for 15 percent of women, the baby blues will develop into depression.

A frightening and debilitating condition, postpartum depression appears to go against everything we ever think about having a baby—the joy, the excitement, the thrill. As a result, many women suffer in silence.

SYMPTOMS

After giving birth, you may have a couple of days before your milk comes in when you feel sad, weepy, and moody. This perfectly normal response may last for a few hours or a few days, and then disappear. Postpartum depression, on the other hand, is much more pronounced: Weepiness may turn to crying all the time and for no particular reason; sadness may become feelings of despair, low self-esteem, and complete inability to cope; and moodiness may turn to extreme outbursts of anger or frustration, obsessiveness, or to a sense of wanting to lock yourself away from the world and reluctance to care for yourself. You'll probably feel deeply anxious and tense, which will affect your sleeping, and probably also your eating habits (you may binge eat, or you may lose your appetite altogether), as well as making you feel confused or panicked in situations that you would normally be able to handle with ease. Physically, you may experience headaches, or back or neck pain.

THE BABY BLUES

If you have been looking forward to the birth of your baby, it may seem irrational to suddenly, when your baby is here, experience symptoms of the baby blues. You may have no idea why you feel weepy or why you're so sensitive to anything family, friends, or medical staff have to say. Try not to be so hard on yourself. Your body has created a new life, and changes in mood may simply be caused by the massive hormonal shifts that occur after delivery. Throughout your pregnancy, hormone levels have shifted to accommodate your baby and by the time your labor begins, your levels of estrogen and progesterone are up to 50 times higher than they were pre-pregnancy. When your baby is born, these levels drop sharply, and within hours are below the levels they were at nine months ago when your pregnancy began.

If you do feel weepy after your baby is born, allow yourself the freedom to cry and to express how you feel to others. If anyone tells you to pull yourself together, speak to someone else who can listen to you and show you understanding. Above all, feel reassured that these feelings are normal and will pass.

If you experience a combination of any of these symptoms, and if they've been with you for more than a week after the birth of your baby, please see your doctor. It's important that you talk to someone, and don't feel guilty or self-critical. If the first person you talk to isn't sympathetic or doesn't take you seriously, find someone who does—for your own well-being and for the well-being of your newborn baby.

Every woman has to find what works best for her and her baby, but during your recovery you can help yourself a lot by being patient and understanding with yourself and by believing that, like the great majority of women who experience this condition, you will get better eventually. Conventional treatment, as well as diet, lifestyle, and supplement and alternative therapy recommendations, will help you through.

CONVENTIONAL TREATMENTS

It's only very rare that a woman with postpartum depression will need treatment with medication, or psychiatric help. It's important to keep reminding yourself that in the great majority of cases, postpartum depression will pass on its own, as long as you have support from your doctor, friends, and relatives. Although decades ago the condition wasn't recognized, doctors and health visitors today are aware that it exists, and there are support structures in place for you.

Your doctor may ask you to fill out a survey to assess whether or not you're suffering from symptoms of postpartum depression. It alarms me how many of the women I see in my clinics confess to masking their true feelings when answering these questions. Please don't be tempted to put on a brave face; please do respond truthfully. Nobody will think any less of you, and you'll not be separated from your baby or family during your illness or recovery.

Medication Occasionally, your doctor may prescribe tranquillizers or antidepressants. These may help lift your mood, but they can also make you feel drowsy and may prevent you from breastfeeding.

Hospitalization If your symptoms are severe, a women's health and wellness clinic may provide the answer. Here, mothers suffering from postpartum depression may be able to get support and treatment, while keeping their babies with them. The focus is on making you feel better so you and your family can get on with enjoying life and your new baby.

YOUR DIET

The most important thing you can do nutritionally to help your mood is to try to keep your blood-sugar levels balanced (see box, p.29). Symptoms of blood-sugar imbalance include fatigue, mood swings, and loss of concentration, and all these will compound the other symptoms of your depression. Make sure you eat little and often (have something at least every three hours), and try to include some healthy protein (such as fish or nuts) in every meal and snack.

SUPPLEMENTS

Don't stop taking a quality multi-vitamin and mineral supplement (see p.320) now that your baby is born (use your prenatal supplement while you're breastfeeding because you know that everything it contains is safe for your baby). Nutritional deficiencies can trigger low moods, so you also need to make sure your nutrient intake is at optimum levels. In particular, pay attention to the following important nutrients. Account for the amounts in your daily multi-vitamin and mineral and then take extra supplements as necessary.

■ ZINC (30mg, daily) Zinc deficiencies can trigger hormonal imbalances and loss of appetite and can exacerbate mood swings.

■ ESSENTIAL FATTY ACIDS (500mg, three or four times daily) Keep taking your omega-3 fish oil supplements (or flax seed capsules) and also take capsules of borage (starflower) oil, which is a wonderful source of omega-6 fats (see p.26). Essential fats build and nourish the membranes of your nerve cells, helping the cells communicate with each other, which is important for mental health.

HERBS

The following herbs have been successful at relieving depression. However, if you're breastfeeding, you must speak to your doctor or healthcare provider before taking either of them.

■ AGNUS CASTUS
(*Vitex agnus castus*) Because postpartum depression can be linked to the hormonal upheaval of pregnancy, agnus castus, a good hormone-balancing herb, can be beneficial. Take 1 tsp. agnus castus tincture in a little water, two or three times daily; or one 300mg capsule, twice daily.

■ ST JOHN'S WORT
(*Hypericum perforatum*) This herb is well known as an important antidepressant (in some trials it has proven to be as effective at relieving depression as some conventional medication). It helps calm anxiety and lift mood. Take 1 tsp. tincture in a little water, or 300mg in capsule form, two or three times daily.

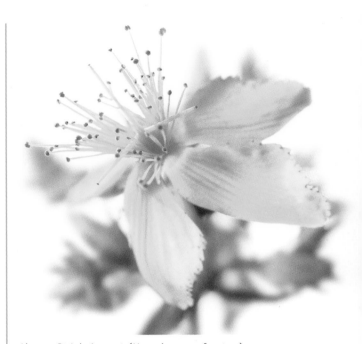

Above: St John's wort (*Hypericum perforatum*)

OTHER NATURAL TREATMENTS

Homeopathy It's especially important that, if you suffer from depression, you see a registered homeopath who can prescribe remedies according to your specific symptoms. In the interim, though, try Sepia (30c) and Pulsatilla (30c), twice daily.

Acupuncture Some studies show that when an acupuncturist stimulates the relevant meridians in the body, symptoms of depression can fall by up to a staggering 44 percent. It's certainly worth giving this natural treatment a go. If you don't like the thought of needles, you could try acupressure instead.

Aromatherapy The essential oils of jasmine, clary sage, and ylang ylang are recommended treatments for postpartum depression. Mix together equal parts of each oil and add one drop of the combined mixture to your bath water. Alternatively, sprinkle a few drops of the blend onto your pillow to breathe in during sleep, or on a tissue to breathe in as a quick fix whenever you feel anxious or nervous.

SELF-HELP

Rest, rest, rest Tiredness makes depression worse, so take every opportunity you can to rest. Sleep when your baby sleeps, and, if you can, ask someone else to help with feeding the baby (using pumped or formula milk), and certainly ask willing friends and family to help with chores. If you have older, pre-school children, think about sending them to a nursery or playgroup at least for a few hours a day to give you some down time. Most of all, don't feel guilty about resting—it's in the interests of all of you that you get better.

Use distraction Leave the big chores to someone else, but find small chores that you can accomplish easily. This helps take away feelings of inadequacy. Simple tasks, such as tidying your wardrobe or polishing your shoes, can restore any lost sense of order.

Join a support group Sometimes talking to other women who have symptoms similar to your own can

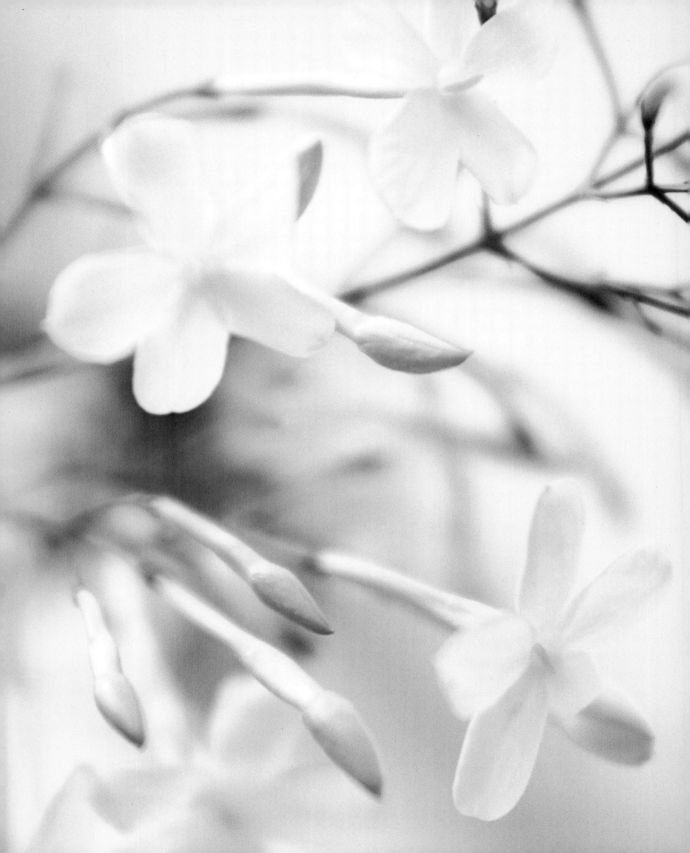

be extremely therapeutic, comforting, and helpful, particularly if you feel like you're the only one who ever feels like this. Ask your doctor to recommend a support group in your area.

Get out of the house If you can, try to get out of the house on your own. Don't feel that you have to be with your baby 24/7. Leave your baby with someone you trust and take the chance to have some time by yourself, even if it's just for half an hour.

Exercise Getting moving may be the last thing you want to do, but regular exercise is proven to beat depression. Aim for gentle exercise for at least 20 minutes a day and, if you can, exercise in the fresh air, so you get all the mood-boosting benefits of daylight.

Don't "bottle things up" It's worth saying again: Talk to somebody. Postpartum depression is an illness, and you're not suffering from it because you're a weak or hopeless mother—and it will get better.

"LETTING GO" MEDITATION

Bottling up your feelings can just make symptoms of postpartum depression worse. Meditation can be a way to help you express and deal with difficult emotions because it's all about letting go of your inner thoughts, feelings, and turmoil in order to empty the mind and find a sense of clarity and peace. Use this exercise every day to help you start recognizing, naming, and letting thoughts and feelings go.

1 Choose a time when your baby is well fed and sleeping, so you can be as confident as possible that you'll be undisturbed for 20 minutes or so. If you're able, ask your partner or a friend or a relative whom you trust to be on hand to deal with any infant grumbling, or with any other children you have, while you have this time to yourself.

2 Sit comfortably in a chair or on the floor and breathe deeply. Try to regulate your breathing so it feels comfortable and natural, not forced or deliberate.

3 Close your eyes and as you feel each emotion rise within in you, give it a label. Try not to make your labels emotive in themselves, make them descriptive, just as you would if you were creating a filing system. If you feel sadness about the baby, label it "baby"; if you feel guilt about changes to your relationship with your partner, label it "relationship"; and so on.

4 As you label each emotion, gently let it go (you could visualize it disappearing into the sky or floating away on a wave), and wait for the next feeling to come along. Do this for 20 minutes or so. Observing your feelings in this empowering way helps you remember that you're in charge of how you feel, not the other way round.

Opposite: Jasmine (*Jasminum officinale*; see Aromatherapy, p.231)

LOSING YOUR BABY

From the earliest beginnings of your pregnancy, you probably felt that the fetus was an integral part of yourself. This instinctive response to pregnancy means that miscarriage or stillbirth can be devastating.

Miscarriage is far more common than you may realize. An estimated one in four women experience miscarriage, and one in three hundred have had three or four miscarriages. Nevertheless, if you lose a baby, your loss will feel both intense and painful. On a physical level, your body went through major hormonal shifts; and, on a psychological level, there had been an immediate bond between mother and baby-to-be. Your instinct may be to rush ahead with another pregnancy, but do give yourself time to mourn. Studies show that unresolved grief may affect your fertility or stop you from fully experiencing the joy of a future pregnancy.

WHAT IS A MISCARRIAGE?

A miscarriage is the loss of your developing baby. The medical profession categorizes that loss according to the point in your pregnancy when you experienced it. At 24 weeks, a live birth is considered "viable"—that is, the baby would stand a chance of surviving (probably with intensive care). If you lose a baby before this milestone, you're said to have suffered a "spontaneous abortion"; after 24 weeks, the loss is called a stillbirth.

When miscarriage occurs it's important that all the "products of conception" are removed from your uterus (the placenta, amniotic sac, and fetus). Often doctors will offer a procedure called a dilation and evacuation (D&E) that confirms your uterus is clear. If you do have a D&E, ask the doctors to test the baby's tissue, as it can sometimes give information as to why you miscarried. In many cases, this information can help the grieving process.

There are three other kinds of fetal loss that aren't strictly miscarriages inasmuch as the body doesn't expel anything spontaneously. These are "blighted ovum," "missed abortion" and "chemical pregnancy." A blighted ovum occurs when an ultrasound shows an amniotic sac, but sadly no embryo within it. A missed abortion occurs when you go for a scan thinking that all is well, only to discover that tragically your baby has died. In a chemical pregnancy, hormone levels have indicated that you're pregnant, but it's thought that the fetus died before it could implant.

SYMPTOMS OF MISCARRIAGE

The symptoms that most commonly alert an expectant woman to the fact that something might be wrong are severe abdominal cramping and/or bleeding from the vagina. This might be heavy or just a few spots that continue to appear over several days. You may experience pain in your lower back, bleeding may contain clots, and vaginal mucus may contain flecks of gray-brown matter. If you're at all concerned at any time during your pregnancy, you must call your doctor.

MOVING ON

Understanding what has happened in your body can be overwhelming when you lose a baby. Doctors may bombard you with information that, at the time, can be hard to absorb. Over the following pages, I'll talk you through all the main causes of miscarriage and stillbirth and give you some information on how to restore your health and how to cope with grief.

First- and second-trimester miscarriage

The great majority of miscarriages occur in the first or second trimester of pregnancy. The experience can be both physically and mentally devastating—but you're not alone.

WHAT CAUSES A MISCARRIAGE?

The women I see in my clinics understandably want to know why they've suffered the devastating loss of their baby. By having this knowledge, they then feel they can do something to prevent a miscarriage from occurring in future pregnancies. Unfortunately, although your doctor may be able to find a tangible reason why you miscarried, in some cases, all your tests results will appear normal and an explanation as to what happened will remain frustratingly elusive. Equally, there may be a single, definable cause for your miscarriage; or it may have been caused by a combination of factors.

The answers are unlikely to be straightforward, but while some of the possible causes and risk factors are out of your control, others (such as smoking, drinking, and weight problems) are not. This goes as much for your partner as it does for you. Here are some of the most common causes and risk factors for miscarriage, and the various treatments that may help reduce or eliminate them.

CAUSES BEYOND YOUR CONTROL

Chromosomal abnormality A chromosomal abnormality is different from an inherited genetic problem and can occur (in the sperm or egg) before or during fertilization—or after it, when the embryo's chromosomes divide. A human being has 46 chromosomes, which make 23 pairs. In a baby, 23 of these chromosomes come from you and 23 come from your partner. If the baby has, say, three chromosomes in a grouping, instead of having a pair, he or she will suffer a trisomy, which will cause a malformation. In some cases, trisomies will cause miscarriage; in others they will not. For example, one of the most common causes of early miscarriage is trisomy 16 (an extra chromosome on the 16th pair); while trisomy 21, which causes the condition Down's syndrome, does not result in miscarriage.

Trisomies are the cause of up to 50 percent of miscarriages, nature's way of ensuring the survival of the fittest. But if you have had a trisomy miscarriage once, you should be reassured that it's unlikely to happen again, although age is a factor. As women get older, their eggs become less healthy, perhaps damaging the 23 chromosomes the woman contributes to the baby. This may explain why older women are more likely to have Down's syndrome babies and are at greater risk of miscarriage (see box, p.236).

Inherited genetic problems If you have recurrent miscarriages, you or your partner might be carrying an inherited genetic problem and should both undergo chromosome analysis (known as karyotyping) to determine if this is the cause.

Fibroids These are benign tumors that can grow anywhere in the body. When they appear in the uterus,

> MORE THAN 50 percent of miscarriages have no known cause.

MISCARRIAGE AND YOUR AGE

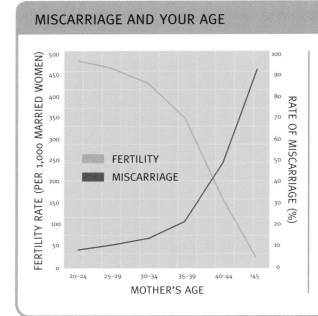

FERTILITY RATE (PER 1,000 MARRIED WOMEN)

RATE OF MISCARRIAGE (%)

FERTILITY
MISCARRIAGE

MOTHER'S AGE

Unfortunately, the rate of miscarriage increases with age because the older you are, the older your eggs are. In addition, older women tend to be more prone to hormonal imbalances that can affect their ability to carry a baby to term. The orange line on this graph shows how fertility declines with age, while the black indicates how rates of miscarriage rise with age. Miscarriage increases more dramatically from the age of 35, which is also when fertility starts to decline more rapidly. But, if you're in your mid-30s or older, don't despair: Although you can't change the quantity of eggs you have, you can definitely improve their quality by following the recommendations on pages 168–173.

they're known as uterine fibroids, and their position is crucial when it comes to your likelihood of miscarrying. If you have fibroids that extend into the uterus cavity, you may have an increased likelihood of an early miscarriage. This is because the fibroids will interfere with the embryo's ability to implant in your uterus lining. The information on pages 114–17 will help you minimize the effects of fibroids on your body and, specifically, your fertility. I also advise that you see a gynecologist to discuss having the fibroids removed.

Bacteria and viruses We come into contact with bacteria and viruses all the time; they surround us, and they frequently cause infection. Unfortunately, there are some infections (such as chlamydia; see p.148) that, caught early in your pregnancy, can increase your likelihood of miscarriage. In fact, I've seen some women in the clinic who have reported having a fever and feeling very unwell and then miscarrying. Always tell your doctor if you experienced any symptoms like this

directly before your miscarriage. In the majority of cases, the link is probably a coincidence, and with any subsequent pregnancy you're likely to be healthy and carry to term. However, if your infection is in the genito-urinary tract, without treatment you may miscarry again. (See also pp.152–3.)

Medication for assisted conception For many women, the fertility drug clomiphene citrate (see p.181) can mean the difference between conceiving and not conceiving because clomiphene triggers ovulation. Unfortunately, clomiphene can also cause your uterus lining to become thinner, making it more difficult for the embryo to attach, which in up to 30 percent of cases will cause a miscarriage.

Problems with hormones The balance of hormones in your body plays a crucial role in your ability to become pregnant. It's also a crucial factor in the safe development of the embryo into a healthy baby. If there are imbalances in your hormones, you may be at greater risk of miscarriage. For example, your pituitary gland releases luteinizing hormone (LH), which controls the development and release of your egg at ovulation. If the levels of LH in your system are too high in the first half of your cycle (which is often the case if you suffer from PCOS; see pp.83–7), unfortunately, you're more likely to miscarry.

Similarly, you have an increased chance of miscarriage if you have lower-than-normal levels of progesterone in your system in the early days of conception. Progesterone is the hormone that the corpus luteum (ruptured follicle) releases after it has expelled its egg—it encourages the lining of your uterus to thicken, in turn helping to maintain your pregnancy in the first delicate weeks. If your doctor tests you for low progesterone and diagnoses a problem, he or she may give you progesterone pessaries or injections in the second half of the cycle to help keep the pregnancy going.

Although you may be predisposed to hormonal irregularities, making them not entirely within your control, you can still take plenty of positive steps to encourage balance. I can't stress enough how important it is to follow my hormone-balancing diet (see box, p.57) before you try for a baby, so as to minimize the risks that hormone irregularities pose for miscarriage.

Autoimmune disorders Your immune system produces antibodies as a natural response to invading bacteria and so on. In an autoimmune problem, such as rheumatoid arthritis and multiple sclerosis, your body produces antibodies that, instead of attacking invaders, start to attack your own cells. Some women can produce blood-clotting antibodies. When these women get pregnant, these antibodies affect the blood supply to the developing baby, terminating the pregnancy.

A doctor will test you for blood-clotting antibodies if you've had three or more miscarriages. He or she will take a blood test to measure levels of the two main antiphospholipid antibodies, anticardiolipin and lupus anticoagulant. If the blood test is positive, your doctor will try to prevent clotting by thinning your blood using medications such as heparin and aspirin.

If you prefer a natural alternative, talk to your doctor about using vitamin E and omega-3 fish oils to thin your blood. In one study, 22 women with antiphospholipid syndrome, who had already had three or more miscarriages, were given fish oil, and they all went on to have a baby without having a further miscarriage.

One controversial area of study suggests that your own immune system attacks the embryo. It's believed that this is because the embryo is half made up of genetic material from your partner, so the body reads it as "foreign." In a normal pregnancy, your immune system has to effectively "quiet down" to accept the embryo, but, for some women, the immune system attacks the cells and the baby miscarries, often before the woman was even aware that she was pregnant. Steroids, lymphocyte immune therapy, or rheumatoid arthritis drugs are all possible medical treatments, but none of them is presently licensed for use in reproductive medicine, and all drugs carry side-effects.

In the nutritional world, an interesting area of research has been into vitamin D. The most important source of vitamin D comes from exposure to sunlight. Vitamin D has an effect on the immune system, and it has been suggested that deficiencies in vitamin D may contribute to autoimmune problems, such as multiple sclerosis and rheumatoid arthritis. It's also thought that vitamin D plays a role in helping the body maintain a pregnancy. So if you've had a miscarriage, ask your doctor to test your vitamin-D levels. If they're low take extra vitamin D in supplement form (as vitamin D3; 400iu, once daily) for two months and then have your levels retested. And when you can, get out into the sunshine—without sunscreen, which will block the manufacture of vitamin D, but only for short periods at a time, to prevent burning.

Problems with anatomy Sometimes a miscarriage is caused by a structural problem. One of the most common problems is an "incompetent cervix," where your cervix does not stay closed, as it should until the beginning of labor. If you suffer a miscarriage before 12 weeks without any bleeding or pain, this may be the cause. In order to rectify it, a medical team can stitch your cervix, usually in early pregnancy, although some doctors offer the procedure before conception. The only concerns that are ever raised about stitching the cervix are that it prevents miscarriage when miscarriage would have happened, for example, as a result of genetic abnormality. I would advise that you have the stitch, but have regular ultrasound scans to monitor the health of your baby throughout your pregnancy.

If you have an abnormally shaped uterus, you may also be prone to miscarriage. A bicornuate uterus, in which the uterus is shaped like a heart rather than a pear, leaves less room for the baby to grow, which can force a miscarriage. If you have a septate uterus, you have a wall of fibrous tissue that effectively runs down the middle of your uterus. If an embryo implants in this fibrous tissue, it can't get the nutrients it needs to survive and develop, so miscarries.

Problems with sperm It takes both a healthy egg and healthy sperm to create a healthy baby. If there are problems with your partner's sperm, you'll be more likely to conceive a fetus that miscarries. He can have a semen analysis test to establish levels of healthy sperm, as well as to assess his sperm count and motility. Make sure your partner follows all the guidelines in my pre-conception plan (see pp.168–73) to boost his sperm health—I've seen big differences in the health of sperm in men who have followed this plan. Remember that it takes at least three months for a man to produce a fresh batch of sperm, so start the plan well before you want to conceive.

CAUSES YOU CAN INFLUENCE

If you have a diagnosis of "unexplained miscarriage," your doctor will probably advise you to wait for a few months and then try again to get pregnant. My advice is for you and your partner to do all you can to reduce your risk of another miscarriage by trying to eliminate as many of the risk factors that are within your control as possible. If you smoke or have a weight problem, for example, you can take steps to put things right.

Your weight As we saw on page 170, to stand the best possible chance of conceiving and staying pregnant, you should not be under- or overweight, but a healthy weight for your height. Studies show that obesity significantly increases the risk of first- and second-trimester miscarriage. In 2008, Stanford University School of Medicine found that more than half the fetuses that miscarried in women who were overweight appeared healthy, showing no congenital abnormalities. The rate of miscarriage for healthy fetuses in women of normal weight is only 37 percent. Researchers believe the difference could be down to the mothers' weight. A BMI of around 22 to 24 (see p.297) is considered ideal for conception and carrying to term.

Your alcohol consumption Alcohol is devastating for sperm, and a man who drinks too much will have higher levels of abnormal sperm. Studies on female animals have shown that alcohol can cause severe damage to the chromosomes the female contributes to the fetus, increasing the rate of miscarriage. The conclusion from a vast number of studies on men and women who drink is that even moderate amounts of alcohol work as a reproductive toxin and increase your risk of miscarrying. I advise you both to abstain entirely from drinking alcohol if you're trying to conceive, and for you to abstain entirely for the whole pregnancy (and throughout breastfeeding).

Your smoking habits If you smoke or your partner smokes, you have a certain increased risk of miscarriage (or chance of having a baby born with abnormalities). Apart from the risks to your own body, and the effects on how well you carry the baby, smoking damages the DNA in sperm, which compounds all the risks, including the risk of losing your baby.

Your caffeine intake Recent research shows that drinking just two cups of coffee a day (which amounts to about 200mg of caffeine) is associated with a 25 percent increased risk of miscarriage compared with 12 percent for women who avoid all caffeine. It's not known whether the higher rate is because caffeine has a stimulant effect causing the uterus to contract, or whether the caffeine may be causing chromosome abnormalities. Caffeine also affects sperm quality.

I advise you to play it safe and avoid caffeine altogether during your pregnancy if you have had a previous miscarriage. If you have not experienced a miscarriage before and are now pregnant, I would suggest that you avoid caffeine where possible, but if you want it on a daily basis, then restrict yourself to only one caffeinated drink a day. Think about all the different ways you might be having caffeine because it's not just found in tea (black and green) and coffee. Certain colas and carbonated drinks contain caffeine, as do chocolate, especially dark chocolate, and some medications. Use decaffeinated coffee to help wean yourself off the caffeine. However, coffee contains two other stimulants, theobromine and theophylline. These remain even after the caffeine has been removed, so eventually you want to be off the decaffeinated coffee as well.

Environmental toxins We know that a number of everyday appliances give off electromagnetic fields (EMFs). These include mobile phones, computers, hair dryers, clock radios, and photocopiers. Research is unclear as to whether exposure to these appliances increases the risk of miscarriage: Some studies show that women who spend a lot of time on computers do have an increased risk. However, other factors, such as stress, working long hours, and sitting still for too long, may also be involved. I recommend that you limit your exposure to these appliances, particularly the length of time you spend on a mobile phone, which emits the most harmful of these types of waves.

As well as avoiding EMFs, try to reduce your exposure to traffic pollution and chemicals. When you buy fruit and vegetables, buy organic where possible, and don't buy them from a stall or a shop where the produce is displayed outside by a busy main road. Also, either reduce your exposure to household and garden chemicals or switch to using more natural products (widely available in supermarkets).

Your stress levels We need to carry out much more research to confirm whether or not stress increases the risk of miscarriage, but, until we know more, I would suggest that you try to limit or manage the amount of stress you're under when you're trying for a baby and during the early stages of your pregnancy.

THE PRE-CONCEPTION PLAN

Everything you do in the pre-conception period affects the quality of your eggs; and the same goes for your partner and his sperm. The better the quality of the egg and sperm, the less likely you are to miscarry. I believe that, if you're prone to miscarriage, following my pre-conception plan on pages 168–73 could make all the difference.

If your doctor has recommended that you take progesterone (because low progesterone levels appear to be causing you to miscarry), follow my pre-conception care supplement guidelines, but do NOT take the herbs at the same time; and if you're taking aspirin and/or heparin for blood-clotting problems, do NOT take extra vitamin E, vitamin C, or essential fatty acids (EFAs), which thin the blood. Rely instead on the amounts of the nutrients already in your prenatal supplement.

YOUR DIET

Eating a healthy, organic diet, according to the guidelines on pages 24–9, is the best way to safeguard your baby's health. In addition, red meat can contribute to abnormal clotting because it increases your body's production of negative substances called prostaglandins. During pregnancy, instead of eating red meat, increase your intake of fish, nuts, and seeds, which contain healthy prostaglandins.

SUPPLEMENTS

The following nutrients are especially important for preventing miscarriage, so make sure your diet is rich in them and that your prenatal supplement (see p.320) contains them in adequate levels—use additional supplements up to the recommended amounts, as necessary.

■ VITAMINS C AND E (500mg vitamin C with bioflavonoids, twice daily, as magnesium ascorbate; and 400iu vitamin E, daily). These vitamins are important antioxidants and will help prevent chromosome damage and abnormal blood clotting. Take them throughout the pre-conception period.

■ FOLIC ACID (400µg, daily) This nutrient isn't just important for preventing spina bifida in your unborn baby, it's also important for preventing miscarriage because, together with vitamin B12 and vitamin B6, it controls an amino acid called homocysteine, which is found in your blood. Women who experience recurrent miscarriage have been found to have high levels of homocysteine.

■ SELENIUM (100µg, daily) This mineral is a powerful antioxidant and so is important for preventing DNA damage to eggs and sperm. Both you and your partner should take it.

■ ZINC (30mg, daily) Deficiencies in zinc can cause chromosome changes in both partners leading to abnormal eggs and sperm. (Make sure your partner takes zinc, too.)

■ CO-ENZYME Q10 (60mg, daily) Research shows that women with low levels of co-enzyme Q10 are at an increased risk of miscarriage. Good levels prevent the uterus from contracting abnormally. Take this supplement for three months before you try to conceive, then stop once you're actually trying.

■ OMEGA-3 FATTY ACIDS (1,000mg fish oil containing at least 700mg EPA and 500mg DHA, daily) Because some miscarriages are linked to increased blood clotting, I recommend that you take omega-3 fatty acids, which can help improve blood flow and prevent abnormal clotting. Take the fish oil in the three-month pre-conception period and continue throughout your pregnancy. (Use flax seed oil if you're vegetarian.)

HERBS

Take the herbs I've recommended below in the three-month pre-conception period only, then stop taking them once you're trying to conceive. Combine equal parts of the tinctures of each of the following herbs. Take 1 tsp. of the combined tincture in a little water two or three times a day; or take 300mg of each herb in capsule form, once or twice a day.

■ AGNUS CASTUS (*Vitex agnus castus*) This herb helps balance your hormones by stimulating the function of the pituitary gland to increase progesterone levels. It's especially helpful to women whose miscarriages are related to low levels of progesterone (see p.237) and also to those who suffer miscarriage and have a short second half to their menstrual cycle (short in this case means fewer than 11 days).

■ BLACK HAW (*Viburnum prunifolium*) Any herb that stops the uterus from contracting inappropriately can be useful for preventing a miscarriage. Black haw is a uterus relaxant, which has exactly this effect.

■ FALSE UNICORN ROOT (*Chamaelirium lutem*) This herb is classed as a tonic for the reproductive system and is therefore helpful for getting and staying pregnant.

Herbalists often combine it with agnus castus (see left) in the treatment of women who have suffered recurrent miscarriages.

SELF-HELP

As well as all the recommendations on the previous pages, I strongly advise you to try to follow a little self-help advice, which will help bring your lifestyle, as well as your body, into balance.

Take your time Don't be tempted to try for a baby right away after you've suffered a miscarriage. Follow my pre-conception care guidelines on pages 178–183 for three to four months after your loss and use natural methods of birth control during this time. Although it can be frustrating to wait, remind yourself that this period is crucial for the health of your future pregnancy and future baby.

Find your natural weight Try to reach your natural weight with a good, healthy diet and extra vitamins and minerals because miscarriage has been linked to obesity and nutritional deficiencies. Finding your natural weight also means you should exercise regularly—but don't overdo it. Remember that exercise places stress on your body, and being underweight can impact your hormones and trick your body into thinking that you're in a period of famine, which in turn encourages the reproductive system to shut down.

Try to relax Stress, like unresolved grief, is bad for you and for your fertility—and for your unborn child. To cope with stress, see the strategies on pages 309–11.

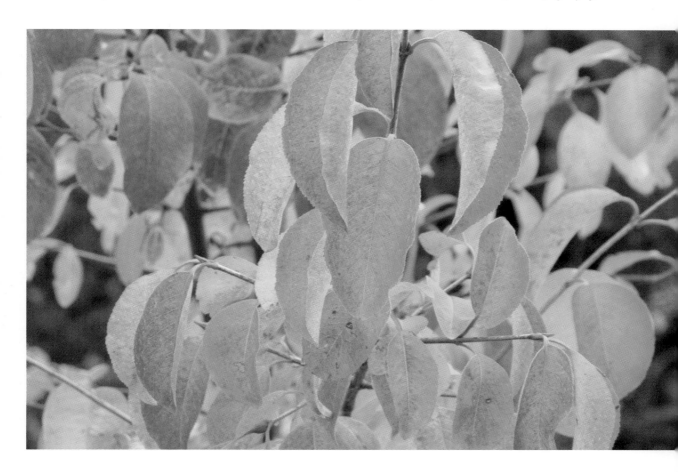

Above: Black haw (*Viburnum prunifolium*)

Stillbirth

About one in 200 pregnancies ends in stillbirth. The baby may die in the uterus (intra-uterine death) or during labor (intra-partum death)—either way, the result for the family is an unfathomable sense of loss.

There are a variety of known causes of a stillborn baby, and several risk factors that we can identify. For example, the risk of stillbirth is higher in women aged over 35 years old; in women with pre-existing medical conditions, such as diabetes; and in those who smoke. Congenital malformations in the unborn baby, placental abruption (or prepartum hemorrhaging, when the placenta separates from the lining of the uterus), pre-eclampsia, birth trauma, infections, and immune disorders are all also risk factors for stillbirth. However, in approximately one-third of cases, even after a postmortem, the cause of stillbirth is indeterminate. Not knowing what happened to your baby can make your loss even harder to deal with.

LOOKING FOR WARNING SIGNS

Stillbirth can occur without symptoms, but if you're past 28 weeks pregnant, your doctor will probably encourage you to track your baby's fetal movements, so that you know he or she is active.

Feeling your baby move inside your uterus is a landmark in your pregnancy and usually occurs between the 15th and 20th weeks. When you start to feel kicks regularly, you know that your pregnancy is going well. If this is your first pregnancy, you may not, at first, even be aware that your baby is moving; many women describe it as a gentle, fluttering sensation. As your pregnancy progresses, the kicks start to feel stronger. Your baby will be very active between weeks 20 and 30. After that, the movements become less frequent but more definite as the baby starts to get cramped.

Many women want to know how many kicks they should feel a day. Studies show that every baby has his or her own individual pattern of waking and sleeping inside the uterus—there's no set pattern or amount of kicks to expect. However, by late in your pregnancy, you'll probably have become attuned to your baby's movements—you'll know at what times of day he or she is most active. Tune in to your baby's pattern and, if there's any kind of change, inform your doctor or midwife immediately. If you have any cause for concern, your doctor may want you to come in for testing to check that your baby is safe.

Other possible warning signs of stillbirth include abdominal or back pain and vaginal bleeding. If you have a lot of bleeding, this may be a sign of abruption, and you should call your doctor immediately. Overall, always err on the side of caution and call your doctor if you're at all concerned.

COPING AFTER THE BIRTH

If you have suffered a stillbirth, you have lost a loved one, and the grieving process is just the same as if you had lost a relative you had known all your life. This is a sensitive time, and you need to treat it with the care and respect both you and your baby deserve. Grief isn't something you can run away from. Symptoms of grief have been observed in women 20 years after they suffered a stillbirth.

Acknowledge your grief The most important thing of all when coming to terms with the loss of a baby is to acknowledge your grief, verbally or nonverbally (see below). Bereavement counselors recommend engaging in some form of grief ceremony. This can be a funeral, or you may also want to write a letter to your baby, or say a prayer. Only when you can acknowledge your grief can you let it go and move on to the next stage of your life.

Try music and art therapy Any way in which you can express your feelings is a positive step on the road to healing. You don't need to be musical to benefit from music therapy, just as you don't need to be artistic to benefit from art therapy. These techniques are merely ways for you to get in touch with your inner self and express your feelings outwardly, but without using words. In making this outward expression, you can gently trigger the healing process.

Keep a journal Studies show that journal-writing can speed up the grieving process, helping you come to terms with loss more swiftly. Because a journal is private, you can be honest with yourself about your thoughts, without fear of judgment or retribution. You also don't have to try to organize your thoughts or make them logical enough for anyone else to understand. Make your journal a free-flow of expression; an open and honest stream of consciousness.

Find support Your partner, friends, and family are your best sources of support during this difficult time. Unfortunately, sometimes those you want to rely on will try to avoid discussing your loss for fear of upsetting you. It's important to be honest with your loved ones and to let them know when you do and when you don't want to talk about your baby. You may prefer to talk to an organized support group. Talking with other women and couples who have experienced the loss of a baby might help you deal with feelings of guilt, isolation, and loneliness. If at any point you feel that you can't cope, seek advice from your doctor, who'll refer you to a bereavement counselor.

Release your guilt Many women feel a huge sense of guilt and self-blame following a stillbirth, believing that their baby's death was caused by something they did, such as drinking the odd glass of wine or working too hard during their pregnancy. I can't stress enough that stillbirth is rarely, if ever, the mother's fault, and it's important to free yourself from feelings of blame and guilt. Visualization and meditation exercises, such as the one in the box below, can help with this important part of the grieving process.

HEALING VISUALIZATION FOR GRIEF

Practice this visualization every day you grieve. Try to lose yourself in it entirely.

1 Sit comfortably and close your eyes. Breathe deeply. Consciously release tension from your body: Start at your feet and work upward, imagining the tension flowing from you.

2 Imagine yourself on a beautiful, warm beach. The sky is cloudless blue, the sand is warm beneath your feet. Ahead of you is a crystal blue ocean. Acknowledge how weighed down you feel—you have a bag on your back. This bag is filled with self-blame and anger.

3 Imagine walking towards the ocean. When you get to the shore, imagine taking the bag from your back, opening it, and pulling out your blaming words and phrases. One by one, imagine throwing these phrases into the ocean—hurl them decisively like heavy stones. When the bag is empty, watch the tide carry your self-blame away for ever.

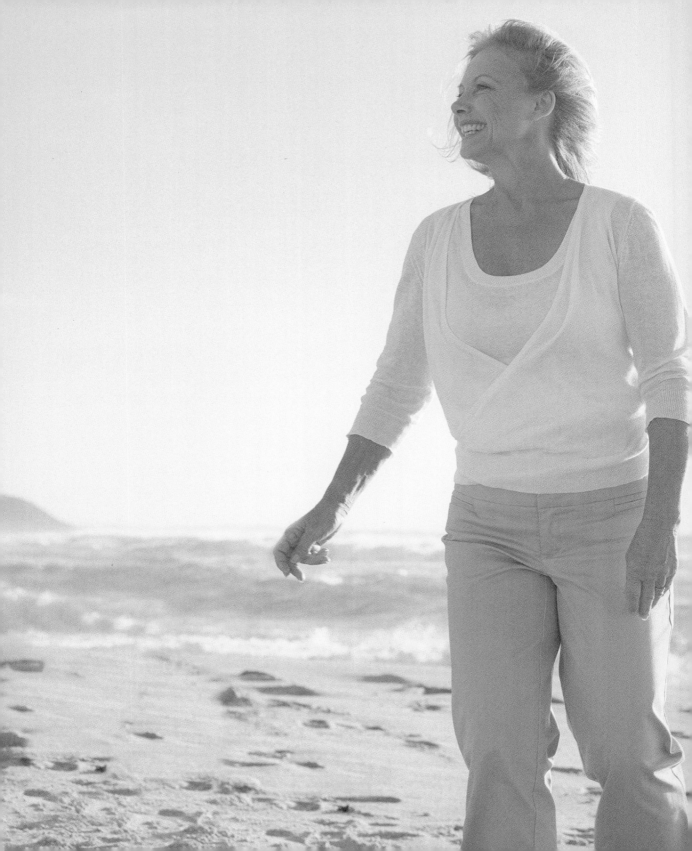

Through menopause 4

In many of the world's cultures, a woman's menopause is a time to be celebrated—a beautiful transition to a new stage of life, a time for joy in which the emphasis shifts from childbearing and chores to becoming "wise women," looked up to by young couples in that society for advice and guidance. In the West, we tend to view menopause as an illness or disorder, something to be "treated" or even ashamed of. However, to me, menopause is no more an illness or disorder than puberty or pregnancy. It's a perfectly natural transition that every woman experiences as she ages, and it's to be celebrated.

Sadly, many of the women I see in my clinic are caught up in the Western view. They see menopause as a time of loss—of periods, of the ability to have children, of youth, and so on. In this chapter, I want to encourage you to have a positive attitude towards menopause. I want to give you the tools that enable you to go through this transition comfortably, easily, and happily, and as naturally as possible.

UNDERSTANDING AND EASING THE CHANGE

Like every natural event in life and nature, menopause doesn't happen overnight. It's a gradual process—a sequence of small changes that together move you towards a new phase in your life.

In the West, the average age for menopause is 51. Your menopause is classed as premature if you're under the age of 40 when it begins.

In the years leading up to menopause, your egg supply diminishes, your ovaries produce less estrogen, and you stop ovulating every month. Your pituitary gland (in your brain) sees this as a signal to release more follicle-stimulating hormone (FSH). It's trying to encourage a follicle to mature in your ovaries and release an egg. This process enables your doctor to run a blood test to see if your menopause has begun—if you have high levels of FSH, the chances are it has.

PROTECTING YOUR BONES

Your bones need estrogen for strength; without it they become brittle and easily breakable. This makes menopause a difficult time for your bones because estrogen production from the ovaries falls. To try to balance this effect, your clever body begins to manufacture estrogen from two other places: your fat cells and your adrenal glands (which produce a back-up form of estrogen called estrone).

SYMPTOMS OF MENOPAUSE

In the West, we have come to expect that our bodies will provide beacons that the change is happening. However, actually, the transition should be subtle: The only thing you should notice is that your periods have stopped. I remember one patient coming to see me who hadn't had a period for six months. She'd noticed no other signs and was confused. "When will the symptoms start?" she asked. She'd had a "model" menopause, and it's this we all need to aim for.

However, some women experience strong menopausal symptoms that dramatically affect their quality of life. Changes in temperature can be one big problem. Night sweats may prevent sleep and cause tiredness, while hot flashes may appear at inopportune moments, such as during meetings, causing embarrassment. But temperature problems aren't all you may experience. Mood swings, irritability, joint pains, lackluster skin and hair, and changes in body shape (the "matronly" shape as one patient called it), as well as a loss of libido or vaginal dryness that makes sex painful, can all impact how easy and happy life feels.

It's easy to blame menopause for these symptoms, but this time in your life may not always be the root of your problems. It's important to bear in mind that an unhealthy diet and lifestyle can cause or aggravate many of the symptoms we automatically attribute to menopause. Any positive changes you make now to how you eat and how you spend your time can significantly ease the way through menopause, as well as keeping you healthy in the long term.

If your doctor suggests that you go on hormone replacement therapy (HRT), I suggest you instead try to sort out your diet and lifestyle to see if you can relieve your symptoms naturally. If you can, you've no need

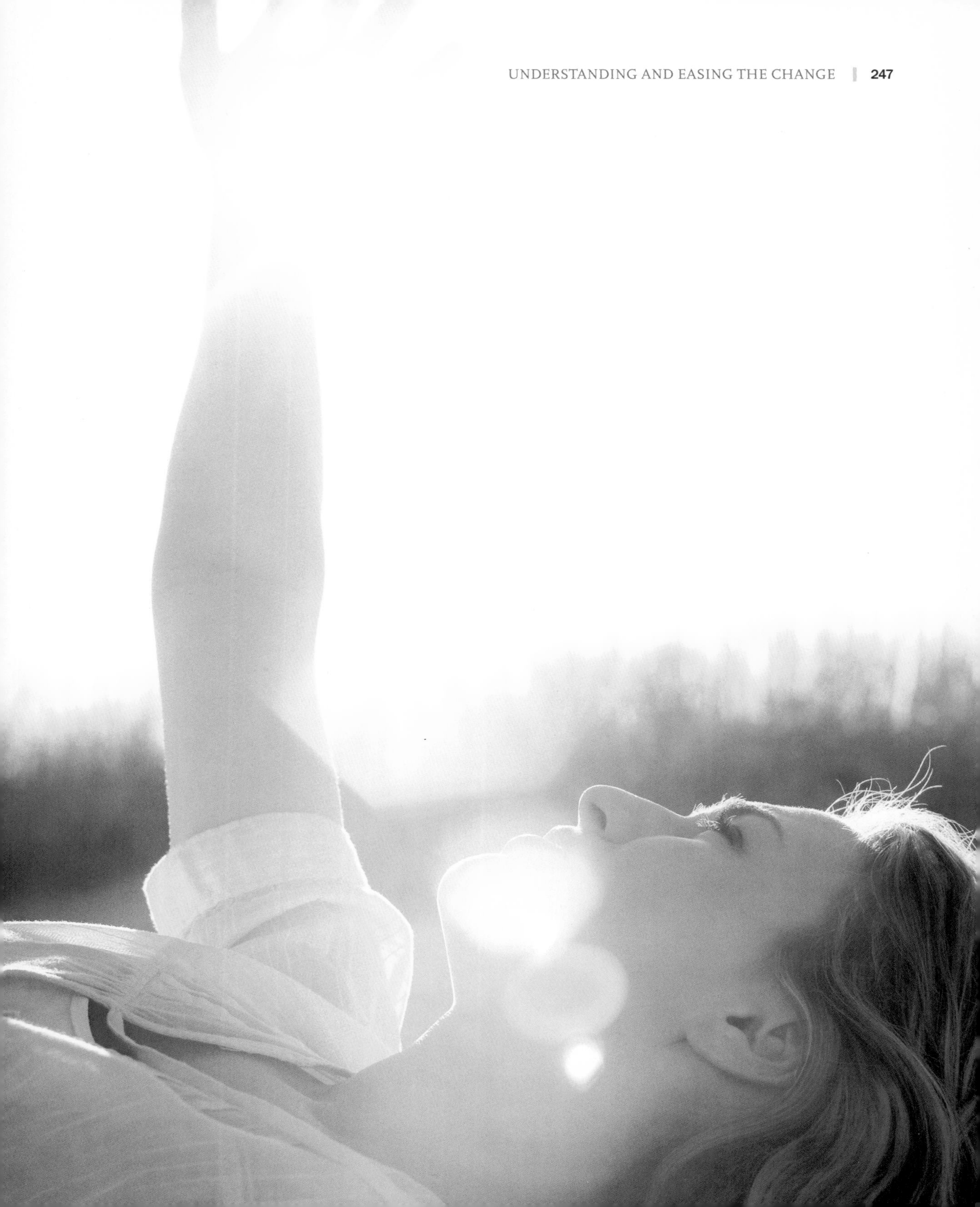

THE PHASES OF MENOPAUSE

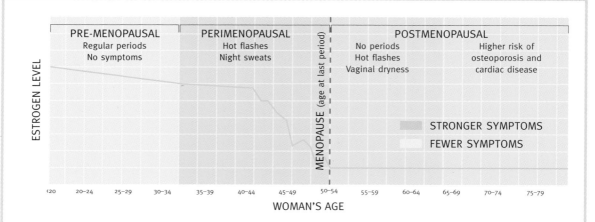

PRE-MENOPAUSAL	PERIMENOPAUSAL	POSTMENOPAUSAL
Regular periods No symptoms	Hot flashes Night sweats	No periods Higher risk of Hot flashes osteoporosis and Vaginal dryness cardiac disease

ESTROGEN LEVEL

MENOPAUSE (age at last period)

STRONGER SYMPTOMS
FEWER SYMPTOMS

<20 20–24 25–29 30–34 35–39 40–44 45–49 50–54 55–59 60–64 65–69 70–74 75–79

WOMAN'S AGE

The transition to menopause actually begins long before you have your last period. To make the process easier to measure, doctors divide it into three phases. The first is the perimenopause, the time leading up to menopause, when your body goes through some of the perceptible changes (see p.247). The second is your actual menopause, the date of your last period. This date is confirmed once you've not had a period for a year. The third is the postmenopause, from the time of your last period onward. This is a time when you need to take care of certain aspects of your health in particular, for example, the health of your heart and your bones.

This graph shows an "average" woman's journey through menopause, and the strength of her symptoms compared with her estrogen levels.

for HRT; if you can't, you can visit your doctor again to discuss the best way forward.

You may continue to have periods even when you've stopped ovulating because your body is still producing weaker levels of hormones that cause a build-up in your uterus lining. But, when your periods begin to appear erratically (one month on, a few months off), or when they become very light over the course of several months, you have a common sign that your estrogen levels are falling and menopause is under way.

TAKING ACTION

Once you think your menopause is starting, visit your doctor for the blood test to measure FSH. Understand, though, that your FSH levels are not a foolproof test. If your periods are erratic, during the months when you don't have one, your FSH levels will be high and menopause is likely. If you get a random period, they would fall again. Make sure your doctor considers your cyclical menstrual symptoms as well as the blood-test results before giving a diagnosis.

Once you've started menopause, think positively about the way forward. You still have choices, not least about what approach to take to ease your transition. For some, HRT provides the answer (see pp.249–51); for others, the natural approach (see pp.252–5) offers an opportunity to bring balance back to the body so that menopause itself is a wholly natural process.

The medical approach: HRT

Hormone replacement therapy (HRT) comes in a dazzling array of creams, pessaries, gels, implants, and tablets. It's the medical approach to dealing with menopause.

So, should you take HRT or not? That's a big question for every woman as she approaches menopause. I hope all the information in this chapter will help you decide what's best for you.

WHAT IS HRT?

When you go through menopause, your body stops producing the hormones estrogen and progesterone. Quite simply, hormone replacement therapy (HRT) puts these hormones back into your system.

When it first appeared in the 1930s, HRT was called "estrogen replacement therapy." The medication was hailed as a wonder drug, an anti-aging miracle that could abolish menopause and keep women "feminine forever." However, in time, research confirmed that giving estrogen on its own increased a woman's risk of developing breast and uterine cancer. Estrogen is a "builder," creating a thick uterus lining that's ready to receive an embryo. In the second half of your cycle, your body produces progesterone so that at the end of the cycle, the uterus lining sheds away and the cycle begins again. Taking estrogen without the balance of progesterone (or progestin, the synthetic form of the hormone), means that the uterus lining can continue to thicken, become abnormal, and lead to uterine cancer. Similarly, a continuous intake of estrogen stimulates breast tissue, again causing cancer.

With this realization, panic set in. Scientists knew that they had to add progestin into the hormone replacement medication in order to make it safer. And that's exactly what they did.

Natural vs synthetic

You may have heard some of the estrogen used in HRT described as "natural." In this case, the word natural means that the estrogens (there are many different kinds) are chemically identical to the hormones produced by your ovaries—but they are still artificial. The "natural" estrogen contained in most HRT is estradiol, considered the most carcinogenic form of synthetic estrogen available. In the USA, special "compounding" pharmacies will make up dosages of HRT according to a doctor's specific instructions, in which case many doctors instruct that the pharmacy use estriol rather than estradiol; while in the UK, doctors may prescribe HRT containing less carcinogenic estriol (the ingredients on the packet will tell you).

THE SIDE-EFFECTS OF HRT

It's easy to imagine that because HRT is simply doing a job your body once did, the medication won't have any side-effects. Unfortunately, HRT can have all sorts of unwanted effects on your system. How many you get and how debilitating they are is unique to each woman. However, overall, around 35 percent of women stop taking HRT because of the unwanted effects.

The most common symptoms that women report to me are breast tenderness and enlargement (up to two cup sizes). I find this particularly alarming—it seems to me that if HRT stimulates breast tissue, it may pose a greater risk of breast cancer (see p.250). If breast changes happen to you, please see your doctor immediately. Other noticeable side-effects are bloating, skin rashes, hair loss, abdominal cramps, and vaginal yeast infections. There are other conditions you may not automatically assume are to do with your HRT but which we know are side-effects of the treatment. These include high blood pressure and thrombophlebitis (vein inflammation caused by a blood clot).

Many women who come to me are concerned that HRT is making them put on weight. Although research concludes that there's no link between HRT and weight gain, my experience with my own patients suggests the opposite. Other women are concerned about the effect HRT has on their psychological health. My patients have described feelings of being "disconnected" or "not there," as if they're watching their lives rather than living them. In some rare cases, these women can become suicidal.

The following are the most serious effects of HRT. I don't include these to alarm you but to give you the opportunity to make an informed decision about whether or not you use this form of treatment. The wonder drug of the 1930s, it seems, may have some serious consequences.

TAKING HRT FOR five years doubles your risk of having a blood clot.

Cancer

Many of my patients come to me with breast cancer at the top of their list of concerns. In 2002, the Women's Health Initiative abandoned their study of 27,000 women after five years instead of eight: It had become clear that the study was putting women on HRT at a 26-percent increased risk of breast cancer. Following the publication of the Health Initiative results in 2002, many women were scared off taking HRT. Researchers then looked at overall breast-cancer rates for 2003 and found that the rate of breast cancer had dropped by 12 percent among 50–69-year-old women—the largest single drop in breast cancer cases in one year. This compounds the link between breast cancer and HRT.

I strongly recommend that you have a breast ultrasound before you consider taking HRT. If the scan indicates that you have any abnormal changes in your breast tissue, avoid HRT. Whereas in natural circumstances these abnormal cells may never have caused a major problem, HRT may act as a catalyst for the cells to multiply, causing cysts or tumors.

You should also bear in mind that the link between HRT and breast cancer is there from the start—it doesn't take several years of cumulative HRT use to become a problem. The good news is that when you stop taking HRT the risk goes down rapidly.

Finally, HRT may make you more prone to uterine and ovarian cancer, especially if these cancers run in your family—heredity is an important factor when assessing your risk.

Blood clots

As well as the cancer dangers, HRT increases your risk of developing a blood clot, which can lead to a stroke, heart attack, or deep vein thrombosis (DVT; where the clot forms in your lower leg). Studies show that taking HRT creates a 41 percent increased risk of strokes and a 29 percent increased risk of heart disease. If you're taking HRT and intend to fly, the increased risk of DVT is a serious one, and I advise you to talk to your doctor before you travel. If the clot moves from your leg, you can suffer a pulmonary embolism, which can be fatal. The simplest solution is to stop taking HRT just before you fly, and resume only once you're back on the ground.

Gall-bladder problems

HRT triples the risk of gall-bladder cancer. In addition, the longer you stay on HRT, the more likely you are to develop gallstones (and you're more susceptible if you've had gallstones in the past).

HRT: THE PROS?

HRT undoubtedly controls the hot flashes and night sweats, and if these symptoms affect your quality of life so badly that you can't function, then HRT can be the solution. In the past, though, many doctors have been extremely enthusiastic about HRT, suggesting that it can boost energy and libido and significantly reduce the health risks and symptoms associated with menopause. Now, however, the Committee on Safety of Medicines in the UK states that women should use HRT only for a maximum of five years and only for the relief of menopausal symptoms such as hot flashes and night sweats. HRT is known to help reduce the risk of bone fracture (a concern for women with osteoporosis), but safety guidelines in the UK and USA state that postmenopausal women over the age of 50 should not take HRT unless they can't take the usual osteoporotic drugs.

The other supposed benefits of HRT treatment also need careful examination. For example, doctors once believed that HRT could help reduce the incidence of Alzheimer's in elderly women. This is because it contains estrogen, which we know can stop the build-up of tangled, damaged proteins in the brain that contributes to the disease. Research now shows that the opposite appears to be true: HRT can contribute to Alzheimer's. Mood swings, depression, and urinary incontinence are all also conditions that early scientific thought or common belief considered treatable with HRT, but which we now know are either unaffected or worsened by the medication.

MAKING A DECISION

We need more randomized, controlled clinical studies—independent of drug companies—on large numbers of women to give definitive answers about the effects of HRT on fractures, heart disease, breast cancer, ovarian cancer, Alzheimer's, and so on. But in my opinion, it's clear that the long-term effects of taking it are not known and that the risks heavily outweigh the benefits. In my experience, the natural approach is immensely successful for treating the symptoms of menopause without risk to your health.

Although I favor the natural approach to coping with menopause, if you're considering HRT you must, in

WHEN YOU STOP TAKING HRT

After you've taken HRT for five years, and sometimes before, your doctor will probably tell you to stop taking the medication; or you may decide to stop taking it anyway. Don't stop the drugs suddenly because doing so can result in withdrawal symptoms that are worse than the symptoms that prompted you to take the HRT in the first place. I recommend that you ask your doctor for a lower dose of the same drug, or a different way to administer it (such as changing from tablets to patches). Gradually reduce your dosage over three months and then switch to the natural approach (see pp.252–5).

consultation with your doctor, weigh the pros and cons yourself to find what best suits you.

If you do decide to take HRT, don't forget that you have options. If you find it difficult to tolerate the side-effects of the first medications you're given, ask your doctor about alternative doses. And, even though you're taking HRT, I still advise you to follow my guidelines for a healthy diet and lifestyle on pages 24–9.

The advice on pages 252–5 on the natural approach to menopause is also relevant because it protects you naturally against osteoporosis, heart disease, and cancer. You should ignore the section on herbs, though, because the HRT is doing their work for you; or if the HRT is not working, they will have an additional hormonal effect that you may not want. (If your HRT isn't working, see your doctor because there are now more than 40 different HRT preparations on the market, so there are others to try.)

If you decide against HRT, or you decide to come off it after trying it, follow my guidelines for natural menopause over the following pages, instead.

Natural menopause

If HRT isn't for you, what's the alternative? Over the following pages, I've set out my guidelines for natural menopause, designed to help you through this transition without the need for drugs.

My natural approach to easing the way through menopause includes dietary and lifestyle recommendations. These will help restore your good health and then nurture it. I've also included herbal and supplement suggestions to help you manage any menopause symptoms you might experience.

YOUR DIET

The first step on your road to natural menopause is to eat a healthy, hormone-balancing diet according to my guidelines in the box on page 57. You should pay particular attention to the following and stock up on the top ten best foods for your menopause (see box, p.254).

Reduce saturated fat Keep down your intake of red meat (such as beef) and cheese because these foods are high in saturated fats—which are not good for your heart. Saturated fats also make your body more acidic. Acidity encourages calcium loss, which in turn can increase your risk of bone disintegration and, ultimately, osteoporosis (see box, p.272).

Boost essential fats Found in nuts, seeds, oily fish, and even eggs, essential fats help lubricate your body from the inside out, so are beneficial for dry skin, vaginal dryness, painful joints, high cholesterol, and a sluggish metabolism.

Stabilize your blood sugar During menopause it's more crucial than ever that you keep your blood sugar stable. As your ovaries produce lower levels of estrogen, your adrenal glands will take over, pumping out an alternative form (there are many types) of estrogen for your body. If you're on a blood-sugar roller coaster, your adrenal glands will have to work harder, tiring them out. See the box on page 29 for tips on how to balance your blood sugar.

Boost natural fiber Have a good intake of natural fiber from fruit, vegetables, and whole grains. In addition to the well-known beneficial effect on your bowels, fiber helps keep your blood-sugar levels stable (see above). Fiber is also important for efficient detoxification because it helps your body eliminate "old" estrogen and other waste products through your bowel.

Eat more phytoestrogens I recommend that you eat phytoestrogens on a regular basis. Changing just ten percent of your diet to include more of these phytoestrogenic foods makes a big difference. In Asian cultures, such as in Japan, women tend to eat more phytoestrogens. Many doctors and nutritionists (myself included) believe that this factor directly contributes to the lower rates of menopausal symptoms (and breast cancer) in Asian countries when compared with those in the West. Certain phytoestrogens, including legumes such as soy, chickpeas, lentils, and so on, contain isoflavones. These seem to work like the menopause drug SERMS (see p.275) in that they stimulate certain estrogen receptors and block others. Soy, in particular, contains two main isoflavones (called genistein and daidzein), which are thought to

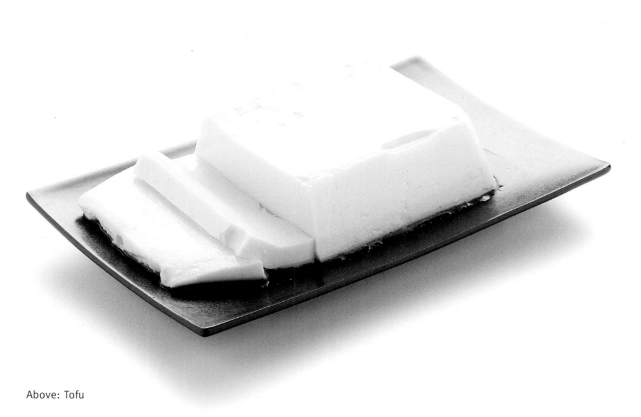

Above: Tofu

have the most significant effect on menopausal symptoms. The strongest and most effective forms of soy are miso and tofu.

The overall result is that phytoestrogens can help balance hormones and reduce symptoms such as hot flashes and vaginal dryness.

SUPPLEMENTS

I recommend that you take a good-quality multi-vitamin and mineral whatever your age, but doing so is especially important during menopause. You need to make sure you have adequate vital nutrients for your bone health, good levels of antioxidants to help slow down the aging process, and other important vitamins and minerals, such as the B-vitamins and chromium,

to help keep your blood-sugar levels balanced. The easiest way to do this is by taking a good, all-around multi-vitamin and mineral supplement designed specifically for menopause (see p.320). Remember, though, that a multi should never replace a well-balanced diet and you must eat healthily, too.

In addition to your multi-vitamin and mineral, you may also want to consider taking the following supplements to help ease the symptoms of menopause. Before taking individual supplements, first check the amount contained in your multi and top up to the total recommended daily amount. If you have specific symptoms (see pp.258–281), add in the supplements (or herbs) listed to treat these symptoms, and also keep taking a multi-vitamin and mineral.

THE TOP TEN FOODS FOR NATURAL MENOPAUSE

1 SOY Singled out as number 1, soy has been proven time and again to have properties that help reduce hot flashes and night sweats. Eat a variety of organic soy foods, including tofu, soy milk, miso, and soy sauce.

2 LEGUMES All the legumes, including soy, are classed as phytoestrogens, so all deserve a place in the natural menopause diet. Go for variety and include chickpeas (good as hummus), lentils, kidney beans, aduki beans, and so on. You can buy organic canned beans, which provide complete convenience.

3 OILY FISH Salmon, tuna, herring, sardines, and mackerel contain omega-3 essential fatty acids that can counteract several symptoms of menopause (see p.252).

4 BRIGHTLY COLOURED FRUIT AND VEGETABLES These foods are rich in antioxidants, which not only slow down the aging process but also help fight cancer and heart disease (risks of developing these diseases increase after menopause).

5 NUTS Like oily fish, nuts contain essential fats (see above), but they also contain antioxidants, including vitamin E (in all nuts) and selenium (particularly in Brazil nuts).

6 SEEDS Nutritional powerhouses, seeds of all kinds contain essential fats, while both pumpkin and sunflower seeds contain good amounts of zinc, which helps keep your hormones in balance. Flax seeds are particularly good because they are also classed as a phytoestrogen.

7 WATER Although water isn't a "food" exactly, it's vital that you keep hydrated at all times of your life, but especially during menopause. Water helps regulate your body temperature, helping to relieve hot flashes and night sweats. It's also important in your body's mission to deliver crucial menopause nutrients to their destinations, and for eliminating waste.

8 CRUCIFEROUS VEGETABLES Broccoli, cabbage, cauliflower, and Brussels sprouts all contain good amounts of antioxidants and also specific substances that can protect against breast cancer. Cabbage is also high in vitamin K, which is known to help prevent osteoporosis.

9 WHOLE GRAINS Rich in fiber, whole grains are not only important for efficient bowel function, but also for helping to prevent heart disease (fiber controls cholesterol) and breast cancer (it also controls estrogen).

10 HERBAL TEAS Sage tea helps control hot flashes and night sweats; dandelion can help with water retention, and nettle tea improves the absorption of minerals, such as calcium and magnesium (these are important for bone health and for preventing osteoporosis).

- B-COMPLEX (containing 25mg of each B-vitamin, daily) If you suffer from severe mood swings, irritability, tension, anxiety, depression, and crying spells, and if your energy levels are low, you could be lacking in B-vitamins.

- VITAMIN C with bioflavonoids (500mg, twice daily, as magnesium ascorbate) Vitamin C can significantly reduce hot flashes, and is needed for your body to produce collagen, a major part of the bone matrix, helping to keep your bones strong. Vitamin C also helps maintain the elasticity of tissue in your skin, vagina, and urinary tract. Bioflavonoids help strengthen the capillaries, improving blood flow and so reducing hot flashes.

- VITAMIN E (400iu, daily) I have found that vitamin-E supplements can help reduce hot flashes and improve vaginal dryness.

- MAGNESIUM (300mg, daily) Take magnesium, which has a calming effect on the body, if you feel anxious or tense, or suffer from insomnia. It can also help if you're getting muscle cramps or twitches.

- OMEGA-3 FATTY ACIDS (1,000mg fish oil, containing at least 700mg EPA and 500mg DHA, daily) Essential fats can help combat dryness in your skin, hair, nails, and vagina. They're also anti-inflammatory, so can relieve aching joints, and they are important for good brain function. (Use flax seed oil if you're vegetarian.)

HERBS

The herb of choice for menopause is black cohosh, a well-known hormone balancer. However, for the most beneficial effects, I recommend you use a combination of herbs. Combining herbs tends to be more effective than taking just a single herb. In my clinic, I recommend Black Cohosh Plus, which combines black cohosh, agnus castus, sage, and milk thistle (see p.320), among other ingredients. However, you shouldn't take any of the herbs listed here if you're already taking HRT because their influence on your hormones could upset your medication levels. If you do take the herbs, aim for 200–300mg dried or powdered herb daily (in a capsule) or combine the tinctures of the relevant herbs in equal parts and take 1 tsp. of the combined tincture in a little water, up to three times daily. Buy organic herbs where possible.

- AGNUS CASTUS (*Vitex agnus castus*) This herb, also known as chasteberry, helps hormone balance. It's particularly useful for the symptoms that occur during perimenopause (see box, p.248), when your periods can seem very erratic and you suffer more mood swings.

- BLACK COHOSH (*Cimicifuga racemosa*) I find this herb to be the best choice for relieving menopausal symptoms such as hot flashes and night sweats. Extensive clinical research shows that it's effective taken around menopause.

- DONG QUAI (*Angelica sinensis*) In Traditional Chinese Medicine, this herb is used as a woman's tonic. It can be helpful for its hormone-balancing effects. It will help ease hot flashes, night sweats, and vaginal dryness.

- GINKGO BILOBA (*Ginkgo biloba*) Take this herb if you feel that your memory and concentration are changing at menopause. Research has shown that ginkgo biloba has a rejuvenating effect on the brain, improving your ability to learn, remember, and concentrate. In addition, it may offer protection against heart disease because it can help prevent clots.

- MILK THISTLE (*Silymarin marianum*) The herb milk thistle is always useful when dealing with any hormone changes in the body. It's important for good liver function, which helps remove old hormones from your system.

- SAGE (*Salvia officinalis*) As well as helping to reduce night sweats (see p.258), according to research in the journal *Pharmacology, Biochemistry, and Behavior*, sage helps improve memory.

OTHER NATURAL TREATMENTS

As well as looking at your diet and adding in supplements and herbs, I've found that other natural therapies can be extremely helpful during menopause. For clarity, I've made individual suggestions for each of the symptoms in the following section. This way, you can tailor your complementary treatments specifically to your own menopause and what works best for you.

MENOPAUSE

What we often think of as menopause is really the "perimenopause," the years leading up to the actual menopause (your last period), which signals the end of your reproductive years.

On a positive note, it also signals a new start. As the anthropologist Margaret Mead said, "There is no power greater in the world than the zest of a postmenopausal woman!" For clarity, I shall use the term "menopause" throughout this section to mean the whole process of change leading up to the last period because this is how we usually talk about it.

Menopause can take anywhere between two and eight years—how long it lasts varies from woman to woman; and when it starts varies, too (see box, p.248).

During the menopausal years, levels of your reproductive hormones (estrogen and progesterone) rise and fall. Apart from intermittent periods (see box, right), the most common symptoms of these hormonal fluctuations are hot flashes, night sweats, and mood swings. These, as well as the menopausal symptoms of reduced libido and hair loss, are featured in this section.

PREGNANCY AND MENOPAUSE

Regular periods typically occur at around the same date each month, but this changes during menopause, and you may find your periods difficult to predict. Your bleeds may also be heavier than you're used to.

Fluctuating levels of progesterone and estrogen during this stage mean that the follicles in your ovaries fail to develop and release an egg. Many of the periods you have during menopause will be "anovulatory," without ovulation. But, during some cycles you may still ovulate and you could still become pregnant. If you aren't trying for a baby, use contraception until you've had no periods for a year if you're over 50, and no periods for two years if you're under 50.

STRESS AND YOUR SYMPTOMS

It's worth reiterating here that stress is a major cause of hormone imbalance. All the symptoms you may experience during these transitional years are caused by hormonal imbalance, so it's important to keep your stress levels down. Don't let yourself get bogged down in any anxiety about being menopausal or not being in control of what's happening to your body. I hope the advice I offer in this section will help show you that you're still master of your own health, even through this change. There are plenty of steps you can take to influence how menopause affects you.

INTERMITTENT PERIODS

These are a normal symptom of menopause and nothing to be concerned about. However, you should see your doctor immediately if:

- Your bleeding is extremely heavy—you're changing tampons or pads every hour
- Your bleeding lasts longer than eight days
- Bleeding occurs between periods
- Periods often occur fewer than 21 days apart

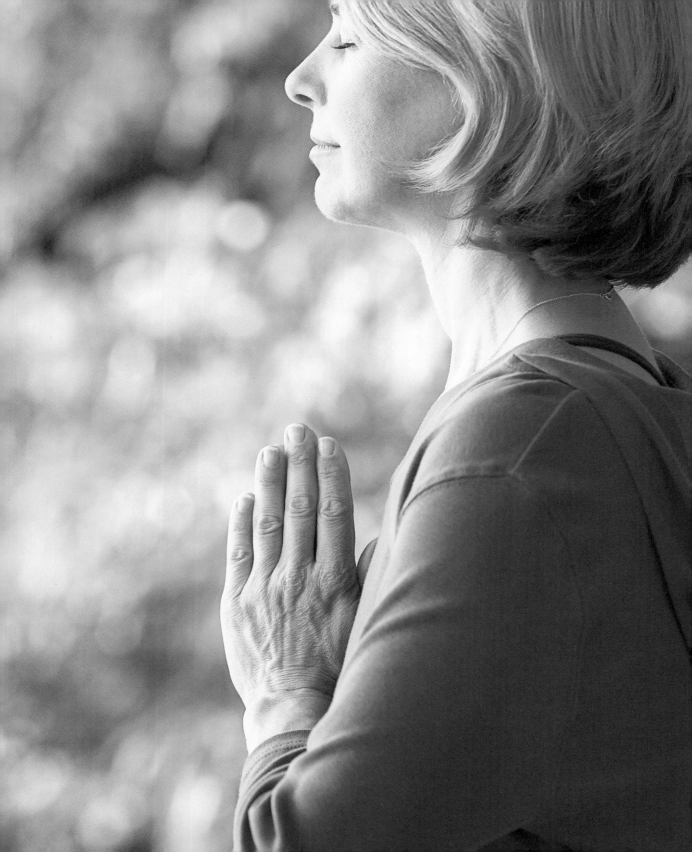

Hot flashes and night sweats

Women complain about hot flashes and night sweats more than any other symptom of menopause. Some women say their hot flashes are so severe that they prevent from them living a normal life.

Hot flashes can appear without warning and make you feel unbearably hot on your face and all over your body. Each flash can last any time between 30 seconds and 30 minutes, and you may experience anywhere between a few a day to up to four an hour. During the night, hot flashes are referred to as night sweats, and they cause immense sleep disruption, sometimes even leading to severe insomnia. Some women have been known to suffer reduced mental agility and even depression as a result of sleep deprivation caused by night sweats.

Day or night, the flash itself will feel hot, usually throughout your body, but afterwards many women complain that they feel cold and shivery. Among the other most debilitating symptoms of a hot flash is the appearance of redness or blotchiness on your face and neck, as well as obvious sweating. You may also feel a tightness or heaviness in your head, and your heart may start to beat faster as the flash begins.

CAUSES

Some experts suggest that falling levels of estrogen (estrogen withdrawal) may cause hot flashes. Others suggest that high levels of follicle-stimulating hormone (FSH; see p.16) are to blame. The flashes themselves occur when your blood vessels dilate (become larger) to let more blood to flow through your circulatory system, aiming to cool you down. This is exactly the same automatic response that lets you to sweat and cool down on a hot day. Some women have a particular trigger for their hot flashes, including spicy food, caffeine, alcohol, hot drinks, and stress. In addition, there appear to be certain risk factors for hot flashes, such as smoking, being overweight, and having a sedentary lifestyle.

YOUR DIET

Research shows that women who eat a diet rich in phytoestrogens report fewer hot flashes and other menopausal symptoms than women who don't. It appears that plant estrogens work to balance hormones, increasing estrogen levels when they're low, but not increasing them unnecessarily when they're high. Essential fatty acids will also help, so eat plenty of oily fish and lots of seeds, such as flax seeds. One small study showed that women taking 4 tbsp. powdered flax seeds daily reduced hot flashes by half.

You should also increase your intake of citrus fruits, which contain substances called bioflavonoids. These strengthen your blood capillaries to regulate blood-flow through your body. In addition, citrus fruits contain plenty of vitamin C, which can help control hot flashes. (As well as eating more citrus fruits, you can supplement. Take vitamin C with bioflavonoids; 500mg, twice daily, as magnesium ascorbate.)

Finally, eat little and often because fluctuations in blood sugar can cause levels of adrenaline to rise, which can trigger flashes. See pages 252–4 for other tips on the foods you should eat during menopause.

FOOD SOURCES OF PHYTOESTROGENS

• Celery
• Garlic
• Grains (such as rice, oats, wheat, barley, rye)
• Fruit (such as apples, plums, cherries)
• Herbs/spices (such as sage, fennel, cinnamon)
• Legumes (such as soy, lentils, chickpeas)
• Seeds (such as sesame, pumpkin, poppy)
• Sprouts (such as alfalfa, mung bean)
• Vegetables (such as broccoli, carrots, potatoes)

SUPPLEMENTS

As well as taking extra vitamin C (see nutritional information, left), take the following supplement.

■ VITAMIN E (400iu, daily) Research shows that vitamin E can be helpful for both reducing hot flashes and also helping overcome vaginal dryness.

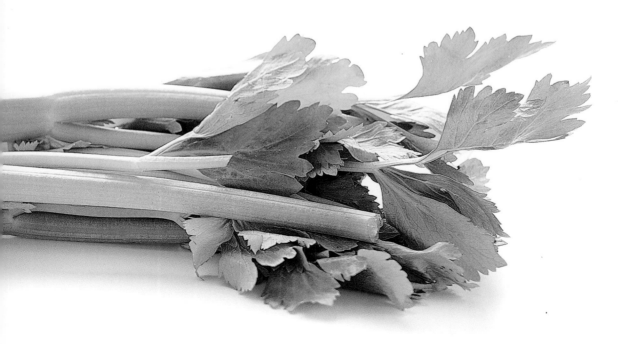

HERBS

Take a combined tincture of the following herbs, mixing the herbs in equal measures. Take 1 tsp. of the combined tincture in a little water, two or three times daily. Alternatively, take 200–300mg of each individual herb in capsule form, daily.

■ AGNUS CASTUS (*Vitex agnus castus*) This herb, also known as chasteberry, is an adaptogenic herb because it has a balancing effect on the body, helping to reduce where there is excess and increase where there is deficiency. It does exactly this for your hormones. You should be able to see results (reduced symptoms) within three months if you take the herb regularly.

■ BLACK COHOSH (*Cimicifuga racemosa*) This herb is really the herb of choice for hot flashes and night sweats. It's thought to work like a SERM (selective estrogen receptor modulator), which stimulates the estrogen receptors in certain parts of the body and does not stimulate those in the breasts or uterus. As a result menopausal symptoms are reduced without risk to your breast or uterine tissue,

unlike the risk with HRT; see p.249–50).

■ DONG QUAI (*Angelica sinensis*) This is a popular herb in Traditional Chinese Medicine and acts as a tonic to the female reproductive organs, helping balance hormones and, as a result, reducing hot flashes and night sweats.

■ SAGE (*Salvia officinalis*) This well-known cooking herb has been shown to help with both hot flashes and night sweats. In one study, it completely eliminated these symptoms in 20 out of the 30 women tested.

■ VALERIAN (*Valeriana officinalis*) This herb has a sedative effect on the body, so if disturbed sleep is making you tired the next day, use black cohosh to get rid of the sweats and add in some valerian to help improve your sleep quality, relieving tiredness.

OTHER NATURAL TREATMENTS

The following are the most useful complementary approaches for treating hot flashes and night sweats. You may also like to try acupuncture, which has been successful in many of the cases I've seen.

Homeopathy A number of homeopathic remedies can help with hot flashes. Take each of the relevant remedies in a 30c potency twice a day. Choose the appropriate remedies from the list below.
• Lachesis is useful if your hot flash starts lower in your body and then moves towards your head. This remedy is good for those women who prefer to wear layers, in order to help them to stay cool in every environment and don't want anything around their necks
• Pulsatilla is useful when there's no consistency to the flushes—they feel different each time they occur
• Sepia if the hot flashes make you feel weak; you may also feel negative and have reduced sex drive

Aromatherapy The best oils to treat hot flashes are Roman chamomile, sage, basil, thyme, and clary sage. Mix any combination of these oils in equal parts, then dilute 15 drops of the blend in 6 tsp. sweet almond carrier oil. Use the combination in a gentle, relaxing massage. Experiment with the blend until you find the right combination for you—that is, the one that gives you the most relief. For an emergency aid while you're out, add a few drops of your blend to a tissue, then put the tissue in a plastic bag and keep it in your handbag. Take out the tissue and inhale the essential oils as soon as you feel a hot flash coming on.

SELF-HELP

Wear layers Layer your clothing so you can pull clothes on and off according to how hot you feel.

Steer clear of triggers For example, if you know a glass of red wine will trigger a flash, drink something else. Apply this approach to all of your triggers.

Breathe through it Many women find that their hot flashes are related to stress. When you feel stress coming on take a deep breath. One study found that when women practiced deep, abdominal breathing (taking six to eight controlled breaths a minute), twice a day, the incidence of hot flashes halved.

Mood swings

In the process of gradual, menopausal change, your hormone levels will rise and fall until they find a new equilibrium. During this time, your moods are likely to fluctuate, too—sometimes dramatically.

Mood swings, when emotions suddenly swing from a stable contentment to irritability, anxiety, and sometimes depression, are among the most common symptoms of menopause. Scientists believe that one reason for this might be that estrogen affects how serotonin (the feel-good hormone) operates in your body. When estrogen levels begin to fall, so levels of serotonin fall, leading to dips in mood. When estrogen levels rise again, so serotonin rises. In addition, blood-sugar imbalances and fatigue (perhaps as a result of night sweats; see p.258) can also trigger dramatic shifts in emotions and temperament. Once your body's estrogen levels have plateaued and you've reached menopause itself, mood usually levels out again.

CONVENTIONAL TREATMENTS

For any symptom related to menopause, your doctor will typically recommend HRT. Although this can ease mood swings for some women, it can also cause them, along with a number of other side-effects and health risks. If your symptoms are extreme, your doctor may offer you antidepressant drugs.

YOUR DIET

Follow my hormone-balancing diet (see box, p.57). Ensure your body gets the nutrients it needs to ease symptoms of menopause by eating lots of fresh, unrefined foods. Follow all the dietary recommendations in natural menopause on pages 252–4 to make sure your hormones stay in balance, and—crucially—you keep your blood-sugar levels stable.

SUPPLEMENTS

For mood swings, the following supplements are the most important of all the recommendations in my natural approach to menopause.

- B-COMPLEX (containing 25mg each B-vitamin, daily) The B-vitamins work together to support the nervous system. They can help ease depression.

- MAGNESIUM (300mg, daily) Known as "nature's tranquillizer," magnesium has a calming effect on the muscles and nervous system, helping to relax you.

- OMEGA-3 FATTY ACIDS (1,000mg fish oil, containing at least 700mg EPA and 500mg DHA, daily) EFAs are important for healthy brain function. (Use flax seed oil if you're vegetarian.)

HERBS

- AGNUS CASTUS (*Vitex agnus castus*) This herb helps ease tension and mood swings. It's one of the best balancing herbs. Take 1 tsp. tincture in a little water, or 200–300mg in capsule form, twice daily.

- ST JOHN'S WORT (*Hypericum perforatum*) This herb is a well-known antidepressant for moderate depression. Take 1 tsp. tincture in a little water, three times daily; or 300mg in capsule form, two or three times daily.

- SIBERIAN GINSENG (*Eleutherococcus senticosus*) This herb helps combat the effects of stress on your mood. Take 1 tsp. tincture in a little water or 250–300mg in capsule form, twice daily.

- VALERIAN (*Valeriana officinalis*) Valerian calms the nervous system. Take 1 tsp. tincture in a little water, or 300mg in capsule form, twice daily.

OTHER NATURAL TREATMENTS

Massage, meditation, yoga, reflexology, and acupuncture are all natural therapies that have had good amounts of success at combating mood swings. See registered practitioners in each field to talk about the possibilities. In the meantime, I advise the following therapies to try at home.

Homeopathy I recommend that you see a registered homeopath to tailor your treatment to your constitution, but in the meantime try Bryonia, Lachesis, and Sepia (all at 30c, twice daily), which are often advised for mood swings.

Aromatherapy The best essential oils for levelling out mood swings are clary sage and geranium. Add about seven drops of each to your bath. If you're feeling down, lavender, bergamot, Roman or German chamomile, and rose can all help boost mood. Add a few drops of each to your bath water or use them in massage. Make sure you dilute the oils in a carrier, such as sweet almond, before applying them (see box, p.48).

HOW TO AVOID COMFORT EATING

It's very easy during this transitional period in your life to reach for comforters to help you feel secure. For some people, comforters may be supportive cuddles from a loved one; for others a comforter may be doing the gardening. For many women I see, though, food seems an instant fix. There's nothing wrong with that—as long as you don't have food cravings for under-nutritious foods.

Problems with food occur when your body and brain don't communicate effectively and the brain doesn't produce enough "calming" chemicals to satisfy food cravings. Put simply, your brain dictates what foods you crave. However, although brain chemicals play a part,

psychological factors are also important. Many women tell me that they eat when they feel lonely, angry, sad, or even happy. Food is seen as both a comfort and a reward. If you're a comfort eater, it's important to:

• Know your triggers: Do you eat when you're sad, lonely, or bored? Look at what else you could substitute instead of food. Find a new hobby, phone a friend, read a book, or busy yourself with some DIY.
• Don't link food and certain activities: Do you automatically open the fridge when you get home or reach for a packet of crisps when you watch TV? Awareness of what you're doing and when is the key. Think,

stop, and ask yourself if you really need to eat right now.
• Go for unrefined complex carbohydrates: Found in rice, potatoes, millet, wheat, rye, oats, and barley, these can help keep your blood-sugar levels balanced, so you don't get food cravings.
• Eat little and often: If you leave a large time lapse between meals, your blood-sugar levels drop and your brain triggers food cravings.
• Be realistic: as long as the main foundation of your nutrition is good, it's fine to treat yourself now and again to chocolate or foods you might consider "naughty." If you deny yourself, you're more likely to end up comfort eating.

Low libido

There are many consequences of a drop in hormone levels at menopause that lots of the women I see simply don't think of— loss of libido, or lack of interest in sex, is one of them.

Fluctuating hormone levels at menopause can contribute to a loss of libido (see below), although this is by no means the only contributing factor. Apart from your hormones, fatigue, stress, illness, relationship problems, a poor diet, too much alcohol, poor body image, and several medical conditions are other factors that can lead to a loss of libido. Happily, you can work on some of these contributory factors to great effect. In addition, a determined effort to make your sex life a priority can be a major step in the right direction.

SEX HORMONES AND SEX

A hormonal roller coaster can also cause vaginal mucus to dry up, reducing lubrication and thinning the vaginal tissue, making intercourse painful. In addition, changes in hormone levels may also decrease the blood flow to your breasts, making them less sensitive to touch and subduing your ability to become aroused.

It's often suggested that lack of interest in sex during menopause is the result of gradually lowering levels of the hormone estrogen. However, in my opinion, this isn't always the case. Your body also produces male hormones and, at menopause, levels of testosterone, which your ovaries produce, can decline, causing lost sex drive.

If you're stressed, your adrenal glands will work overtime producing stress hormones, and it does this at the expense of androgens. This compromises your libido still further, and it's another good reason to watch your stress levels and take time to relax as you approach menopause. Yet, male hormones can also

have the opposite effect. In some women, falling estrogen leads to a preponderance of testosterone in the system, increasing sex drive, rather than dulling it. You may also find your sex drive improves because you feel liberated by your inability to get pregnant—sex with your partner can be carefree and contraception-free.

CONVENTIONAL TREATMENTS

Hormone replacement therapy (HRT) If your only symptom of approaching menopause is a loss of sex drive, your doctor is unlikely to prescribe you with HRT. However, if you're also suffering from hot flashes, mood swings, and irregular periods, HRT will probably be the medical answer. Although HRT can boost sex drive in some women, in others it has the opposite effect. Studies show that when taken orally, the artificial hormones in HRT are metabolized by your liver, which releases a protein that binds to testosterone, leaving less testosterone free to circulate in your system, rather than making any impact on your sex drive.

Estrogen pessaries If you're suffering from lack of lubrication or vaginal dryness (see p.278–81), your doctor may prescribe estrogen pessaries or creams to make intercourse easier and more enjoyable. These go directly into the vagina to soothe vaginal tissues.

YOUR DIET

In my view, and for many of the women I see, feeling healthy and feeling sexy go hand in hand. So, as a first step, make sure you eat a healthy diet as set out on pages 24–9. Although it's important to make sure you have a healthy intake of good fats, try to reduce your intake of saturated fats (from animal products). Not only are these unhealthy, they'll also make you feel sluggish and encourage you to put on weight. Good-quality unsaturated fats come from oily fish, eggs, nuts, and seeds. These foods are important for overcoming low libido because sex hormones (such as testosterone) are manufactured from the cholesterol contained within them. Also good fats help keep soft tissues, such as those in the vagina, lubricated and supple.

Snack on bananas, berries, and almonds. Bananas are a good source of vitamin B6, which is important for the manufacture of sex hormones. Berries are rich in the mineral zinc, which helps your body produce sex hormones, and they're also high in antioxidants, which help optimize blood flow to the sex organs. Snacking on a handful of almonds will help keep up your intake of essential, healthy fats, which we already know are vital for your production of sex hormones.

SUPPLEMENTS

- VITAMIN B6 (50mg pyridoxal-5-phosphate, once daily) Your body uses this B-vitamin in its manufacture of sex hormones.

- VITAMIN E (300iu daily) Studies on menopausal women show that vitamin-E supplements can improve hot flashes, vaginal dryness, and other menopausal symptoms. (As well as taking a supplement, include plenty of vitamin-E-rich foods, such as vegetable oils, whole grains, seeds, and nuts, in your diet.)

- MAGNESIUM (300mg, daily) This nutrient helps to relax and calm your system, making you more receptive to sex.

- ZINC (15mg, daily) Zinc is essential for hormone balance and sex drive, hence the age-old belief that oysters (which are high in zinc) are an aphrodisiac.

- OMEGA-3 FATTY ACIDS (1,000mg fish oil, containing at least 700mg EPA and 500mg DHA, daily) Boost your intake of essential fats (see above). (Use flax seed oil if you're vegetarian.)

HERBS

- AMERICAN GINSENG (*Panax quinquefolium*) This herb can increase stamina and may aid sex drive. Take 1 tsp. tincture in a little water, twice daily; or 300–600mg in capsule form, daily.

- DAMIANA (*Turner aphrodisiaca*) In Central America, where this herb is grown, women take it as a traditional remedy for low libido. Take 1 tsp. tincture in a little water, or 300–600mg in capsule form, twice daily.

- GINKGO BILOBA (*Ginkgo biloba*) This herb can improve blood flow to the sexual organs, making them more responsive. Take 1 tsp. tincture in a little water, twice daily; or 400mg in capsule form, daily.

- ST JOHN'S WORT (*Hypericum perforatum*) Well known for its ability to combat depression, St John's wort contains L-tryptophan, an essential amino acid that the brain uses to manufacture serotonin (a mood-enhancer), melatonin (thought to help regulate the reproductive cycle), and zinc, which is essential for the production of sex hormones. As a result researchers believe that it can help boost libido. Take 1 tsp. tincture in a little water, three times daily; or 300mg in capsule form, two or three times daily. (Note: St John's wort can interfere with other medications, so consult an herbalist.)

OTHER NATURAL TREATMENTS

Aromatherapy massage Try a sensual massage with your partner using essential oils with known aphrodisiac qualities. Massage itself will promote improved blood-flow and energy levels. Combine 15 drops of any combination of the following oils in 6 tsp. sweet almond oil: damiana, sandalwood, jasmine, rose, neroli, bergamot, and ylang ylang.

SELF-HELP

Cut out the libido-lowerers Cut out smoking and alcohol, which have all been shown to lower sex drive.

Exercise This can boost your mood and body image, while pelvic-floor exercises (see box, p.127) can tone your muscles to increase your enjoyment of sex.

Devote more time to foreplay A crucial part of arousal, foreplay should feature highly in your sex life. It starts even before you touch each other: Most sex therapists agree that good sex begins in the head. Set the mood for sex: Use romantic music, dimmed lighting, a candle-lit bath, or a raunchy movie. And, if you haven't felt sexy in a while, masturbation and touching yourself can be a good way to reconnect with your sexuality and release sexual tension.

Make time for sex Research shows that the less a woman has sex, the lower her libido. If you think you haven't got time for sex—make time. Put it higher on your list of priorities and, however busy you are, make time for your partner: Intimacy can only take place when you're close. Women who have regular sex at least once a week have more regular menstrual cycles; and a satisfying sex life can ease stress and keep your organs healthy.

Make time for your relationship Relationship troubles can contribute to problems in the bedroom. If you don't feel listened to or respected, it's natural to respond with dampened sexual enthusiasm. If the problem is too big to sort out alone, consult a relationship or marriage therapist.

Feel beautiful If a poor body image is inhibiting your libido, stop focusing on what the media tell you is beautiful or desirable and concentrate on the bits of you that you find beautiful and pleasing. Ask your partner what he or she loves about you and why he or she desires you, and love those things about yourself, too.

Touch each other Don't underestimate the importance of non-sexual touch. Being hugged is essential for your physical and emotional well-being.

Ask for help Depression is a well-known inhibitor of sexual desire. If you feel you can't cope alone, ask for the support of family and friends, or a counselor.

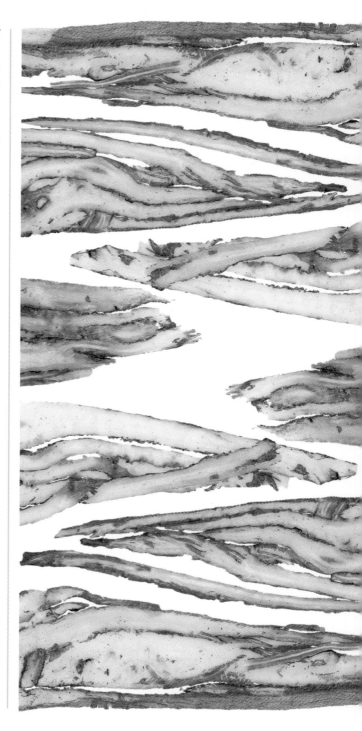

Right: American ginseng (*Panax quinquefolium*; see Herbs, opposite)

Hair loss

Your hair follicles need estrogen to function properly and for your hair to grow. As estrogen levels fall during menopause, you may find that you have increasingly regular bad-hair days.

A gradual loss or thinning of the hair, or ironically the growth of unwanted facial hair, is common during menopause. In addition, it's one of the menopausal symptoms that can get worse postmenopausally. Although to other people the difference is probably imperceptible, running your hands through your hair, you may find your hair feels generally thinner all over. Alternatively, your hair may visibly appear thinner at the front of your scalp. Other problems with hair include dullness, dryness, split ends, poor hair growth, and dandruff. You may find that your body hair, including your pubic hair, thins or disappears; some women also discover that their hair grows in unwanted places, such as on their face.

CAUSES

As you go through menopause, the levels of estrogen in your body fall. Although this means you're not necessarily producing more male hormones, your body interprets that it has more male hormone (such as the androgen testosterone) in circulation. Actually, what has happened is that the counterbalance of the estrogen is no longer there. As androgens begin to dominate your system, you can experience symptoms that are more often associated with male characteristics, such as male pattern baldness, acne, and increased facial hair (particularly on your upper lip).

You may be genetically predisposed to hair loss. In a condition called androgenic alopecia, you may have inherited—from your mother or father—a tendency towards imbalance in your hormones, particularly in later life. According to research, up to 13 percent of women have some degree of this sort of hair loss prior to menopause. After menopause, the condition becomes even more common, with one study showing that as many as many as 75 percent of women over the age of 65 are affected by it.

If you notice a considerable amount of hairs on your pillow in the morning, or if your hairdresser mentions to you that your hair has become thinner, you should see your doctor for a check up. Although the condition might simply be related to menopause, there can be other medical conditions that result in hair loss, including anemia (low iron in the blood) and thyroid problems. Stress, too, can cause you to lose your hair—at any age.

CONVENTIONAL TREATMENTS

If you've entered menopause and your hair is thinning, your doctor is most likely to offer you HRT, or one of two other medical options.

Hormone replacement therapy (HRT) For most women, the thought of going bald, even partly bald, is terrifying. Some women have told me that they have considered going on HRT just to stop hair loss in its tracks. Although HRT raises levels of estrogen in your system, it doesn't always solve the problem. For some women it does make a difference, but, ironically, one of the listed side-effects of HRT is hair loss itself. Unfortunately, there's no way to predict how your body will respond until you try it.

Minoxidil First developed for treating high blood pressure, minoxidil has now been found to thicken the hair. Your doctor will offer the drug orally, as a pill, or as a lotion to apply directly to your hair and scalp. As with any drug, minoxidil has side-effects, the most common one being an itchy scalp. Other side-effects can include acne, headaches, very low blood pressure, irregular heartbeat, chest pain, and blurred vision. Most importantly, though, this medication does not address the cause of the problem, and as soon as you stop using it, your hair loss will return.

Spironolactone This medication has mild diuretic properties and interferes with your body's ability to bind male hormones to the receptors in the hair follicle, so preventing hair loss. It has been linked to an increased risk of bleeding from the stomach, as well as irregular periods, rashes, and drowsiness.

YOUR DIET

I prefer to think of things rather differently from the more usual viewpoint that your hair is affected by your menopause. I like to think that your hair is a barometer of your overall health (along with your skin and nails, too). Think about a cat or dog—when an animal is unwell, a glossy, sleek fur coat becomes dull, limp, lifeless, and thinner. This gives you a key to how you might slow down the deterioration of your hair— namely, by taking care of your whole self by eating well and making sure you have your full quota of essential vitamins and minerals.

As well as making the choice to eat healthy foods, make sure you eat regularly throughout the day, including mid-morning and mid-afternoon snacks, and don't skip meals. This will help keep your blood-sugar levels balanced and in turn manage your hormone levels, helping to prevent an excess of the male hormone testosterone in your system.

Protein Your hair follicles need good-quality protein in different forms in order to grow. Stock up on legumes, nuts, seeds, and fish. In your body, protein is broken down into its constituent parts, known as amino acids. The most important amino acids for preventing hair loss are arginine, cysteine, lysine, and tyrosine, which are found in all protein-rich foods.

Essential fats If you have dry hair that breaks easily and lacks shine, you may lack the necessary levels of essential fatty acids. Boost your intake by eating plenty of oily fish (such as salmon, tuna, and sardines), nuts, and seeds.

Biotin Egg yolk, brown rice, lentils, oats, soy beans, sunflower seeds, walnuts, and green peas are rich in biotin. This important vitamin helps metabolize essential fats and is crucial for healthy hair and for the overall health of your skin and nails.

Iron Eat plenty of iron-rich foods, such as dark green vegetables, and stock up on vitamin-C-rich foods, too, which will help your body absorb the iron better.

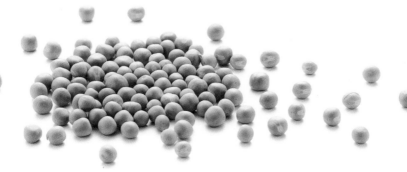

SUPPLEMENTS

■ B-COMPLEX (containing 25mg of each B-vitamin, daily) This is essential for your nervous system, so if your hair loss is stress-related, take this, too.

■ VITAMIN C with bioflavonoids (500mg, twice daily, as magnesium ascorbate) This vitamin helps in the manufacture of collagen, which holds hair tissue together, preventing splitting. Vitamin C also aids iron absorption.

■ VITAMIN E (600iu, daily) This vitamin is thought to help reduce testosterone in women.

■ ZINC (50mg as zinc citrate, daily) Zinc deficiency can weaken hair, causing it to break and stopping it from growing back at its normal rate. Zinc helps the oily glands on the follicles to prevent hair from shedding.

■ OMEGA-3 FATTY ACIDS (1,000mg fish oil, containing 700mg EPA and 500mg DHA, daily) Take this for three months. (Use flax seed oil if you're vegetarian.)

HERBS

■ HORSETAIL (*Equisetum arvense*) The outer skin of the stems of this herb contains large amounts of silica, a chemical compound that improves the formation of connective tissue in the body, and so improving the health of the hair (and of the skin and nails). Take 300mg in capsule form, twice daily.

■ SIBERIAN GINSENG (*Eleutherococcus senticosus*) If stress is contributing to your hair loss, take Siberian ginseng to support your adrenal glands. Take 1 tsp. tincture in a little water, 250–300mg in capsule form, twice daily.

OTHER NATURAL TREATMENTS

Homeopathy See a homeopath for a constitutional remedy, but at home you can try the following. Take a 30c potency of the appropriate remedy, twice daily.
• Nat mur is the ideal remedy if your hair falls out when it's brushed, combed, or even touched
• Phosphorous is suitable when you have bald spots, and your hair comes out in clumps

---

HERBAL HAIR RINSE

Make a rosemary hair rinse by steeping 1 cup rosemary leaves and stems in 2 cups water for 20 minutes. Wash and rinse your hair normally, and then do a final rinse using your rosemary "tea." Rosemary is believed to encourage hair growth from the follicles. Do this every time you wash your hair. For extra shine, you can add a cup of nettle tea, too.

• Sepia is the one to use when your hair loss is accompanied by fatigue and chronic headaches

Acupuncture According to Traditional Chinese Medicine, hair loss (and premature graying) is linked to a deficiency in the kidney meridian. You may want to visit an acupuncturist to have the relevant meridians stimulated in order to promote hair growth.

Aromatherapy massage Massaging essential oils into your scalp can increase the circulation to your head and reduce stress (through the massage). You can also capitalize on some of the beneficial properties of certain oils for hair health. For example, rosemary essential oil is believed to stimulate the activity of the hair follicles. Dilute 3 to 6 drops of essential oil in 3 tsp. carrier oil, such as jojoba or grapeseed oil, and massage the blend into your scalp. Alternatively, use clove oil (in the same dilution), which contains eugenol, known to stimulate hair growth; or cedar of Lebanon oil. Aim to massage your scalp two to three times per week, using the technique in the box on the opposite page. If you can bear to, leave the diluted essential oil in your hair overnight and wash it out normally in the morning. (Cover your hair with a shower cap to protect your bed linen during the night.)

SELF-HELP

Be gentle Use a soft brush and avoid blow drying, straightening, or curling your hair as much as possible. If you do use straighteners or curling tongs, use a heat-resistant hair protector spray, too, made from natural products (also use natural shampoo and conditioner). To prevent breakages, comb your hair carefully when wet, teasing out tangles rather than pulling.

Avoid stress As I've already said, stress can worsen hair loss, so keep your stress levels to a minimum. Find a relaxation routine that suits you, be it meditation, visualization, or a breathing exercise. The meditation on page 51 is a good start. Make sure you spend at least part of each day, even if it's just 30 minutes, doing something you enjoy for yourself—perhaps reading a book, or listening to your favorite pieces of music.

FOUR-STEP SCALP MASSAGE

Massage your scalp using the technique below for a few minutes, twice a day. You can also use this technique when you want to massage in essential oils (see opposite).

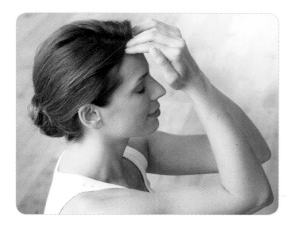

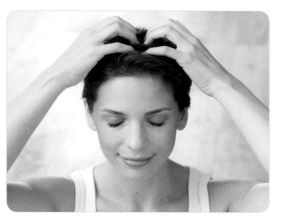

1 (above left) Use your fingertips to make small circular movements along your hairline. Begin in the middle of your forehead; work down the sides, around your ears, and to the back.

2 Using the tips of your thumbs and fingers of both hands, pinch your scalp all over your head, being careful not to pull too hard at your hair as you do so. Make the movements quick and fluid. Your scalp should tingle when you've finished.

3 Make your hands into claws and place your fingertips at your hairline on your forehead (palms over your head). Use your fingertips to "comb" your whole scalp from front to back.

4 (above right) Finally, beginning at the center of your head, work outward and around using your fingertips to make small circular movements that gently manipulate your skin over your scalp. Use firm pressure. Do this over your whole head.

POSTMENOPAUSE

You've been through the hot flashes and intermittent periods, your mood swings have abated, and, while menopause symptoms may still come and go for a while, generally things have settled down.

When you've had no periods for a year, the date of your last period was also the date of your actual menopause. In the medical view, from that date of your last period, you're classed as being postmenopausal. The medical profession chooses to wait a year before deciding on the date of your menopause because of the erratic nature of your periods as your ovaries wind down.

For many women, this last period typically occurs around the age of 51, but it can happen earlier or later, depending on your genetic predisposition, your body clock, and whether you've had reproductive surgery.

Although the majority of women go through menopause as a natural process when they get older, age isn't the only trigger for the winding down of your reproductive system. Other causes include surgical removal of your ovaries (known as oophorectomy), radiation therapy to your abdomen or pelvis, and chemotherapy to treat cancer. Whether nature or surgery have stopped your periods, once they've stopped permanently, you're postmenopausal.

While the problems associated with the menopausal process, such as hot flashes, can continue for several years after menopause itself, there are other symptoms more typical of the post-transitional period. These include vaginal dryness and irritation, memory problems, osteoporosis, stress incontinence, and heart disease. These are the conditions that I want to focus on in this section of the book. And the great news is that, although your doctor is likely to want to prescribe you HRT for many of them, there are plenty of natural solutions to them all.

Osteoporosis

Statistics suggest that one in six Western women suffer a hip fracture at some point in their lives. The highest risk is for postmenopausal women because low estrogen increases the risk of osteoporosis.

A woman came to my clinic who was only in her 50s, but she'd been out walking and had lightly stubbed her toe, resulting in a fracture. Another had broken a rib when she sneezed. Both these women were suffering from osteoporosis, a condition in which the bones become porous and fragile.

A breakage in a bone is a diagnosis of the condition—once your bones are so fragile that they break from the slightest knock or trauma, the chances are that osteoporosis is already quite advanced. In bodies without osteoporosis, the rate at which we lose and form bone (a process called bone remodelling) is equal, so that we have a constant bone mass, or density. Osteoporosis occurs when the rate of bone loss is greater than the rate of bone formation.

As a woman, you reach your peak bone mass between the ages of 25 and 30. This density remains stable until you reach menopause. At this time in your life there can be a rapid decline in bone mass as a result of the drop in estrogen levels in your body. What's interesting is that not all women have the same drop in bone density around menopause. Some women have very little loss of bone, while others can lose up to a fifth of their bone mass in the first few years after their last period. As you're unlikely ever to know how fast you're losing your bone, it's vital that you think about osteoporosis prevention.

LEARNING FROM HISTORY

Studies on the remains of 18th-century women have taught us that the bones of modern women are far less strong and dense than those of our ancestors. Clearly something in today's lifestyle affects the health of our bones. In this section, I'll explain how simple diet and lifestyle changes can go a long way to keeping your bones in top condition, and even to prevent osteoporosis altogether.

CAUSES

Certain risk factors can make you more prone to osteoporosis. Top of the list is a family history of the disease, followed by lifestyle factors (such as little exercise, poor diet, drinking too much of certain drinks, and smoking), digestive problems, some medications, and weight changes. Problems that you experienced when you were younger, such as an eating disorder or irregular periods, can also increase your risk.

Family history If your mother or grandmother suffered from osteoporosis, your risk of developing the condition increases, perhaps by as much as 80 percent. Talk to your relatives and find out whether osteoporosis runs in your family.

A sedentary lifestyle The strength of your skeleton works on a system of supply and demand. If you demand lots from it, it will supply the bone density to accommodate your demands; if you make few demands on it, your bone density will reduce proportionately. The answer? To move more. Studies show that women who are active for at least 24 hours a week have a 55 percent lower risk of hip fracture than those with sedentary lifestyles. The reduced risk is 41 percent even in those who walk for just four hours a week. Also, any exercise that keeps you fit, flexible, toned, and coordinated (such as yoga, Pilates, dancing, and so on) means you're less likely to fall and have a fracture.

Smoking You'll be aware of the negative effects of smoking in relation to lung cancer and emphysema, but you may not know that smoking can also affect the density of your bones, reducing their density by up to a quarter. Smoking affects your female hormones, particularly estrogen, which when lowered can contribute to osteoporosis.

Food and drink It stands to reason that a healthy diet is important for your bone health, because your food should supply good levels of vital bone-building nutrients, such as calcium. But it's also important to know that certain things that you eat or drink can actually have a negative effect on your bones. For example, alcohol has a diuretic effect and causes you to excrete valuable nutrients, including calcium, in your urine. The most important foods to avoid, however, are acidic foods (see box, below left).

Irregular periods If you stopped menstruating for up to six months (not including pregnancy or breast-feeding) before the age of 40, you may have an increased risk of osteoporosis. This is because amenorrhoea (see pp.106–9) can be caused by hormonal problems, and if you didn't have the right levels of hormones for your cycle to function effectively, you didn't have the right levels to protect your bones either.

Early menopause Termed premature ovarian failure (POF), early menopause is a menopause that occurs before the age of 40, often with no medical reason. Your increased number of years without estrogen compounds your likelihood of developing osteoporosis. In this case, it may help to go on HRT. This can artificially restore your levels of estrogen, until around the age of 50 when you can allow yourself to enter menopause at a more "normal" stage of life.

Changes in weight Being underweight increases your risk of osteoporosis—a thin frame makes you more at risk of fractures. On the other hand, fat cells produce estrogen, which helps protect your bones as you go through menopause. However, being overweight isn't the answer either. See the Body Mass Index (BMI) chart on p.297 and, using the healthy diet and lifestyle information in this book, try to stabilize your weight at its natural levels.

Digestive problems You need vital nutrients to keep your bones healthy, and this relies upon the health of your gut. If your gut doesn't absorb nutrients from your food effectively, your body can't benefit from

ACID–ALKALI BALANCE

Nutritionists often talk of the acid–alkali balance in the body. This is because a healthy body should be slightly alkaline. However, in the West most of us veer towards the acidic end of the scale. When your body becomes too acid, it leeches calcium from your bones and teeth to neutralize the acidity and correct the imbalance. To help prevent this, try to avoid too many acidic foods, including too much meat protein (research shows that vegetarians are much less likely to develop osteoporosis) and sugar. Cut out caffeine altogether if you have a family history of osteoporosis; otherwise drink no more than two cups of coffee, or equivalent in other caffeinated drinks, daily. Keep to a minimum drinks containing phosphoric acid (it's used to give a tangy taste to carbonated soft drinks).

them. The best way to boost your digestion is to eat a healthy, balanced diet and to take time chewing your food carefully—digestion begins in the mouth.

Certain medications If you're on steroids for problems such as rheumatoid arthritis or ulcerative colitis, or if you've had to take steroids in the past for any other reason, you need to be aware that these drugs can have a negative effect on your body's ability to absorb calcium. Low levels of calcium will decrease your body's bone-building activity. Remember also that diuretics and laxatives can cause you to flush out vital nutrients and so can have a negative effect on your bones. Avoid them if you can.

DIAGNOSING OSTEOPOROSIS

As always, the more information you have, the easier it is to make informed choices about what you need to do to keep yourself healthy and well. Checking for the risk of osteoporosis is no different. If your bone density is good, you need only work on prevention; but if you already have a problem with your bone density, you have to look at taking action to strengthen your bones now. Osteoporosis is a silent condition, so you can't tell you have it by symptoms, unless it has gone so far that you suffer a fracture. However, it is now relatively easy to assess whether or not a woman is at risk of the condition, by using a number of tests. These tests include:

DUAL ENERGY X-RAY ABSORPTIOMETRY (DEXA)
This X-ray machine is able to pick up changes in bone density far sooner than ordinary X-ray equipment, and it is the most reliable and widely used machine for diagnosing osteoporosis. It makes an image of your bones using two X-ray beams set at different frequencies. The machine can calculate the bone-mineral density by the rate your bones absorb each beam. The World Health Organization defines osteoporosis by what is called a "T score," which is a measurement compared to a young adult. So a T score of more than minus 1 (-1) is considered normal; between minus 1 (-1) and minus 2.5 (-2.5) is classed as osteopenia (low bone density); and a score lower than minus 3.5 (-3.5) is categorized as osteoporosis.

ULTRASOUND BONE SCANNER
An ultrasound is passed through the bone in the heel of your foot to give a reading of bone density. Research shows that ultrasound is as good as DEXA scans at predicting who will go on to have a fracture. It's the technique I use in my clinics. You'll be given a "T score" according to the same system as the DEXA machine.

BONE TURNOVER ANALYSIS
This test does not measure the density of your bone or its quality, but its turnover—how quickly your bone is breaking down. It's a useful test for mon-itoring how well you're doing with exercise, diet, supplements, or even drug treatment for osteoporosis. You'll be asked to provide a urine sample, which is sent to a lab. Here, technicians use the sample to assess the speed with which you lose bone. You can usually have the test repeated every three months to make sure your bone turnover is not too rapid.

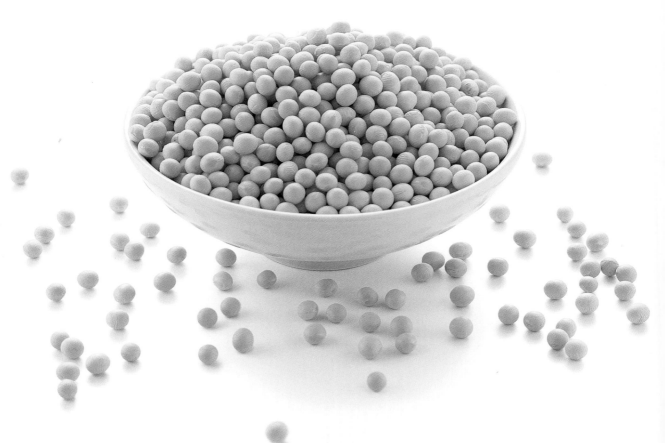

CONVENTIONAL TREATMENTS

In the past, the usual recommendation for preventing and treating osteoporosis has been hormone replacement therapy (HRT). In the USA, pre-menopausal women can still use HRT (or HT, hormone therapy) to prevent osteoporosis. However, the country's Food and Drug Administration (FDA) recommend that, because of the side-effects of HRT, women should, where possible, use other medications to prevent osteoporosis. It also states that doctors should not prescribe estrogen as a preventative, unless the patient can't take osteoporotic drugs. In the UK, the Committee on the Safety of Medicines has stated that women who are undergoing a normal, natural menopause should use HRT for a maximum of only five years, and only for the relief of symptoms such as hot flashes and night sweats. They don't advocate it to prevent osteoporosis, unless you can't tolerate osteoporotic medication.

Although HRT is effective in most cases against osteoporosis, as soon as you stop taking the medication, your bones break down as before. This means that you would have to be on HRT for the rest of your life to permanently prevent bone loss. Prolonged use of HRT poses considerable health risks, and so now there are several other medications for osteoporosis.

Selective estrogen receptor modulators (SERMS) These drugs aim to stimulate the estrogen receptors in your bones and brain—but not your breasts and uterus because doing so may increase your risk of cancer in these areas. In other words, the drugs make certain parts of your body more sensitive to estrogen; and other parts less sensitive.

Bone-saving medications You may be offered one of two drugs that help preserve your bones. Biphosphonates work by stopping bone breakdown: you won't lose "old" bone, so your bone density will increase. However, there are concerns about the usefulness of keeping old bone. Strontium ranelate is a newer drug that has a dual action, stopping the break-down of old bone and helping to build new bone, too. Both drugs carry side-effects: The bisphosphonates cause digestive problems and strontium ranelate can cause nausea, skin irritation, and blood clots.

YOUR DIET

A healthy, balanced diet (see pp.24–9) helps ensure strong, healthy bones. Reduce those foods and drinks that are known to increase your risk of osteoporosis (see p.272) but also watch the amount of dairy products you eat. Although cheese is a good source of calcium, it also encourages the excretion of calcium (cheese is more acidic than milk). And remember that tea contains caffeine—and tannin, which can hamper calcium absorption. Increase your intake of boron-rich foods (see p.276), too, by eating soy beans, apples, pears, raisins, broccoli, hazelnuts, and almonds.

Avoid bran Avoid adding bran to your food or having it as a breakfast cereal. Bran is a refined food, which means that the best part of the grain has been stripped away. It also contains phytates, which have a binding effect on crucial minerals, including calcium, and can stop your body absorbing them.

Sweeten naturally Try using a natural sweetener called xylitol in place of sugar. Found in fruits and berries, especially raspberries and strawberries, plums, and cauliflower, xylitol has a low glycemic index and does not cause blood-sugar swings. It may also directly benefit osteoporosis. Incredibly, studies on animals show that xylitol can increase bone calcium and bone density and prevent bone loss. Xylitol should be available in health-food stores and you use it in exactly the same way that you would sugar.

See the light Try to boost your intake of vitamin D, which is essential for your body's absorption of calcium. Eat plenty of oily fish and eggs, which contain this vital nutrient, and spend time outdoors. Sunlight encourages your body to manufacture vitamin D.

Opposite: Soy beans

SUPPLEMENTS

- B-COMPLEX and FOLIC ACID (containing 25mg of each B-vitamin and 400µg folic acid, daily) B6 and B12 help reduce levels of homocysteine, a hormone that may increase the risk of osteoporosis.

- VITAMIN C with bioflavonoids (500mg, twice daily, as magnesium ascorbate) This vitamin is essential for the formation of healthy collagen, the cement that holds your bone structure together. Take it in the form of ascorbate (such as magnesium ascorbate) rather than ascorbic acid, which is too acidic for bone health.

- BORON (1mg daily, in a multi-vitamin and mineral) This mineral is concentrated in bone and improves calcium absorption. It's also found in a number of different foods (see p.275).

- CALCIUM and MAGNESIUM (combined supplement containing 500mg calcium citrate and 900mg magnesium citrate, daily) The most difficult form of calcium for your body to absorb is calcium carbonate, so I advise supplementing with calcium in the form of citrate, which is 30 percent more absorbable. For the best effects combine it with magnesium, which is just as important for your bone health: Magnesium deficiencies can make your bones more fragile.

- ZINC (15mg, daily) This vital nutrient is often found to be deficient in women with osteoporosis, and we know that it's important for healthy bone metabolism. Take a supplement to make sure you keep your levels up.

HERBS

Use herbs that provide you with valuable bone-strengthening minerals or those that help improve your absorption of these nutrients. Blend equal parts of the dried herbs to make an herbal tea infusion and drink it up to three times a day.

- ALFALFA HERB (*Medicago sativa*) and OAT STRAW (*Avena sativa*) Both these herbs are thought to help with osteoporosis because of their high calcium content.

- HORSETAIL (*Equisetum arvense*) This herb contains the highest amount of silica of any herb. Silica is important for healthy skin, ligaments, and bones. It helps with the formation of collagen, which is part of your bone structure, and it's thought that it can help keep bones flexible.

- NETTLES (*Urtica* spp) Nettle contains good amounts of the minerals calcium and boron, but it can also help improve the general absorption of nutrients from your food.

OTHER NATURAL TREATMENTS

Homeopathy Constitutional homeopathic treatments are best, but if you can't visit a homeopath, Calc carb and Calc phos can help your body to absorb calcium. Take both in a 30c potency, twice daily.

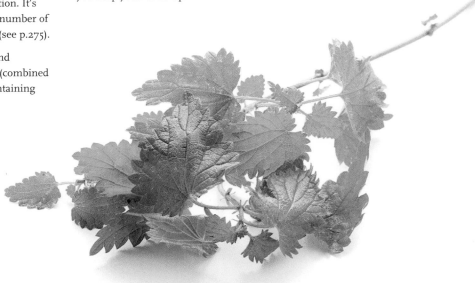

SELF-HELP

Increase the demand on your bones Do some weight-bearing exercise; for example, walking, jogging, dancing, aerobics, and racket sports. Aim for 30 minutes to an hour of activity, five times a week.

Watch your stress levels When stress levels are high, your adrenal glands have to work overtime, exhausting them so they can't produce the replacement estrogen your body needs at menopause. Also, when you're stressed, your digestion suffers, which will affect your nutrient intake.

Balance your weight Make sure you're not underweight, which can reduce estrogen levels in your body, contributing to bone loss.

BONE-STRENGTHENING YOGA POSE

The Camel pose works on strengthening the bones in your spine and pelvis. It's a deep stretch that may take time to perfect—only go as far as is comfortable. Practice daily.

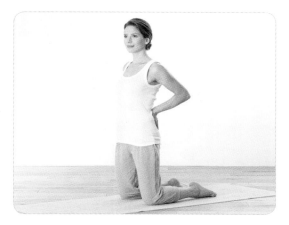

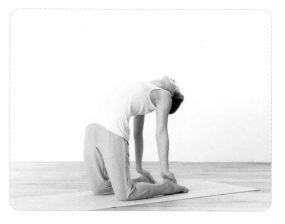

1 Kneel, legs hip-width apart, toes pointing behind you. Keep your back straight, your tailbone lifted, and your head erect. Imagine a cord is pulling you up from the top of your head, gently lengthening your spine. Place your hands at the tops of your buttocks, fingers pointing downward. Keep your thighs at right angles to the floor. Move your shoulder blades towards each other, feeling a stretch across your chest.

2 Breathe in through your nose. As you breathe out through your mouth, bend backward. Keep your thighs upright, arch your lower back, and slide your hands down your legs until they reach your ankles, heels, or soles of your feet. (Turn your toes under if it helps.) Drop your head backward; keep your throat soft. Lift your pelvis to relieve pressure from your lower spine. Hold the pose for 30 seconds; release and repeat.

Opposite: Nettles (*Urtica* spp)

Vaginal dryness

Affecting half of all postmenopausal women (although it can occur at any time in a woman's life), vaginal dryness is perhaps the most distressing and least talked about symptom of menopause.

Vaginal dryness is medically known as "atrophic vaginitis," and although this may sound very much like a disease, it's important to remember that it's not. Nor is it an inevitable symptom of menopause.

Vaginal dryness can make your vagina feel not only dry, but also itchy and at times tender. It may take you longer to become lubricated during lovemaking, which can make sexual intercourse feel uncomfortable, or even painful. And not only can vaginal dryness cause pain and bleeding during intercourse, it can also increase the possibility of developing a vaginal infection, which itself compounds the problem.

CAUSES

Normally, mucous membranes (the vaginal epithelium), located at the mouth of your uterus, keep the vagina moist. Estrogen helps these membranes produce lubrication and stay plump and soft. The lubricant is slightly acidic, which helps protect the vagina from foreign bacteria, keeping it free from infection. After menopause, when estrogen levels are low, all these benefits are at risk. Low levels of estrogen also cause the vagina and surrounding connective tissue to lose elasticity and the tissue that lines the vagina to become thinner and more fragile.

Although hormone imbalance, in particular low estrogen, is the most probable cause of vaginal dryness, stress and fatigue play a part, too. More rarely, a condition known as Sjögren's syndrome (which is an autoimmune condition that causes dryness throughout the body, including in the eyes and skin, as well as the vagina), cancer medications, and chronic yeast infection can also be causes.

CONVENTIONAL TREATMENTS

Vaginal dryness occurs sometimes transiently and at other times permanently. If the condition is persistent and makes intercourse too painful and uncomfortable for you, your doctor may suggest conventional HRT, or a cream or pessary that contains estrogen, which you should use vaginally.

Hormone replacement therapy (HRT) HRT increases vaginal lubrication and thickens the vaginal lining, but the treatment has health risks (see pp.249–51), and, in my opinion, is not appropriate if vaginal dryness is your only postmenopausal problem.

Estrogen creams and pessaries If you prefer not to take HRT, your doctor can prescribe vaginal creams or pessaries containing estrogen. There are a variety of products made up of different types of estrogens, but the least carcinogenic of these estrogens is estriol. One study found that a dosage of only 0.1mg vaginal estrogen daily (given as recommended by your doctor; see below) provided effective relief from vaginal dryness. You'll have to use an applicator to insert the cream or pessary directly into your vagina to

LEFT UNTREATED vaginal dryness can devastate a love life.

soften and tone it, and so make intercourse more comfortable. When you start using vaginal cream, you apply the dosage just inside your vagina daily for three or four weeks. Then you can reduce your use to once or twice a week. Once everything is working smoothly, you can move over to using a drug-free lubricant (see p.280).

YOUR DIET

Women who eat a nutritious diet generally experience fewer problems with their vagina in the menopausal years, so do follow my guidelines for a healthy, balanced diet on pages 24–5. For hormone balance, it's especially important to make sure you eat enough essential fatty acids (EFAs) and to supplement with fish oil (see below). A low- or no-fat diet can make your whole body drier, including the vagina. It's also important to eat plenty of phytoestrogens, as research shows that phytoestrogen-rich foods, such as soy, chickpeas, lentils, and flax seeds, can change the cells of the vagina so that they become softer, moister and more elastic. Eating plain, organic yogurt with active cultures four or five times a week may also help maintain healthy intestinal flora and vaginal balance.

SUPPLEMENTS

- VITAMIN C with bioflavonoids (500mg, twice daily, as magnesium ascorbate) This is essential for collagen formation, to give tissue its elasticity.

- VITAMIN E (400iu, daily) This powerful antioxidant is known for its anti-aging properties. Research shows it can significantly reduce vaginal dryness.

- OMEGA-3 FATTY ACIDS (1,000mg fish oil containing at least 700mg EPA and 500mg DHA, daily) You need these for hormone balance and to keep the cells of your vagina lubricated. (Use flax seed oil if you're vegetarian.)

- PROBIOTICS (one capsule containing at least ten billion organisms, daily) Probiotics help keep unhealthy bacteria and yeasts (flora), such as candida, in check, reducing your susceptibility to vaginal infections.

HERBS

- AGNUS CASTUS (*Vitex agnus castus*) The women's wonder herb, agnus castus has hormone-regulating and relaxant properties, and so can help combat vaginal dryness both by helping to balance your hormones and helping you to relax, if your dryness is partly caused by stress. Take take 1 tsp. tincture in a little water, or 200–300mg in capsule form, twice daily.

- DONG QUAI (*Angelica sinensis*) In Traditional Chinese Medicine, the root of the dong quai plant is used to treat several symptoms of menopause, including vaginal dryness. Take 1 tsp. tincture in a little water, or 300mg in capsule form, twice daily.

- MOTHERWORT (*Leonurus cardiaca*) Motherwort helps relax the smooth muscles of the body, and can help plump up the vaginal walls and make them more flexible. It has been used in Traditional Chinese Medicine for centuries as a hormone regulator. Take 1 tsp. tincture in a little water, or 200–300mg in capsule form, twice daily. Studies show that with regular use like this, you can increase vaginal lubrication and the thickness of the vaginal wall within a month. (Taking 1 or 2 tbsp. flax seed oil daily can have the same effect, if you prefer.)

OTHER NATURAL TREATMENTS

Homeopathy Although I recommend seeing a registered homeopath for constitutional remedies that can be tailored to your individual symptoms, at home you can try the following. Take those remedies that are most relevant to your particular problem in a 30c potency, twice daily, until the problem appears to have rectified itself.

• Bryonia, Lycopodium, and/or Belladonna for general vaginal dryness, with few other symptoms
• Nat mur if you have vaginal dryness is accompanied by water retention
• Staphysagria if your dryness is accompanied by thinning in the vaginal wall and severe pain and soreness during sexual intercourse

Acupuncture In Traditional Chinese Medicine, the symptoms of menopause are believed to be related to imbalances (in particular, a sluggishness) of *qi* energy in the kidney and spleen meridians. Expect your practitioner to treat these energy pathways to relieve vaginal dryness.

Aromatherapy Relaxing and sexually stimulating essential oils can help put you in the mood for love-making and encourage lubrication. Put a few drops of a relaxing oil, such as lavender, into an essential oil burner, turn the lights down low, and let the calming mood fill the room. You can combine the lavender with any of the oils on page 264, too, to increase desire. Alternatively, try a sensual aromatherapy massage using 15 drops of lavender essential oil in 6 tsp. of sweet almond oil; or use 5 drops of lavender oil in your bath.

Reflexology The ovary, pituitary, and adrenal reflex points on the soles of the feet are those most likely to be treated in a reflexology session to overcome vaginal dryness (because of their influence on your hormone balance). These points are located in the middle of the heels and in two points in the middle of the soles, respectively. A reflexologist will also look at other contributory factors in your lifestyle and may treat other reflex points, too.

SELF-HELP

Drink water Check you're drinking enough water. You should consume six to eight glasses of water or herbal tea daily. This keeps your tissues (those in the vagina as well as in the skin and so on) hydrated and plumped up, preventing drying and cracking.

Get moving Regular exercise can help keep your vagina supple and lubricated. Aim for at least 30 minutes of moderate exercise five to six times a week. In addition, practice pelvic-floor exercises (see box, p.127) regularly because these can help strengthen your pelvic floor muscles, making sex more enjoyable.

Have more sex Regular sex and masturbation can help—women who have sex once or twice a week tend to lubricate more rapidly when aroused. Spend longer on foreplay, too. You may find it helpful to use a good-quality, natural lubricant before sex. I like to recommend Sylk, a product from New Zealand that is natural and water-soluble, derived from the vine of the kiwi; and also Yes, an organic lubricant that contains no preservatives or chemicals and is made from cocoa and shea butter.

Take care of your vagina Avoid douches, talcum powder, hot baths, and perfumed toilet papers, bath oils, and foams as they can irritate the vagina. Don't wash the inside of your vagina with soap, as this will dry out the skin. The vagina is self-cleansing and, in most cases, warm water is all that you need to wash it.

Avoid tampons If you're still menstruating, wear pads instead of tampons, which can dry out the vagina. If you want to wear a tampon, use an organic cotton one and change it every three to four hours. Avoid wearing panty liners between periods unless absolutely necessary because they can dry and irritate the vagina.

Use probiotic pessaries You can buy acidophilus (probiotic) pessaries to insert vaginally to help prevent yeast infections and help with lubrication. Vaginal infections can cause irritation to the vaginal opening and make sex painful, so refer to the relevant section in this book if this applies to you.

Communicate with your partner Insufficient lubrication can be connected to feelings about your partner and your relationship. If you have repressed anger or resentment towards your partner, you may have trouble getting aroused and sufficiently lubricated. Deal with problems as they come along, instead of letting them accumulate. Try to talk about how you feel, rather than apportioning blame or guilt. Use plenty of "I" statements. (See also box, p.157.)

Opposite: Motherwort (*Leonurus cardiaca*; see Herbs, p.279)

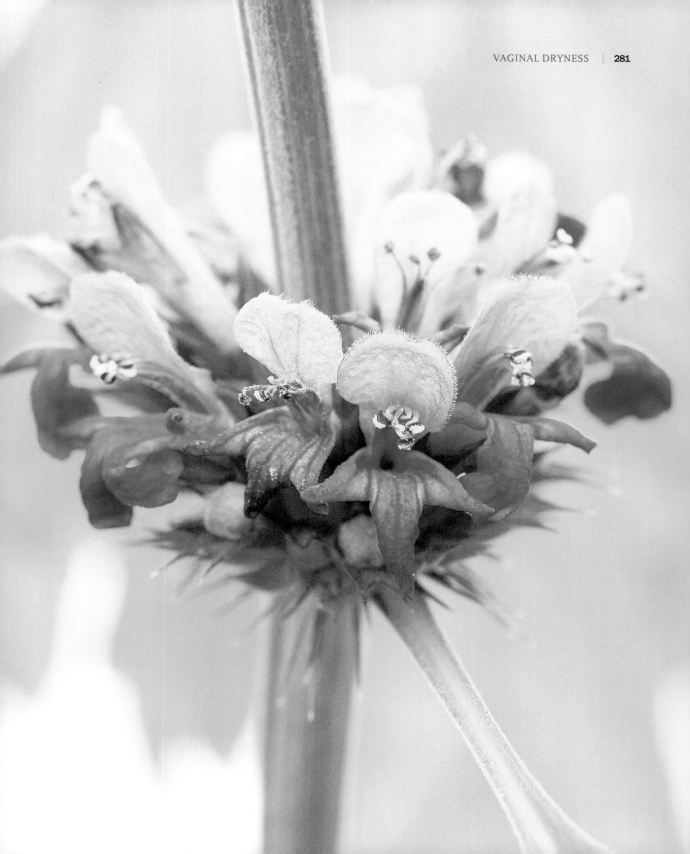

Memory loss and poor concentration

It was once assumed that brainpower automatically decreased with age, but research now shows this simply isn't true. Your brain is able to acquire new skills and store information well into old age.

In other words you can have an agile mind and can increase your knowledge and intelligence well into menopause and beyond.

SUPPLY AND DEMAND

Just as with your bones and muscles, the strength of your brain is all about supply and demand. If you make demands on your brain cells, they'll keep on strengthening your neural networks. This means they'll go on creating pathways that make information evermore readily accessible, in turn improving your ability to retain and recall information.

We do have to work harder on our memory and concentration as we go through menopause, though. Your brain contains estrogen receptors. When these are stimulated with estrogen, they're thought to help maintain cognitive function. Estrogen levels fall during menopause and remain low in the postmenopausal period. It's easy to assume that this means your brain function will fall into decline and that this is an inevitable, irreversible process. However, research now proves that if you keep your brain active, there's no inevitability about a decline in brain function at all.

OXYGEN SUPPLY

As well as constant use, a healthy brain needs a good supply of blood to bring it lots of oxygen. This means your circulation needs to be in good order. Chilblains or very cold hands and feet are an indicator that your circulation isn't as good as it could be, and that means that the circulation to your brain isn't so good, either.

CONVENTIONAL TREATMENTS

If your memory loss is related entirely to your age, your doctor is likely to offer you nothing more than advice on how to restore your brain power by using your brain more. Occasionally, you may be offered HRT, but be aware that this carries significant potential side-effects (see pp.249–51). If you start to notice that changes in memory are affecting how you function each day, it would be a good idea to see your doctor. If you can't remember how to get to a familiar place or can't follow the steps in a recipe, you need to have a check up.

YOUR DIET

Food nourishes your brain as well as your body; what you eat and drink affects your mental performance, as well as your physical. If you don't eat properly, your brain won't be getting the nutrients it needs to function efficiently. Whatever your age, a poor diet causes foggy thinking, forgetfulness, and poor concentration.

Your brain is a greedy organ and requires a constant supply of oxygen, energy, and glucose. As a first step, try to follow my guidelines for a healthy, balanced diet on pages 24–9. In particular, ensure your diet is rich in fiber by eating five portions of fruit and vegetables a day and stocking up on whole grains, nuts, and seeds.

Providing glucose

Of all nutrients, your brain needs glucose more than any other, but the supply of glucose throughout the day must be a steady one. This means making sure you eat plenty of unrefined carbohydrates, such as wholegrain

BRAINY BREAKFASTS

BREAKFAST ONE Have an egg (scrambled or poached) on wholewheat or rye bread. The bread in this breakfast gives you unrefined slow-releasing carbohydrate, while the egg is a first-class protein, which slows down the carbohydrate-release even more, provides essential amino acids (see below), and contains valuable omega-3 fats, which help keep your brain cells well lubricated.

BREAKFAST TWO Blend together some mixed berries (fresh or frozen) with soy, rice, or oat milk and with your choice of nut (for example, almonds or cashews) and seeds (such as flax seeds or pumpkin seeds). Experiment with the quantities until you get your desired consistency. The berries provide antioxidants (to protect your brain from free-radical damage), and the nuts and seeds provide protein (for brain power) and good levels of essential fats to lubricate your brain cells.

bread, rice, and pasta, and vegetables and that you avoid eating highly refined products, such as those made with white flour and lots of sugar. You can choose to refer to glycemic index (GI) lists, if you like, but I prefer to advocate one simple rule: The more fresh and unprocessed a food is, the more likely it is to have a steadying effect on your blood sugar.

Make sure you eat every few hours because, if you skip meals, there'll be too little glucose in your bloodstream, and you'll feel sluggish and find it hard to remember or concentrate properly. You can even feel lightheaded or dizzy. Aim for five or six nutritious and balanced meals and snacks a day and make sure that each one of them contains a little high-quality protein—a sprinkling of nuts and seeds, for example.

Eating breakfast is a brain-boosting essential. Your brain never rests—even when you're asleep—so a good, healthy breakfast (see box, above) is the best way to replenish your energy after a night's sleep and help you stay alert all morning.

Providing protein

Protein provides the building blocks for essential amino acids, such as tryptophan, which the brain uses to make neurotransmitters, including serotonin (often called the "feel-good" chemical, because it has pain-relieving properties). In addition, protein foods help control the release of sugar or glucose into the bloodstream. To ensure you get a full range of essential amino acids, include a wide range of high-quality protein in your diet in the form of nuts, seeds, oily fish, soy products, peas, beans, lentils, quinoa, eggs, and (in moderation) dairy products.

Providing fats

The amount and type of fat you eat is important for brain function, too. You need to reduce saturated fat in your diet because saturated fat, which is found mainly in animal products, clogs up your arteries, impeding the all-important circulation to your brain (see opposite). You also need to avoid hydrogenated fats (see p.26) because they can harden brain cells, preventing the neural pathways, which boost your information storage and recall, from making healthy connections.

All that said, your brain is 70 percent fat and needs certain types of fat to function optimally. These necessary fats (which nourish all the cells in your nervous system, not only those in your brain) are essential fats.

Foods rich in essential fats contain actual components of brain-cell membranes. They include oily fish (sardines, mackerel, and so on), nuts and seeds (particularly walnuts and almonds), and some leafy green vegetables (such as kale and cabbage).

ANTIOXIDANTS AND YOUR BRAIN

Antioxidants are substances found in food that help maintain the health of your cells (see p.28) by protecting against free-radical attack. They also encourage healthy brain function, including improvements in memory. If you're already eating five portions of vegetables and fruit a day, as well as plenty of whole grains and other fresh food, your intake of antioxidants is likely to be good. Just in case, here's a diet checklist to make sure you have a high intake of the following crucial antioxidants:

• Beta-carotene, found in orange and yellow fruits and vegetables, such as carrots
• Vitamin C, found in citrus fruits, such as oranges, and in berries, green and red peppers, and leafy green vegetables
• Vitamin E, found in nuts, seeds, whole grains, and oily fish
• Selenium found in nuts, eggs, and whole grains
• Zinc found in fish, legumes, and almonds

You can also boost your antioxidant intake by using supplements. Consider taking vitamin B6 (25mg, daily), vitamin C (500mg, twice daily), vitamin E (300iu, daily), magnesium (300mg, daily), and selenium (100µg, daily).

And finally ...

Increase your intake of phytoestrogens, which are found in soy products and lentils, because studies show that eating a phytoestrogen-rich diet can result in significant improvements in both short- and long-term memory. And remember that water is crucial for a healthy brain. If you don't drink enough, you're liable to suffer from dehydration and accompanying headaches and poor concentration. The solution is simple: Make sure you drink six to eight glasses of water a day—more on hot days or if you're exercising and sweating a lot. Don't wait until you're thirsty to drink because thirst is a sign that you're already dehydrated. As for caffeine, one or two cups of coffee a day seems to have a stimulating effect on the brain, but any more than that and you'll decrease blood flow to your brain.

SUPPLEMENTS

■ BORON As well as taking antioxidant supplements (see box, left), you should make sure that your daily multi-vitamin and mineral supplement includes boron (1mg, daily). Studies show that boron is important for healthy brain function, particularly for concentration and short-term memory function.

■ OMEGA-3 FATTY ACIDS Supplement with a good-quality fish oil (1,000mg, daily), containing at least 700mg EPA and 500mg DHA; or with flax seed oil (1,000mg, daily).

HERBS

■ GINKGO BILOBA (*Ginkgo biloba*) This herb comes from one of the world's longest-living trees. It is without exception *the* "memory herb." I have seen it help sharpen focus and improve memory in women of all ages. The herb helps keep blood vessels flexible, improving blood flow to the brain, and so its supplies of oxygen and glucose. Ongoing research is currently attempting to determine if supplementing with gingko can delay or alleviate dementia. Take 400mg ginkgo biloba in capsule form daily, or 1 tsp. tincture in a little water, twice daily.

OTHER NATURAL TREATMENTS

Homeopathy As always, I recommend a constitutional consultation with a homeopath. However, remedies you can try at home are Lachesis and Sulphur. Take either or both in a 30c potency, twice daily.

Acupuncture To improve memory and concentration, an acupuncturist will usually concentrate on the heart-channel meridian, as well as other meridians specific to your overall general health.

Full-body aromatherapy massage A full-body massage with a qualified aromatherapist, especially with the stimulating essential oil rosemary, can boost circulation so that your brain gets a good supply of oxygenated blood. If you're using rosemary essential oil in a massage at home, make sure you dilute it in a carrier oil such as sweet almond using a dilution of 15 drops of rosemary oil to 6 tsp. of carrier.

SELF-HELP

Moderate your alcohol The odd glass of wine or two a week won't hurt, and may actually boost your brain power, but too much alcohol can destroy brain cells, so try to limit your intake.

No smoking Nicotine causes your blood vessels to constrict, hampering blood flow to your brain. Avoid smoking and passive smoking alike.

Keep fit Regular exercise can boost circulation to the brain and also release mood-enhancing endorphins into your body, making you feel more alert.

Sleep well Quality sleep is crucial for a healthy brain and nervous system—but not too much sleep! You should be aiming for between six and eight hours a night. Any more or less than that can lead to poor concentration, fatigue, and memory loss.

MEMORY EXERCISES

Exercises, such as the ones below can help keep your memory agile. In addition, do crosswords, play word and number games, and make a point of reading a newspaper, magazine article, or chapter of a book every day.

EXERCISE 1: CAN YOU REMEMBER?
Every day try to recall the following:
• What you were thinking about five minutes ago
• What you were thinking about one hour ago
• What you were doing this time yesterday
• What you wore last weekend

EXERCISE 2: KIM'S GAME
Try this variation on a children's classic party game.
• Ask a friend or your partner to gather ten items on a tray. They should be random, unrelated.
• Look at the tray for 1 minute. Memorize everything you see. Then, cover the tray and write a list of everything you remember was on it. When you've finished, turn your paper over.
• Next, ask your friend to take away one undisclosed item from the tray. Uncover the tray and note which item has gone.
• Check your list against the items on the tray. Did you remember them all? Were you right about the missing item? Next time you play (this time with new items), reduce your memorizing time by 5 seconds, and keep reducing it each time you play until you can memorize ten different items in 15 seconds.

Heart disease

Once you've been through menopause and the levels of estrogen in your blood have decreased, your risk for heart disease increases. Protecting your heart helps safeguard your old age.

Heart disease is the world's biggest killer. Although a woman's risk of heart disease, also known as coronary disease, does not reach the same level as a man's until she is 75, it's still a leading cause of death for women. In heart disease, the arteries that supply your heart with oxygen and nutrients become narrowed by atherosclerosis (commonly known as "hardening of the arteries"). This restricts the supply of blood and oxygen to your heart. Unfortunately, for many women the first indication that something's wrong is a heart attack.

It's important to appreciate that heart attacks rarely strike suddenly. In the great majority of cases, your heart and circulation will have been unhealthy for a long time, even if you didn't know it. Heart disease is a degenerative condition: It builds up over a number of years. In addition, most experts—myself included—agree overwhelmingly that heart disease can be caused (and prevented) by your diet and lifestyle. If your diet and lifestyle are healthy, your risk of developing heart disease decreases significantly, compared with a woman whose diet and lifestyle are unhealthy.

CAUSES

Most of us know the main risk factors for heart disease already: a lack of exercise coupled with a diet that is high in saturated fat and sugar; being overweight or overstressed; smoking; diabetes; high blood pressure, or a family history of heart disease; and stroke. Essentially, of those risk factors within your control, leading an unhealthy, sedentary life puts a strain on your heart and potentially shortens your life.

Increased risk for coronary disease is also associated with the process of aging, and there's also a relationship between heart health and a woman's midlife transition through menopause. Before menopause, a woman's hormones (especially estrogen) offer some protection for her heart and blood vessels.

To understand how you can reduce your susceptibility to heart disease, it's important to look in more detail at the risk factors within your control.

UNDERSTANDING CHOLESTEROL

Although the word cholesterol has negative associations for most of us, cholesterol has a positive function in your body as well as a negative one. Cholesterol is a type of fat that exists in all your cell membranes. Eighty percent of cholesterol is produced by your liver, and only 20 percent comes directly from your diet. It's essential to the healthy functioning of your body, and you could not live without it. Cholesterol is the starting point for many of your hormones, including the sex and stress hormones; and it's vital for nerve transmission, the formation of vitamin D (which you need for healthy bones), and the formation of bile. Problems occur only when you take in excess cholesterol from foods that are naturally high in cholesterol, or when your body starts to produce too much.

You may be surprised to learn that foods with fats do not have to contain cholesterol; it's found only in animal products (meat, dairy products, butter, and eggs). Vegetable products are cholesterol-free: An avocado and olive contain fat, but neither contains cholesterol.

HOW YOUR HEART WORKS

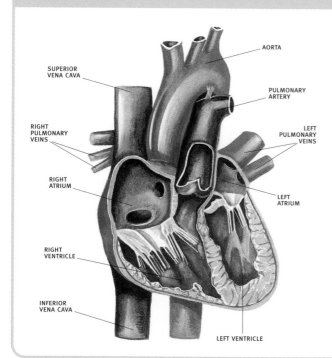

AORTA

SUPERIOR VENA CAVA

PULMONARY ARTERY

RIGHT PULMONARY VEINS

LEFT PULMONARY VEINS

RIGHT ATRIUM

LEFT ATRIUM

RIGHT VENTRICLE

INFERIOR VENA CAVA

LEFT VENTRICLE

About the size of your fist, your heart lies just to the left of your breastbone and is a complicated pump responsible for circulating blood, oxygen, and nutrients through your body. It's divided into four chambers: The right atrium and left atrium are the upper chambers of the heart, and the right ventricle and left ventricle are the lower chambers. The heart muscle contracts in two stages to squeeze blood out of the heart. This is known as systole. When the heart relaxes—known as diastole—blood fills up the heart again, and the whole process (which takes a fraction of a second) is repeated.

The heart has arteries that carry blood away from the heart. Capillaries (small blood vessels) connect arteries to veins. The veins then carry blood back to the heart. Heart disease can occur when arteries clog up with plaque.

Furthermore, foods such as shellfish contain very little fat but a high level of cholesterol, and nut butters (such as peanut butter), which we often perceive to be unhealthy, are high in fat but low in cholesterol.

In order for cholesterol to travel in the bloodstream, it has to combine with a protein, after which it's known as a lipoprotein. There are two main types of lipoprotein that carry cholesterol around your body. Low-density lipoproteins (LDL, or "bad" cholesterol) are responsible for carrying cholesterol via the arteries to the cells of your body. High-density lipoprotein (HDL, or "good" cholesterol) collects cholesterol from the tissues and returns it to the liver for disposal. When you have high levels of LDL, cholesterol can deposit on damaged and inflamed arterial walls. These deposits, which also consist of saturated fats and calcium (that's why cardiolo-

gists talk about calcification of arteries), are called arterial plaque or atheroma. These cause atherosclerosis (hardening), which can lead to blocked arteries and, as a result, high blood pressure.

Checking your cholesterol

To check your cholesterol, your doctor will give you what's known as a "lipid" test. You need to know not only your total cholesterol level but also the separate levels of LDL and HDL (so that you know how much of your cholesterol is good and how much is bad). You also need to know your level of triglycerides (blood fats) because high levels of these have been linked to a higher risk of strokes and heart disease. Make sure you haven't eaten or drunk anything (except water) from 10pm the night before your tests. (See box, p.288.)

LEVELS OF CHOLESTEROL

Below are the low- and high-risk values for the five lipid measurements taken in a cholesterol test. They indicate your relative likelihood of developing heart disease (HD). (Both US and UK systems of measurement are given in the table.)

	LOW HD RISK	HIGH HD RISK
TOTAL CHOLESTEROL	USA: 200mg/dL and below UK: 5.0 mmol/L and below	USA: over 200mg/dL UK: over 5.0 mmol/L
HDL	USA: over 60mg/dL UK: Over 0.9 mmol/L	USA: 60mg/dL and below UK: 0.9 mmol/L and below
LDL	USA: 100mg/dL and below UK: 3.0 mmol/L and below	USA: over 100mg/dL UK: over 3.0 mmol/L
CHOLESTEROL/HDL	More than 20%	Less than 20%
TRIGLYCERIDES	USA: less than 150mg/dL UK: Less than 2.3 mmol/L	USA: In US over 150mg/dL UK: Over 2.3 mmol/L

Cholesterol and iron

Generally, your body needs iron for energy and to nourish your muscle cells. Without good levels, you'll become anemic, which can cause you to feel tired all the time. However, having too much iron in your system and supplementing with iron can also be bad for you. Iron oxidizes LDL "bad" cholesterol; only once it's oxidized, does LDL seem to damage the arteries.

The fact that after menopause you'll no longer have periods means that iron can build up in your system (you lose iron when you bleed). For this reason, I recommend that you have regular blood tests to assess your iron levels, as well as the tests to establish your levels of cholesterol. Take iron supplements only if a blood test reveals that your blood levels are low. Many breakfast cereals are fortified with iron—avoid eating these after menopause, too. (However, don't try to cut iron-rich foods out of your diet.)

YOUR DIET

Quite simply, the best thing you can do for your heart is to eat a healthy, balanced diet according to my guidelines on pages 24–9. It's especially important to increase your intake of oily fish, nuts, seeds, and oils—because these foods are good sources of essential fatty acids (EFAs), which are known to prevent heart disease. The omega-3 fish oils are particularly important because they not only help prevent abnormal blood clotting, they can also help lower bad cholesterol (LDL) and increase the levels of good cholesterol (HDL). Phytoestrogens (see p.31) are another food group that has this effect on LDL and HDL. They have the added benefit of helping to lower your body's levels of triglycerides (blood fat).

Try to boost your intake of antioxidants (see p.28), which are found in brightly colored fruits and vegetables. These important nutrients reduce your risk of heart disease by attacking the harmful free radicals that cause cell damage in your body. If you have a family history of heart problems, I strongly advise you to take a good antioxidant supplement (see opposite).

Fats and your heart

There are two kinds of fat that are particularly bad for your heart health.

Saturated fat Regardless of your age and time of life, you should try to reduce your intake of foods that contain saturated fat, such as animal products and deep-fried foods, which clog up your arteries.

Trans fats For a healthy heart, you need to avoid trans fats altogether. These harmful fats, found in hydrogenated products such as margarine, as well as in ready-made meals, cookies, and other processed foods, can't be properly broken down in the body, so they remain in the system, like a sort of plastic. Increasing your consumption of trans fats by only two percent can increase your risk of heart disease by a massive 30 percent overall.

SUPPLEMENTS

■ VITAMIN D3 (400iu, daily) If you have high cholesterol, have a blood test to check your vitamin-D levels. The body uses cholesterol to make vitamin D, so if you're deficient in it, your liver may pump out more cholesterol to try to increase levels of the vitamin in your system. If you correct the deficiency through supplementation, your liver won't have to produce so much cholesterol. (Don't use vitamin D2 supplements because it's not as efficient as D3 in helping to correct a deficiency.)

■ ANTIOXIDANTS (one capsule daily, containing at least 10mg vitamin A, 400iu vitamin E, 500mg vitamin C, 100µg selenium and 15mg zinc) A good-quality antioxidant supplement protects the heart because it improves circulation and can prevent abnormal clotting. It also "mops up" the free radicals that damage cells in your body and cause disease. Taking vitamin C and vitamin E in combination is more powerful for heart health than taking either vitamin on its own.

■ CO-ENZYME Q10 (100mg, daily) A powerful antioxidant, co-enzyme Q10 may be able to help the heart pump more efficiently, reduce blood clotting, and lower cholesterol. In one US study, patients who were given co-enzyme Q10 within three days of having a heart attack had a dramatically reduced incidence of repeated heart failures.

■ GARLIC (1,000mg, daily) Garlic is a superfood when it comes to the heart. It's best eaten in its raw form, but if you find this difficult (not least for social reasons), you can take it in a concentrated organic form as a supplement. The best form to take is aged garlic. Research shows that aged garlic supplements can reduce total cholesterol levels by five to seven percent, reduce "bad" cholesterol, increase "good" cholesterol, and reduce blood pressure. Clinical trials in the USA have shown that aged garlic can reduce arterial plaque by more than 50 percent.

■ OMEGA-3 FATTY ACIDS (1,000mg fish oil, containing at least 700mg EPA and 500mg DHA, daily) This can help prevent abnormal blood clotting by reducing the "stickiness" of blood platelets. (Use flax seed oil if you're vegetarian.)

THE GOODNESS OF GRAPES

All grapes contain high amounts of antioxidants, among the most important of which is resveratrol, which has a strong heart-protecting effect. The grapes produce this antioxidant to protect themselves when they are under attack from insects or bad weather. In humans, resveratrol helps prevent narrowing of the arteries and stops blood platelets sticking together, therefore decreasing the risk of clots. It's this action that's recently led to a surge in people drinking red wine for medicinal purposes! It's true that red wine contains more resveratrol than white wine. This is because the grape skins are left in contact with the wine for longer during the wine's fermentation process. But actually, wine (alcohol) has nothing to do with it. Eating grapes is considerably better for you— as they contain less sugar and no alcohol. Try to eat a handful of red or white grapes daily to give a boost to your heart.

HERBS

■ GINGER (*Zingiber officinale*) Ginger has a stimulating effect on the body, helping to boost circulation. It also helps lower cholesterol. Drink a cup or two of ginger tea, daily.

■ HAWTHORN (*Crataegus oxyacantha*) The most-often recommended herb for high blood pressure, hawthorn is a vasodilator— it can keep blood vessels open to ease blood flow and so lower blood pressure. Take 1 tsp. tincture in a little water, twice daily; or 300mg in capsule form, daily. You could also try the herbs ginkgo biloba (*Ginkgo biloba*) and devil's claw (*Harpogophytum procumbent*). Take them at the same dosage as hawthorn.

HOMOCYSTEINE AND HEART DISEASE

When you eat protein, your body creates a toxic amino acid called homocysteine. Your body has to detoxify it, render it harmless, and excrete it through your urine. If this process goes awry, the homocysteine builds up in your blood, leading to abnormal blood clotting and to narrowing of your arteries. I advise all my patients to ask their doctor for a homocysteine test as well as a cholesterol test. If you find your levels are too high, get plenty of exercise, which can lower levels of homocysteine in your blood. In addition, B-vitamins (B6, B12, and folic acid) help detoxify homocysteine, so supplement at these dosages:

- Vitamin B6 (25–50mg)
- Vitamin B12 (500µg)
- Folic acid (0.5–5mg)

OTHER NATURAL TREATMENTS

Homeopathy In homeopathy, heart disease and high cholesterol are a constitutional problem and so need individual treatment. Using the appropriate remedies, the homeopath will aim to lower cholesterol, stop the formation of plaque in the arteries, and work on lowering blood pressure.

Acupuncture Acupuncture has been used in clinical trials to successfully lower cholesterol, so it's definitely a treatment worth exploring for heart disease in general. In Traditional Chinese Medicine, the left side of the heart connects to the liver meridian, and the right side of the heart connects to the lungs. Don't be surprised if your acupuncturist appears to be working on many organs in order to strengthen your heart.

SELF-HELP

Stop smoking Smoking not only causes lung disease, it causes heart disease, too. Stop.

Limit alcohol Too much alcohol can increase the triglycerides levels in your blood. Aim for no more than one glass of wine on two or three days of the week.

Get fit Exercise is important for the health of your heart because it improves circulation and can improve the ratio of good (HDL) to bad (LDL) cholesterol. Aim for 30 minutes of moderate to vigorous exercise daily.

Reduce stress Stress and anxiety can contribute to an increased risk of high blood pressure. Use the information on pages 309–11 to reduce your stress levels.

Weigh in It's never healthy to be overweight, but this is especially true when it comes to the risk of heart disease. However, a good indicator of the relative risks to your heart is where you store fat on your body. If you carry more weight around your middle, rather than on your hips, you're at a higher risk.

Most women who have been through menopause notice that they put on a few extra inches around their waist. Your body will be reluctant to lose this extra weight because fat is a manufacturing plant for estrogen, which helps protect your bones from osteoporosis. While this is good news for your bones, it's not such good news for your heart.

The BMI (body mass index) isn't the best test or measure for fat around the middle. Instead, to assess your susceptibility to heart problems, find your waist-to-hip ratio. Take a tape measure and compare your waist measurement (at the narrowest point) with your hip measurement (at the widest point). Then divide your waist figure by your hip figure. For example: 34in. waist divided by 37in. hip = a hip to waist ratio of 0.9. If your result is greater than 0.8, you're "apple shaped" (carrying weight around the middle) and you need to take action.

YOGA FOR YOUR HEART

Yoga tones muscles, helping with the breakdown of cholesterol. This is the Warrior pose.

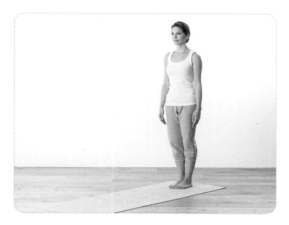

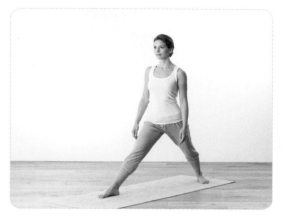

1 Stand, feet together, arms by your sides. Breathe deeply, in and out, to focus your mind. Feel your feet connecting with the floor.

2 Breathe in, turn your left foot outward, and step forward with your right foot about 3 feet. Breathe out. Try not to wobble.

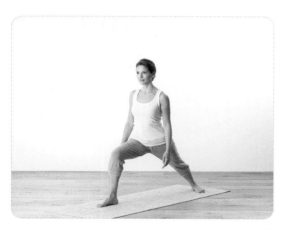

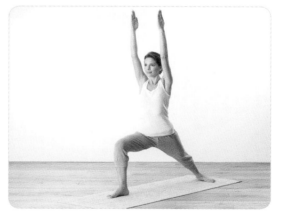

3 Breathe in; as you breathe out bend your right knee keeping your left heel grounded. Aim to get your right thigh parallel to the ground.

4 Breathe in. As you breathe out, raise your arms over your head, palms facing. Hold for 6–8 breaths. Breathe in. Exhale and straighten your right leg; bring your arms to your sides. Step your right leg back. Repeat, left leg forward.

Stress incontinence

Although stress incontinence is most typically associated with pregnancy, declining levels of estrogen during and after menopause can lower muscular tone, increasing the risk of leakage.

Most of the causes of stress incontinence are to do with a weakening of the tissues that support various structures in your body, in this case your bladder. It's all about your internal strength.

If you've been through menopause and you experience leaking when you cough, laugh, sneeze, exercise, or lift, or if you get an urge to go to the toilet that comes without warning, you probably suffer from stress incontinence. You may even leak without realizing it.

CONVENTIONAL TREATMENTS

Although many women simply live with this condition, I urge you to see your doctor so that he or she can rule out any serious cause. Your doctor will typically offer you one of two techniques for providing relief.

Surgical techniques If you're offered surgery, it's likely to come in one of two forms. The first is a sling operation. This takes around half an hour and usually requires only a local anaesthetic. Two incisions are made: one in your groin and another in your vagina. Through these, a surgeon inserts a piece of surgical tissue to form a sling to support your urethra and vagina, essentially doing the work of the weakened muscles. You'll usually be out of hospital within 24 hours. Or, you may be offered colposuspension. Performed under general anaesthetic, this operation requires an incision just above your bikini line. Surgeons tighten the pelvic floor muscles with stitches, lifting the neck of the bladder. Surgery for stress incontinence has a good success rate, but in some cases the problem returns.

OTHER TYPES OF URINARY INCONTINENCE

Stress incontinence is not the only type of urinary incontinence you may have. The others include:

URGE INCONTINENCE
This occurs when women can't hold their urine long enough to get to a bathroom. Healthy women can have the condition, but it occurs most often in women with diabetes, stroke, Alzheimer's disease, Parkinson's disease, or multiple sclerosis. It may also be an early sign of bladder cancer.

OVERFLOW INCONTINENCE
This is when small amounts of urine leak from a full bladder, and it's typically caused by diabetes and spinal cord injury.

FUNCTIONAL INCONTINENCE
This occurs in women with normal bladder control, who can't get to a bathroom in time because of a disorder, such as arthritis, which stops them from moving quickly.

Collagen bladder-neck injections Your doctor will recommend these if your incontinence is caused by a weak outlet valve in your bladder, or if you've tried surgery and it didn't work. You'll be given a local anaesthetic, and your surgeon will fill your bladder with water and then inject collagen (the connective tissue for bones and skin) into several places along the bladder neck. This plumps up the bladder wall and makes the urethral tube smaller, so you experience more resistance to passing urine. The procedure has a good success rate (up to 70 percent). The only side-effects are those from the operation (passing blood or stinging when urinating), which subside in a few days.

YOUR DIET

Your muscles, ligaments, and soft tissues all need vital nutrients to perform at optimum levels. This means revising your diet so it's as healthy as it can be is an essential first step to overcoming stress incontinence. See my tips on pages 24–9 to decide where you might need to make changes.

Try drinking a glass of unsweetened cranberry juice daily. Although this is most well known as a successful natural remedy for urinary tract infections and cystitis (see p.153), it can also help prevent incontinence. (You can take it in capsule form, if you prefer (200–300mg, once a day).

SUPPLEMENTS

You can use supplements to help improve muscle control and strengthen collagen in your body.

- VITAMIN A (25,000iu daily, as beta-carotene) This vitamin can help the body to produce collagen and enhance the strength of your cartilage, which keeps the organs in your pelvic area in position.

- VITAMIN C with bioflavonoids (500mg, twice daily, as magnesium ascorbate) This can also help encourage the formation of collagen in your tissues.

- CALCIUM (1,000mg, daily) and MAGNESIUM (500mg, daily) Take these minerals together to improve urinary muscle control.

HERBS

Take 300mg of each of the following herbs, in capsule form, twice daily; or combine the tinctures of each in equal parts and then take 1 tsp. of the combined tincture in a little water, twice daily.

- HORSETAIL (*Equisetum arvense*) This herb has a high silica content. This compound is important for healthy ligaments and it helps provide good amounts of collagen.

- LADIES' MANTLE (*Alchemilla vulgaris*) Ladies' mantle has an astringent effect on the body, helping to tighten up tissue and ligaments.

OTHER NATURAL TREATMENTS

Homeopathy Take the appropriate remedies from the following list at 30c potency, twice a daily. Consult a practitioner for a constitutional treatment plan, too.
• Causticum is useful if you feel you need to go to the toilet frequently
• Nat mur helps balance the changes to your hormones following menopause

Acupuncture An acupuncturist inserts needles along meridians, including the urinary bladder and liver meridians, to help strengthen the pelvic floor.

SELF-HELP

Tighten your pelvic floor The single, most important thing you can do for yourself is to tighten up your pelvic floor muscles, using Kegel exercises (see box, p.127). Practice these exercises at least once a day.

Monitor your fluids It's important to drink between six and eight glass of water a day, but it's also important not to drink too much. Try to keep a note of how much water, juice, and herbal tea you are drinking because these all count towards your fluid intake. Once you've reached eight glasses of liquid in a day, think twice before drinking any more. Experiment with the amount you drink and see how your fluid intake affects the stress incontinence until you find a happy medium.

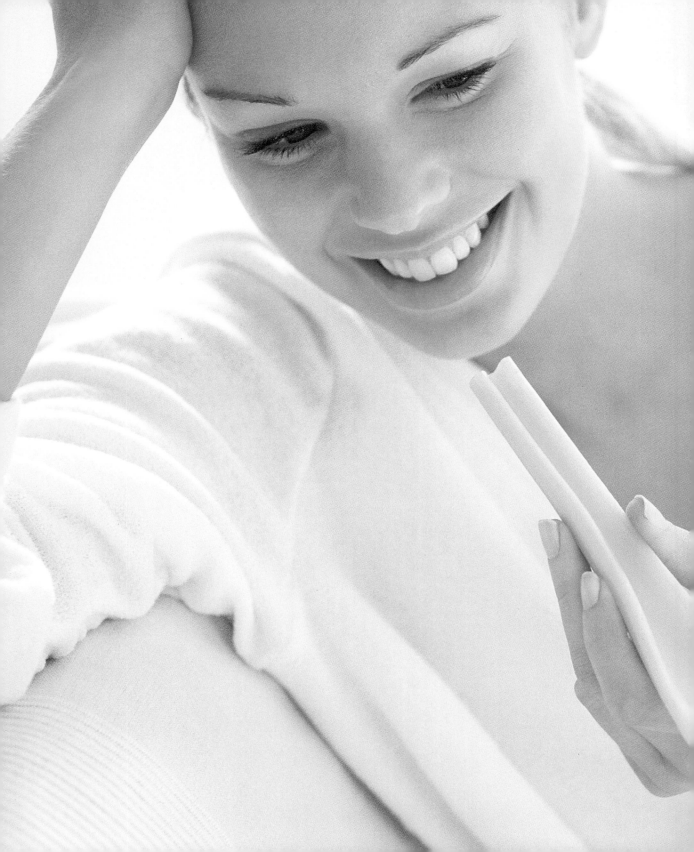

Optimum healthcare 5

Many of the health problems women face throughout their lives are caused by an unhealthy diet, a lack of exercise, an overload of stress, and the hormonal imbalances and body-system malfunctions that these poor lifestyle choices cause. But it doesn't have to be this way. As I hope this book has shown you, there are many, many things you can do to optimize your health and to balance your hormones so every system in your body is functioning at its peak.

This chapter is all about taking care of your whole self—helping you feel and look great so that you naturally start to make healthier lifestyle choices, giving you a long, happy, beautiful life. We start by looking at weight, then your immune system, then the signs of aging, and, finally, the importance of dealing with stress. Optimum healthcare is about using natural approaches to find both your inner and outer beauty and well-being. My hope is that you'll use this chapter at every stage of your life to look and feel great.

Optimizing your weight

Millions of women follow diets, visit diet clubs, read weight-loss books, and look for low-calorie and low-fat foods when they visit the supermarket. We seem to be preoccupied with weight loss.

We're far more likely than men to go on a diet. But being thin, or weighing little, isn't always the answer—it's more important to be the right weight for your height and build, whatever that weight might be.

WHY DO WE FOCUS ON WEIGHT SO MUCH?

We all have an inbuilt image of the "body beautiful"—a mind's-eye projection of what it would be like to be "perfect." I don't think there's a woman who comes into my clinic who wouldn't change something about herself—a thinner waist, more toned arms, a smaller bottom, skinnier thighs, bigger eyes, or glossier hair. I think, partly, this is to do with the media, but not just today's newspapers and magazines. Throughout modern history, painters and then photographers have captured beauty and held their images up as icons of perfection—visions we mere mortals should aspire to. In addition, fashion gurus have drawn our eye and attention not just to how to look but to what to wear. It's been a bit of an obsession—often not a healthy one.

Medically, women are more likely than men to suffer from conditions such as an underactive thyroid (see pp.58–61) and PCOS (see pp.83–7), which can lead to weight problems. We're also more likely to lose weight as a result of an eating disorder. Any medically triggered weight problem needs help from your doctor—to balance hormones in the case of thyroid and PCOS and to seek counseling if you suffer from anorexia, bulimia, or other eating problems. These conditions can have serious consequences for organ function.

In this section, though, I'll focus on what tends to be the bigger issue—that of being overweight. I want to look at restoring your healthy weight, using natural methods for long-lasting (permanent) results. The truth is that beauty is about being healthy. Once you're healthy, your skin glows, your hair shines, your eyes sparkle, and your weight optimizes. You'll feel perfect, regardless what any modern "ideal" seems to be.

WHAT SHOULD YOU WEIGH?

In my opinion height and weight tables are unreliable methods of assessing a healthy weight. Throughout the book, you'll have found that I've asked you to check your BMI—body mass index. Although this is a standard measure of whether your weight is right for your height, it really is just a ratio of height to weight and doesn't tell you how much body fat you're carrying. So, for example, you could have a completely sedentary lifestyle and weigh the same as an athlete. You'd have the same BMI score, but you'd have completely different percentages of body fat, and you'd be considerably less healthy. A rugby player, who's made almost entirely of muscle, might find himself in the obese category on a BMI chart, even though he has very little body fat and is, in fact, perfectly healthy.

However, if you don't have access to scales that can calculate your percentage of body fat (see box, p.298), your BMI is the next-best tool at hand. It will give you some indication of whether or not you need to lose or gain weight. Then, just try to be honest with yourself as to whether that weight is made up of fat or muscle.

HOW TO CALCULATE YOUR BODY MASS INDEX (BMI)

Use this chart to give yourself a rough idea of whether or not you need to lose weight. Calculate your BMI by multiplying your weight in pounds by 703, then dividing that number by the square of your height in inches. So, if my weight is 140lb. and my 5ft. 6in., my BMI is 140 x 703 / 66^2 = 22.5.

A BMI score of less than 18.5 indicates that you're underweight for your height; 18.6–24.9 represents normal weight for your height; 25–29.9 is an overweight reading; 30–39.9 is obese; and 40 or more is dangerously obese (meaning that this level of weight is putting your health dangerously at risk of heart disease and diabetes).

WEIGHT (LB)

HEIGHT (FT)	100	105	110	115	120	125	130	135	140	145	150	155	160	165	170	175	180	185	190	195	200	205	210	215	220	225	230	235	240	245	250	HEIGHT (CM)
5'0"	19	20	21	22	23	24	25	26	27	28	29	30	31	32	33	34	35	36	37	38	39	40	41	42	43	44	45	46	47	48	49	152
5'1"	18	19	20	21	22	23	24	25	26	27	28	29	30	31	32	33	34	35	36	36	37	38	39	40	42	43	44	44	45	46	47	155
5'2"	18	19	20	21	22	22	23	24	25	26	27	28	29	30	31	32	33	33	34	35	36	37	38	39	40	41	42	43	44	45	46	157
5'3"	17	18	19	20	21	22	23	24	24	25	26	27	28	29	30	31	32	32	33	34	35	36	37	38	39	40	41	42	43	43	44	160
5'4"	17	18	18	19	20	21	22	23	24	24	25	26	27	28	29	30	31	31	32	33	34	35	36	37	38	39	40	40	41	42	43	163
5'5"	16	17	18	19	20	20	21	22	23	24	25	25	26	27	28	29	30	30	31	32	33	34	35	36	37	37	38	39	40	41	42	165
5'6"	16	17	17	18	19	20	21	21	22	23	24	25	25	26	27	28	29	29	30	31	32	33	34	34	35	36	37	38	39	40	40	168
5'7"	15	16	17	18	18	19	20	21	22	22	23	24	25	25	26	27	28	29	29	30	31	32	33	33	34	35	36	37	38	38	39	170
5'8"	15	16	16	17	18	19	19	20	21	22	22	23	24	25	25	26	27	28	28	29	30	31	32	32	33	34	35	36	37	37	38	173
5'9"	14	15	16	17	17	18	19	20	20	21	22	22	23	24	25	25	26	27	28	28	29	30	31	31	32	33	34	35	35	36	37	175
5'10"	14	15	15	16	17	18	18	19	20	20	21	22	23	23	24	25	25	26	27	28	28	29	30	31	32	32	33	34	34	35	36	178
5'11"	14	14	15	16	16	17	18	18	19	20	21	21	22	23	23	24	25	25	26	27	28	28	29	30	31	31	32	33	34	34	35	180
6'0"	13	14	14	15	16	17	17	18	19	19	20	21	21	22	23	23	24	25	25	26	27	27	28	29	30	31	31	32	33	33	34	183
6'1"	13	13	14	15	15	16	17	17	18	19	19	20	21	21	22	23	23	24	25	25	26	27	27	28	29	30	30	31	32	32	33	185
6'2"	12	13	14	14	15	16	16	17	18	18	19	19	20	21	21	22	23	23	24	25	25	26	27	27	28	29	30	30	31	31	32	188
6'3"	12	13	13	14	15	15	16	16	17	18	18	19	20	20	21	21	22	23	23	24	25	25	26	26	28	28	29	29	30	31	31	191
6'4"	12	12	13	14	14	15	15	16	17	17	18	18	19	20	20	21	22	22	23	23	24	25	25	26	27	27	28	29	29	30	30	193
	45	48	50	52	54	57	59	61	63	66	68	70	73	75	77	79	82	84	86	88	91	93	95	97	100	102	104	107	109	111	113	

WEIGHT (KG)

UNDERWEIGHT BMI LESS THAN 18.5   **HEALTHY WEIGHT** BMI 18.6–24.9   **OVERWEIGHT** BMI 25–29.9   **OBESE** BMI 30–39.9   **DANGEROUSLY OBESE** BMI 40 AND ABOVE

BODY-FAT SCALES

In view of the fact that a BMI reading is really only one indicator of your health, you can now buy scales that not only give you your weight, but can also give you a measurement of your body-fat percentage. While you stand on the scale, a small electric current passes through your feet. The current takes longer to travel through fat than it does to travel through muscle, so the speed at which this impulse makes it through your body enables the machine to calculate how much fat you carry.

WHAT CAUSES WEIGHT GAIN?

It's easy to think that weight gain is controlled only by the mechanism of calories in and energy out. Although this is mostly the case, and you certainly won't lose weight unless you burn more calories than you consume, there are a number of other reasons for weight gain—and you may find some of them surprising.

Dieting

It's official! Studies now prove conclusively that dieting makes you fat. It's simple really. When you restrict your food intake, your body thinks there's a shortage of food and it doesn't know how long this "famine" is going to last. As a result, it does a number of things.

First, your body slows down your metabolism so you don't burn so many of the calories it thinks are scarce; and, second, it lets go of muscle and water first to preserve your fat reserves. The overall result is that it looks as though you're losing weight, but in reality, you're losing water and muscle and slowing down your metabolism. The result is that you eat like a bird, but after an initial loss, your weight plateaus. When you eat normally again, the weight piles on—as fat.

Overeating and under-exercising

As I've already mentioned, "calories in" have to be fewer than "calories out" for you to lose weight; if they're greater, you'll gain weight. However, it isn't quite that simple. To lose weight sustainably, you need to consider not just how many calories you consume, but what type. You need to eat healthy food from the three food groups: fats (mainly unsaturated fats), carbohydrates (mainly unrefined carbohydrates and healthy simple carbohydrates, such as fruit), and protein (such as fish, eggs, nuts, seeds). Omit one of these three important food groups and you'll hamper your efforts at weight loss.

Many overweight women simply eat too much bad fat and too many refined carbohydrates (such as cookies and cakes). Low-fat and no-fat diets don't work, either because they restrict the essential fats that help boost your metabolism. In addition, no-fat and low-fat foods often contain other unhealthy ingredients (often salt or sugar) to make them tastier. Anything that contains extra sugar triggers blood-sugar imbalances (see box, p.29), encouraging weight gain.

Nutritional deficiencies

You need good levels of vitamins, minerals, essential fats, and amino acids for your body to be in good health and for it to burn off excess fat when appropriate. If your body registers that you have an increased need for certain nutrients, it can create cravings. Or, if you have a particular nutritional deficiency, it may increase your appetite in the hope of plugging the gaps. If you respond by eating food that's of poor quality and lacking in nutrients, your body may continue to prompt you to eat in order to get enough nourishment—the cravings go on, and so does the weight.

Food intolerances and allergies

A food intolerance is a reaction to certain foods that doesn't involve your immune system—perhaps you lack certain enzymes that permit your body to process a food correctly, resulting in abdominal pain or nausea.

A food allergy, on the other hand, involves an immune reaction. Your immune system thinks you've eaten something harmful and releases histamine to defuse the harmful substance. Common allergic reactions include hives, rashes, and throat swelling. Perversely, reactions as a result of some food intolerance can lead to a slight addiction to the culprit food, leading you to crave and then overeat that food and so gain weight.

Prescription drugs

Some drugs can cause weight gain. The most obvious culprits are steroids—although never be tempted to come off steroids suddenly, always talk to your doctor first. The Pill, hormone replacement therapy, and anti-depressants may also cause weight gain.

Artificial sweeteners

Sugar is fattening, and many women use artificial sweeteners to help them to cut calories. Ironically, though, artificial sweeteners can actually increase your appetite, causing you to gain weight. The problem is that because they give you a sweet taste without the calories, your brain gets confused and starts looking for the "missing" calories by triggering your appetite.

Candida infection (yeast overgrowth)

If you suffer from a yeast infection, such as candida (see pp.144–7), your digestion is compromised because the proportion of "healthy" bacteria in your gut is low in comparison to "unhealthy" bacteria. If your digestion is poor, you aren't getting the nutrients you need to lose weight.

CONVENTIONAL TREATMENTS

There are three main ways in which your doctor is likely to suggest you lose weight. The first is by suggesting that you diet. Then, if the problem is severe, he or she may suggest one of the following two options.

HOW TO FIT IN REGULAR EXERCISE

Healthy eating is crucial for optimum weight loss, but it must be combined with regular exercise. Exercise lowers your risk of breast cancer, boosts your immunity, keeps your digestion functioning efficiently, helps balance your blood sugar and your hormones, and boosts your metabolism. Include both aerobic exercise and weight-training for the most effective weight loss.

THREE OR FOUR TIMES A WEEK, TRY TO:
• Do 40 minutes' aerobic exercise (such as swimming, cycling, jogging, or running)
• Do 30 minutes of weight, resistance, or strength training. Push ups, pull downs, lunges, and squats are all good muscle-builders that burn fat.

EVERY DAY, TRY TO:
• Walk 10,000 steps. Invest in a pedometer—you'll be amazed at how quickly the steps build up if you simply get off the bus one stop early, or walk the children to school
• Do 30 minutes of something vigorous, such as gardening or power-cleaning the house.

If you're new to exercise, start slowly and never push yourself too far. Aerobic exercise should make your heart beat faster, but not make you breathless (runners say that you should be able to hold a conversation while you run). Increase the time you spend exercising, rather than the speed. Gentle for longer is better than short, fast bursts.

Weight-loss medication If you're clinically obese, your doctor may offer you medication, such as the drug orlistat. This medication inhibits the enzyme that enables your body to break down fat, absorb it, and store it. As a result, the fat in your food simply passes through your digestive system and out again without entering your body. Although this sounds like a marvellous solution, the medication will also stop your body absorbing fat-soluble vitamins such as vitamins A, D, E, and K, which are essential for your general health. You may also suffer "anal leakage" (the leaking of an oily, sometimes fecal discharge from the anus), which is prevented only if you adopt a strictly low-fat diet.

Surgery This is typically the last option your doctor will offer you, when all other attempts at weight loss have failed. Surgical options include stomach stapling or gastric bands (to physically reduce the size of your stomach so that you feel full quicker), liposuction (which sucks fat from your body), and jaw wiring (in which your jaw is wired so that you can't open your mouth wide enough to eat solid food; the wire is removed only once you've reached your target weight). None of these approaches is necessarily permanent, and all of them carry risks.

YOUR DIET

The only way to successfully and permanently lose weight is to change your eating habits for the rest of your life. Follow my advice on healthy eating on pages 24–9, paying particular heed to the sections on eating unrefined carbohydrates and keeping your blood-sugar levels balanced.

Avoid sugar, artificial sweeteners, and refined foods and try to follow the principles of a low glycemic index (GI) diet. GI measures how fast sugar hits your bloodstream. A faster sugar-hit is more likely to raise your body's insulin levels, in turn preventing it from breaking down stored fat. To lose weight you need to be eating foods that give you a steady, slow sugar release so that fat is burned as energy. Whole grains, vegetables, nuts, and seeds that are close to their natural state have a low GI. In addition, add protein to each meal. The combination of protein and carbohydrate slows down the rate of your digestion, which means that this combination keeps your blood sugar more stable, making it easier to lose weight. Finally, make sure you get enough essential fatty acids from oily fish (such as anchovies and sardines) and nuts and seeds because your body needs essential fats for weight loss.

SUPPLEMENTS

- B-COMPLEX (containing 25mg of each B-vitamin, daily) These essential weight-loss nutrients help the body produce energy, help control fat metabolism, and are important for blood-sugar and hormone balance.

- CHROMIUM (200µg, daily) Your body needs this nutrient to regulate insulin and control levels of blood sugar, fat, and cholesterol.

- MAGNESIUM CITRATE (300mg, daily) and MANGANESE (5mg, daily) Both of these supplements are important for blood-sugar balance, while manganese also helps produce energy and metabolize fat.

- ZINC (15mg, daily) This mineral is important for balancing your hormones and controlling appetite.

- CO-ENZYME Q10 (25–30mg, daily) This antioxidant supplement is vital for energy production and has been shown to help boost weight loss.

HERBS

When you're trying to lose weight, herbs that boost liver function (see box, p.43) are important because a healthy liver is essential for detoxifying the body and for efficient digestion. In addition, try the following.

- DANDELION (*Taraxacum officinale*) This herb can boost weight loss because it's a natural diuretic. It encourages your body to release fluids without making it lose vital minerals and other nutrients. Take 1 tsp. tincture in a little water, twice daily; or 200–400mg in capsule form, daily.

Opposite: Sardines

OTHER NATURAL TREATMENTS

Homeopathy Homeopathic remedies are usually tailored to your individual needs (visit a homeopath for a unique treatment plan), but some good remedies for weight loss include the following, and you can try these at home. Take those that are relevant to you in a 30c potency, twice daily for one week.

• Argentum nitricum if you have problems with cravings for sweet and sugary foods
• Calcarea carbonica if you tend to eat when you're stressed; it calms down your body
• Graphites if you're finding that you're gaining weight because you're going through menopause

Acupuncture As long as you have good nutritional help at the core of your treatment, acupuncture can give a significant boost to weight loss. It can stimulate the body to release endorphins, the "feel-good" neurotransmitters that help control appetite and, therefore, cravings and overeating. Although a practitioner is likely to focus on your spleen and thyroid meridians (see p.47) to help improve your metabolism and blood-sugar balance, he or she will also tailor your therapy to take into account the root cause of your weight gain (whether the cause is physical or emotional).

Massage Most natural therapies could be recommended for weight loss, but I particularly recommend massage because it can help boost circulation and detoxification. Cleansing your system helps remove fat reserves. If you can, treat yourself to a full-body massage once a month, or even once every two months.

Aromatherapy Grapefruit essential oil may be especially potent for weight loss because research shows that its primary component (limonene) can reduce appetite. Add 15 drops grapefruit essential oil to 6 tsp. carrier oil, such as sweet almond. Use it in a massage at home. Abdominal and thigh massages are particularly straightforward for self-practice. Gently knead the flesh over your abdomen and thighs (back and front), working the oil into your skin.

SELF-HELP

Chew your food Take your time when you eat and make sure you chew properly—digestion begins in the mouth, and it's essential that you mix your food properly with saliva. Also, remember that it takes 20 minutes for your brain to register that you've eaten enough—if you eat too quickly, your brain hasn't had time to notice that you're full, leading you to overeat.

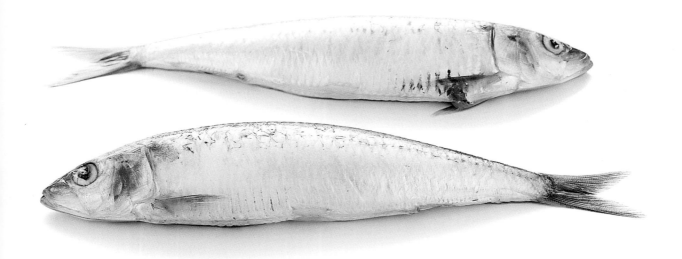

Boosting your immunity

Like an invisible army, your immune system diligently patrols your body, working around the clock to fight bacteria, viruses, or other enemies that can poison your system.

For good health, I cannot stress enough how important it is for your immune system to be working at optimum levels. Only then can it protect you from infection and heal you quickly when you're ill.

SYMPTOMS VS ILLNESS

The first step towards strong immunity is to change how you think about symptoms. Contrary to popular belief, common symptoms, such as a cough, high fever, runny nose, a discharge, or a stomach upset, are signs your immune system is doing its job. Using drugs to ease symptoms of illness compromises your immune system, hampering its natural healing ability.

Treating your symptoms is not the goal of natural medicine. The premise of preventative medicine and the foundation stone of all natural health techniques is to ensure that your immune system is strong when you aren't ill, so that it can fight invaders properly.

WHAT AFFECTS YOUR IMMUNITY?

A number of factors can affect your immune system. The most common offenders include the following:

Lack of sleep

While you sleep your body is busy repairing, rejuvenating, and healing. It's also the time when your natural killer cells get on the move, fighting infection from foreign invaders. If you don't sleep enough, this important aspect of your immunity can't do its work, and the number of killer cells in your body falls, making you more generally prone to infection.

A poor diet

In no sense is the phrase, "you are what you eat" more true than with regard to protecting your body's immune defences. Good nutrients are essential for every part of your immune system. When you eat healthily, you give your body the basic building blocks it needs for renewal, repair, and defence against illness.

Stress overload

When you're under stress, your adrenal glands release too much cortisol, which hampers your immune response, increasing your risk of infection and inflammation, and, according to some studies, diabetes, cancer, autoimmune problems, early aging, and arthritis.

Overuse of antibiotics

The regular use of antibiotics upsets your gut's balance of healthy bacteria, which help fight off invaders.

Too many toxins

Environmental toxins (in the air and water, and in your food) compromise your immune response because they divert precious energy from fighting infection to eliminating these harmful substances.

Emotional upset

Depression, unhappiness, anxiety, and a negative attitude to life all seem to have an inhibiting effect on immunity. Scientific studies consistently show that people with an upbeat, positive outlook have more robust immune systems.

It stands to reason that if all these factors weaken your immunity, avoiding them or working to overcome them will help boost your immunity. The most important immunity-boosters are to eat a healthy, immunity-boosting diet; to learn to relax (see pp.309–11); and to avoid environmental toxins by getting plenty of fresh, unpolluted air and eating organic foods.

YOUR DIET

A good diet will keep you generally healthy, but you can also consume or avoid certain foods to specifically help your body fight off bacteria, yeasts, and viruses.

Avoid sugar Studies show that diets high in sugar can reduce the ability of neutrophils (white blood cells) to engulf and destroy bacteria and inhibit the ability of infection-fighting lymphocytes to produce antibodies that neutralize invading microorganisms. It's estimated that just 24 tsp. of added sugar a day can hamper your white blood cells' ability to kill bacteria by up to 40 percent. You may think that 24 tsp. sounds like a lot, but sugar can mount up easily because it's added not only to sweet foods but to savoury foods, such as soups and sauces, too. It's thought that generally we consume around 30 tsp. sugar daily.

Eat in color My mother always used always to tell me to "eat your greens." Now, though, we should eat a rainbow. Colourful fruits and vegetables contain antioxidants, which protect your cells from free-radical damage and strengthen your immunity. The well-known antioxidants are beta-carotene, vitamins A, C, and E, and also the minerals selenium and zinc. By choosing a variety of foods in different colors, you'll be sure to get a range of antioxidants.

For greens, go for broccoli and kale (which you should steam rather than eat raw or heavily cooked). Try watercress, too, as it's packed with powerful anti-oxidants, including those essential for healthy eye function. Then, think of all the other brightly colored fruit and vegetables you can include in your diet: toma-toes, pumpkin, corn, sweet potatoes, apples, citrus fruits, kiwi fruit, papayas, strawberries, blackcurrants, red, yellow, and green peppers, and so on. When choosing berries, go for blueberries, which have the strongest antioxidant effect of all the berries.

Boost beneficial bacteria Your gut is home to 70 percent of your immune system. It's your body's largest barrier between you and the outside world. The stronger that barrier, the stronger your immune defences. The gut's defences come in the form of beneficial bacteria (probiotics). One such probiotic is lactobacillus acidophilus, which is also found in yogurt with active cultures. In order to colonize the gut, probiotics "feed off" prebiotics, making it important that you eat plenty of prebiotics, too. Prebiotics occur naturally in foods such as garlic, onions, leeks, asparagus, Jerusalem artichokes, chicory, peas, beans, lentils, oats, and bananas.

WHEN TO HAVE AN IMMUNITY BOOST

Your body sends you several signs if your immune system is in danger. Among these are:

- Fatigue
- Listlessness
- Repeated infections (healthy adults get two or three colds a year; if you get sick more than four times a year, your immunity's in trouble)
- Inflammation anywhere in the body
- Allergic reactions
- Slow wound healing
- Chronic diarrhea
- Yeast infections, such as oral thrush, candidiasis (candida overgrowth in the body), or vaginal yeast infections

IMMUNITY SUPERFOODS

I think all healthy foods are superfoods, but some have extra-special immunity-boosting powers. These include garlic, which contains antimicrobial compounds (see opposite); and nuts and seeds, which provide antioxidants including zinc, selenium, and vitamin E, and essential fats. Seaweeds contain zinc and selenium and may have anti-cancer effects. Experiment with the different seaweed varieties: add kombu to soups; or toast some nori and sprinkle it on rice or oatmeal. Mushrooms, especially shiitake mushrooms, are antiviral and antibacterial because they may enhance the activity of your immunity's white blood cells.

Boost omega-3 Essential fatty acids increase the action of you body's phagocytes, white blood cells that engulf bacteria. Eat oily fish, such as mackerel, sardines, salmon, trout, and fresh tuna, at least three times a week. If you don't like fish or are vegetarian, you can use flax seed oil in your diet instead. Add it to salad dressings or mix it into a smoothie. Always use this oil raw (don't cook with it) because heating it up damages it, making it harmful.

YOUR DRINKING HABITS

As important for your immune system as it is for your general health, water transports nutrients to your cells and carries away toxins, helping to make you less vulnerable to infection. Aim for six to eight glasses of water or herbal tea a day. To get a double benefit, you could start your day with a glass of warm water mixed with the juice of a lemon. Like all citrus fruits, lemons contain antioxidants called bioflavonoids. These help improve immune function.

Although you should drink enough to flush out toxins, try to avoid drinking substances (diuretics) that cause you to lose valuable immunity-boosting nutrients, such as zinc. So avoid alcohol and drinks containing caffeine as much as you can. Save alcohol for special occasions and drink green rather than black tea, and instead of coffee. Although green tea does contain some caffeine, it also contains powerful antioxidants—called polyphenols—that may inhibit the growth of cancer cells.

SUPPLEMENTS

Take these supplements on a daily basis, especially during winter. You can break over the summer, but take them again if you feel illness coming on, or if a "bug" is going round.

■ B-COMPLEX (containing 25mg of each B-vitamin, daily) B-vitamins help produce antibodies and are needed for the proper function of lymphocytes (a type of white blood cell), which help fight infection and disease.

■ VITAMIN C with bioflvonoids (500mg, twice daily, as magnesium ascorbate) Take this antioxidant as a separate supplement because the amount in a multi is usually too low. Vitamin C is essential for the production of white blood cells, which fight off disease.

■ ANTIOXIDANTS Every woman, however healthy, would benefit from making sure their daily multi-vitamin and mineral contains adequate amounts of the following powerful antioxidants: vitamins A (2,500iu) and E (400iu) and the minerals zinc (15mg) and selenium (100μg).

■ OMEGA-3 FATTY ACIDS (1,000mg fish oil, containing at least 700mg EPA and 500mg DHA, daily) Omega-3 fatty acids are anti-inflammatory and can boost immune-system function (see far left). (Use flax seed oil if you're vegetarian.)

■ PROBIOTICS (containing at least ten billion organisms per capsule; one capsule daily) This supplement helps increase the friendly bacteria in your gut, which help keep yeast, unhealthy bacteria, and other invaders in check, protecting you from infection.

HERBS

■ ASTRAGALUS (*Astragalus membranaceus*) Studies show that astragalus is a tonic to the immune system, and it's particularly good for fighting off colds and flu. When you feel illness coming on, take 1 tsp. astragalus tincture, twice daily; or 500–900mg in capsule form, daily, until you feel your immune system is stronger.

■ ECHINACEA (*Echinacea purpurea*) This immunity-boosting herb enhances lymphatic function and is antiviral. It works best when you take it with breaks (say, for example, ten days on, three days off, ten days on, and so on). Begin taking the herb as soon as you feel you're coming down with something and then take it through the duration of the illness and for a couple of weeks afterward. During the cold season, you may want to supplement generally with echinacea once or twice a week. Whatever frequency you use, each day take 1 tsp. tincture in a little water, three times a day; or 300–400mg in capsule form, twice daily.

■ GARLIC (*Allium sativum*) Garlic contains allicin, which is antibacterial, antiviral, and antifungal. Take an aged garlic supplement (1,000mg, daily) as a preventative.

OTHER NATURAL TREATMENTS

Homeopathy A homeopath chooses immunity-boosting remedies according to your physical and emotional health, but you can try the following at home. Choose the most appropriate remedies from the list below and take 30c twice daily when you're fighting an infection. Stop when your symptoms improve.

• Arsenicum album is the remedy to use if you're restless and often worry about your health; you feel that everything has to be in its place; and tend to be generally negative in your approach to life

• Nux vomica is for you if you're competitive and highly strung; you easily fly off the handle and are impatient

• Pulsatilla is useful if you're shy and gentle; you may find it difficult to make decisions and may not express anger easily; you tend to avoid confrontation and often cry easily

Acupuncture An acupuncturist will assess your general condition and then make the decision as to which acupuncture points to stimulate and which meridians to balance. Research shows that balancing just the stomach meridian can improve general immune function. If you have an acute immunity problem, such as a cold or the flu, the practitioner may stimulate your gall-bladder meridian.

SELF-HELP

Apart from avoiding toxins and learning to relax, try the following to boost your immune system naturally.

Exercise A number of studies have found a clear link between moderate, regular exercise and a strong immune system. It seems that during exercise physiological changes occur in your body's defences that encourage your immune cells to circulate through your body faster and more efficiently. When you've finished exercising, though, your immune-system function returns to normal within a few hours. If you undertake consistent, regular exercise you can help make the changes more long-lasting.

Although exercise is undoubtedly an immunity-booster, it's important not to go overboard. Exercising too hard and for too long can have the opposite effect on your immune system, lowering it. In one study, more than an hour and a half of high-intensity endurance exercise a day made athletes susceptible to illness for up to 72 hours after the exercise session. My advice is to aim to do 30-minute exercise sessions at least five times a week. If you can, try to make these sessions (or as many of them as possible) in the open air, rather than in a gym. Walking, cycling, and running or jogging are the obvious choices.

Have fun! Last, but by no means least, remember that one of the best ways to boost your immunity is to enjoy your life. Many studies have found that happiness and a positive attitude are linked to a healthy immune system.

Beating the years

There's no need to accept that weight gain, wrinkles, dry skin, and a whole host of other problems are inevitable aspects of aging. Natural healing offers plenty of solutions to beat the clock.

Research shows that poor diet, too much sun, lack of exercise, and stress can speed up the aging process. On the other hand, you can combat the wear-and-tear factor by stalling the action of free radicals on your body.

FREE RADICALS AND AGING

Highly reactive compounds, free radicals are produced during your body's normal metabolic processes, and also by such things as air pollution and overheating certain oils. They can attack and damage the genetic code and memory of your cells and prevent your cells from producing energy.

This all sounds deeply complex, but the effects of free radicals are around us all the time. Have you ever seen what oxygen does to certain metals? Rust is a product of oxidization, triggered by free radicals. What about wrinkles? Free radicals are the culprits of those, too. They also contribute to cancer and heart disease.

You can't do anything to prevent free radicals, but your body does have defence mechanisms that can clear them away. Your major line of defence is through your diet. In addition, you can make certain lifestyle changes that can help you fight free-radical attack.

IT'S UP TO YOU

Age happens (free-radical attack seems to escalate over the age of 30), but how it happens and whether or not you look older than you should is—to a certain extent—up to you. You know you can avoid weight gain, heart disease, osteoporosis, and high cholesterol through diet and exercise. You know you can minimize wrinkles by taking care of your skin. Keeping your mind active can keep your brain young. You know that extra weight, aches and pains, memory loss, and so on can make you look and feel old. In other words, visible aging is at least partly a product of how you live your life and, particularly, how well you treat yourself.

In my opinion, it's never too early to start thinking about how well you're aging, and it's never too late to make positive changes. So, whether you're in your teens or your seventies, I urge you to start taking care of your body and your mind, and develop a battle plan to slow down the aging process in your body, so you can start to hold off the years with success.

YOUR DIET

A healthy diet is your front line of defence against aging, so follow my recommendations on pages 24–9. These will help prevent weight gain and poor health by keeping your blood-sugar levels and hormones balanced and by ensuring that every system in your body gets the nutrients it needs to function at optimum levels. It's especially important to make sure you eat at least five portions of vegetables and fruit, preferably organic, every day.

All vegetables are longevity foods, but perhaps the ones with the most power to prevent premature aging are leafy green vegetables, such as broccoli, Brussels sprouts, and kale. Leafy greens are loaded with nutrients that can help prevent free-radical attack. Studies show they can help block cancer, prevent heart attacks and obesity, and keep osteoporosis at bay.

HOW TO STAY BEAUTIFUL

The following are my top tips on how to maintain beautiful skin, hair, and eyes in as natural a way as possible. Make them the staples of your beauty routine.

YOUTHFUL SKIN
As you age, your skin naturally loses its elasticity, giving you a few lines. However, as well as eating healthily and avoiding over-exposure to the sun, there's plenty you can do to keep your skin smooth.
DRINK PLENTY OF WATER Water keeps your skin hydrated and helps flush out harmful toxins.
USE A CLEANSER Cleanse the skin on your face twice a day with a product suited to your skin type. Some cleansers contain good exfoliating ingredients. Then use a good moisturizer or face oil to keep wrinkles at bay. Choose products with the most natural, preferably organic, ingredients.
SMILE! Smiling takes years off your face. Keep smiling and try not to get too stressed or anxious, so that you keep frowns at bay.

BEAUTIFUL HAIR
Falling estrogen levels do affect the quality of your hair as you age, but dull hair needn't be an inevitability. Try the following to help your hair keep its shine.
USE GENTLE PRODUCTS Shampoos containing sodium laurel sulphate can dry out your hair. Use those made with essential oils, herbs, and vegetable oils. Essential oils such as rosemary and ylang ylang stimulate hair growth; lavender and tea tree help fight dandruff; and vegetable oils such as soy bean, safflower, and corn help condition the hair shaft.
MASSAGE YOUR SCALP Head massage nourishes the roots of your hair to stimulate hair growth.

USE A MULTI Take a multi-vitamin and mineral supplement that contains vitamins C and E, B-vitamins, and biotin to improve hair condition.

SHINY EYES
A nutritional deficiency can cause age-related eye problems. Bright eyes are a tell-tale sign of youth.
GET YOUR ANTIOXIDANTS These can reduce your risk of cataracts and macular degeneration (in which cells in the central retina die). Vitamin A can help protect against blindness; and lutein, vitamin C, and zinc may help alleviate glaucoma. Bioflavonoids and selenium are also important antioxidants for eye health. Here's where to find all these nutrients:

- Vitamin A: orange and yellow fruits and vegetables, such as carrots, sweet potatoes, and butternut squash; and fish
- Vitamin C: sweet peppers, kale, strawberries, broccoli, oranges, and cantaloupe
- Vitamin E: sunflower seeds, almonds, and hazelnuts
- Selenium: whole grains, eggs, garlic, and seafood
- Zinc: quinoa, lentils, and whole grains
- Bioflavonoids: cherries, grapes, and plums
- Lutein: leafy green vegetables, such as kale and collard greens

FEAST ON FATS Essential fatty acids may help ease symptoms of dry-eye syndrome and guard against macular damage. Find them in coldwater fish (salmon, mackerel, trout), hemp or flax seeds.

Boost antioxidants Although a well-balanced, nutritious diet is key to staying young, nutrients called antioxidants—vitamins A, C, and E, as well as zinc and selenium—are the key players in an anti-aging diet. Found in vegetables, nuts, and fruits, antioxidants are your body's defence against free-radical attack. Make sure you eat a rainbow of fruits and vegetables (see p.303) because different antioxidants are found in differently colored foods. For example, leafy green vegetables, berries, carrots, beets, and so on all contain different antioxidants, but all with the same free-radical fighting benefits.

Increase fats and B-vitamins Essential fatty acids (found in oily fish, nuts and flax seeds) and B-vitamins (found in whole grains) can help balance your hormones and keep your skin supple.

SUPPLEMENTS

In an ideal world, you would get an adequate intake of the above (and all) nutrients from the food you eat. However, because modern farming and processing techniques deplete the nutritional power of much of your food, I urge every woman to take a good-quality multi-vitamin and mineral every day—not as a replacement for a healthy diet, but as an insurance policy.

SELF-HELP

Build up a sweat Aside from a healthy diet, there is perhaps nothing of more benefit to your anti-aging plan than moderate exercise. Study after study shows that exercise can reverse many of the physiological changes that are normally associated with aging. Don't overdo it, though, as exercising too hard and for too long can have the opposite effect.

"Moderate" means about 30 minutes of aerobic exercise, five times a week. In addition, weight-bearing exercises, such as brisk walking, jogging,, and dancing can help keep your bones strong and prevent osteoporosis; stretching and yoga can help keep you flexible (there's nothing more aging than seized-up joints). Aim to do 30 minutes of weight-bearing or suppleness exercises two or three times a week.

Other research has found that exercise can help prevent age-related increases in weight, cholesterol, and blood pressure. As you get older, your metabolic rate (the rate at which your body burns fat), gradually slows down. However, regular exercise can help give your metabolism a boost. If you're over 60 and find the idea of regular workouts unappealing, consistent low-level exercise, such as taking the stairs instead of the elevator, parking the car far from the entrance to the supermarket, walking round the block for ten minutes, gardening, and housework, can also be beneficial and help prevent many of the problems that make women feel old before their time.

No smoking Not only does smoking damage your fertility, lower your immunity, and increase your risk of cancer and heart disease, it gives you dry skin and yellow teeth. The facial contortions required to puff on a cigarette leave you with unsightly wrinkles around your nose, mouth, and eyes. In fact, smoking is one of the fastest ways to accelerate the aging process. If you want to stay young-looking, you have to quit.

Enjoy the sun in moderation Lying in the sun for long periods of time or spending hours under a tanning machine may give you what you think is just a tan, but dermatologists call it "photoaging." This is because exposure to ultraviolet rays (from the sun or a sunbed) can cause wrinkles, age spots, and even cataracts. With overexposure, your skin eventually thickens and becomes leathery and harsh. The fairer your complexion, the more your skin will suffer.

This doesn't mean you should spend your life indoors. Studies show that you need at least 30 minutes of natural light every day so you don't become deficient in vitamin D. A deficiency can increase your risk of osteoporosis, heart disease, breast cancer, and, ironically, premature aging. As with everything in life, expose your skin to the sun in moderation.

Overcoming stress

There are two kinds of stress. Short-term stress is what you feel when you, say, miss a train, and it can have an energizing effect on your body. Long-term (chronic) stress can damage your health.

Long-term stress is often triggered by serious life events—you may be experiencing financial worries, job pressures, bereavement, or relationship issues. You know the stress is long-term when you have some of the symptoms listed in the box below. Thankfully, there are many natural approaches and coping strategies you can put in place to help you through the worst and overcome chronic stress altogether.

CONVENTIONAL OR NATURAL?

Most doctors treat the symptoms of stress rather than the underlying cause. Your doctor may offer you medication for, say, depression or high blood pressure. Although the medication may help you feel better in the short term, it won't solve the stress itself.

For this reason, the natural approach to stress-busting tends to be more effective. Natural medicine is designed to strengthen all your body systems so your stress response becomes more resilient. The following natural therapies can all help you beat stress. Bear in mind, though, that if your life is stressful, you also need to devise strategies to reduce your load. You may need to ask for practical help from someone else, overhaul your lifestyle, or simply find someone to talk to openly. Without positive action, no treatment plan will be as effective as it could be.

THE SYMPTOMS OF CHRONIC STRESS

If you experience two or more of the following symptoms for three months or more, you may be suffering from chronic stress.

- Sleep problems
- Tension (including neck, head, back, and shoulder pain)
- Digestive disorders
- Hair loss
- Fatigue
- High blood pressure
- Palpitations
- Chest pain
- Skin problems (such as hives, eczema, psoriasis, and rashes)
- Jaw pain
- Infertility
- Menstrual problems
- Sexual difficulties
- Immune suppression (making you prone to recurrent illness and infections)
- Nervousness, anxiety, and panic attacks
- Depression and moodiness
- Irritability and frustration
- Memory problems and lack of concentration

YOUR DIET

Follow my recommendations on pages 24–9 for a healthy, balanced diet. Also take into consideration the recommendations for taking care of your adrenal glands (see pp.66–9), which take a beating as they pump out adrenaline when you're under stress.

In addition, a stressed body uses up B-vitamins very quickly, so you need to make sure you get enough B-rich foods, such as whole grains, oily fish, eggs, brown rice, beans, sunflower seeds, and nuts.

Antioxidants can help repair the damage stress does to your cells. Try to eat lots of fresh, preferably organic, brightly colored fruits and vegetables. In particular, zinc is an essential antioxidant for any woman with a stressful lifestyle. Your body needs it for cell repair, efficient digestion, strong immunity, and fortified emotional health. You also need zinc for the production of the adrenal hormones. Natural sources of zinc include yeast, eggs, legumes, pumpkin seeds, seafood, and whole grains. A shortage of essential fats (EFAs) has been shown to trigger symptoms of stress, so add plenty of nuts, seeds, and oily fish to your diet.

Bear in mind, too, that unstable blood-sugar levels can trigger symptoms of stress, so follow the advice on balancing your blood sugar in the box on page 29. Avoid stimulants such as coffee, tea, nicotine, and sugar and keep alcohol intake to a minimum.

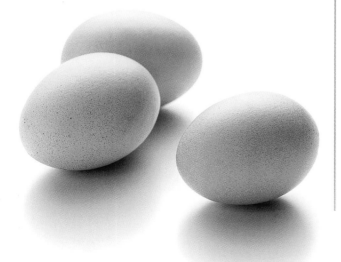

SUPPLEMENTS

Take a good-quality multi-vitamin and mineral supplement (see p.320) daily and add in the following to meet my recommended amounts for each.

■ B-COMPLEX (containing 25mg of each B-vitamin, daily) Low levels of B-vitamins can contribute to feelings of anxiety, stress, and even depression. It's important not to become deficient during times of stress, when your body is using up B-vitamins especially quickly.

■ ANTIOXIDANTS These help mop up the free radicals created when you're stressed. Your multi should contain the most important antioxidants; if not, top up.

You need: vitamins C (with bioflavonoids; 1,000mg as magnesium ascorbate) and E (400iu) and the minerals zinc (25mg) and selenium (100µg).

■ OMEGA-3 FATTY ACIDS (1,000mg fish oil, containing at least 700mg EPA and 500mg DHA, daily) Your nerve cells need essential fats in order to function effectively, and you need good nerve function to overcome stress. (Use flax seed oil if you're vegetarian.)

HERBS

As well as taking the following to help you cope with the effects of stress, try rhodiola and valerian for boosting adrenal-gland function (see p.68).

■ SIBERIAN GINSENG (*Eleutherococcus senticosus*) The herb of choice for stress, Siberian ginseng is an adaptogen, which means it can help your body adapt any way it needs to in order to cope with stress. Studies show that it can improve energy levels, stamina, and endurance and boost immunity. Take 1 tsp. tincture in a little water, or 250–300mg in capsule form, twice daily.

■ Other stress-relievers include: borage (*Borage officinalis*), damiana (*Turnera aphrodisiaca*), gotu kola (*Centella asiatica*), lemon balm (*Melissa officinalis*), lime flowers (*Tilia officinalis*), oats (*Avena sativa*), Roman chamomile (*Chamaemelum nobile*), skullcap (*Scutellaria lateriflora*), and vervain (*Verbena officinalis*). Blend the tinctures equally; take 1 tsp. of the combined tincture in a little water, twice daily.

OTHER NATURAL TREATMENTS

Virtually every complementary therapy is designed to help balance your body's systems, boost immunity, and encourage relaxation, so anything from massage and reflexology through to osteopathy and acupuncture should have a positive effect on stress symptoms.

Homeopathy I advise that you visit a homeopath to receive constitutional treatment, but for self-help try the following, all in a 30c potency. Choose the remedy or remedies that seem most appropriate for you and take each three times a day for three days.

• Aconite for anxiety and panic
• Belladonna for hot, tense, throbbing headaches
• Chamomilla when you're irritable and agitated
• Ignatia for grief and emotional upset
• Nux vomica when you've pushed yourself too hard
• Pulsatilla when you feel tearful and under pressure

Aromatherapy Essential oils used in massage, baths, or by burning or vaporizing may have an uplifting and relaxing effect. Try basil, bergamot, Roman or German chamomile, geranium, jasmine, lavender, marjoram, neroli, and rose. To strengthen the adrenal glands, try ginger, lemongrass, and rosemary. For an aromatherapy bath, use 1 or 2 drops of each of the oils in the bath water and relax in it for 20 minutes or so. Or, for a restorative aromatherapy massage oil (ask your partner to give you a back or neck and shoulder massage), use a total of 15 drops of essential oil or blend of essential oils in 6 tsp. of carrier oil, such as sweet almond.

SELF-HELP

Have a home spa Relaxing in a warm bath relieves sore muscles and joints, reduces stress and tension, and promotes a good night's sleep. Add some soothing music, soft lighting, and essential oils (see above).

Make time to relax Find time to zone out from the distractions of everyday life. Meditation may help because its aim is to free your mind from the daily pressures and demands that weaken your resistance to stress. If meditation isn't for you, you could spend 20 minutes a day writing in a journal; lose yourself in a piece of music for half an hour; or paint a picture, focusing on the details. It doesn't matter what activity you choose as long as it helps you to unwind.

Sleep well To cope with the stresses and demands of life, every woman needs around eight hours of good-quality sleep every night (see box, p.39).

Get your 30-a-day Research shows that regular, moderate exercise is linked to a reduction in the stress hormones that cause poor health. Make sure you get 30 minutes of exercise a day, five times a week. Try running, brisk walking, cycling, swimming—or anything else that raises your heart rate over its resting levels.

Get your priorities right If you feel the symptoms of stress coming on, learn to prioritize. There's nothing in your life more important than your health. Learn to say no if you feel that you've taken on too much. Being assertive is invigorating and empowering. Make lists to give you a sense of control over your life.

Have fun There's truth to the saying that laughter is the best medicine. Laughter reduces the body's levels of stress hormones and can boost immunity. Try to find humor in all the little things life throws at you. In addition, several studies show that making love, stroking a pet, being good to yourself, and seeking out pleasurable experiences have a beneficial and measurable physiological and psychological effect on your body.

Look on the bright side Optimism can counteract the negative impact of stress on your well-being because it's often how you perceive things that determines whether or not they overwhelm you. Having a positive attitude enhances your ability to manage stress. Try to look at life through "rose-colored glasses" every now and then.

Glossary

Bold type indicates another entry in the glossary.

acid–alkali balance using diet to achieve a more alkaline and less acid effect in the body

adaptogen herb that has a balancing effect on the body, either correcting a deficiency or reducing an excess

adhesions bands of scar tissue that can make structures in the body stick together when normally they would be separate

adrenaline "fight-or-flight" hormone released by the adrenal glands when the mind or body experiences stress

androgen "male" hormone, which, in women, is produced by the ovaries and the adrenal glands

anovulation menstrual cycle in which ovulation does not take place

antibodies specialized proteins found in the blood that act like an army to ward off and destroy foreign invaders

anti-mullerian hormone hormone produced by the ovaries, which is measured to check the level of **ovarian reserve**

antioxidants substances found in food that help control the damage caused by **free radicals**

autoimmune disorder condition in which the body produces **antibodies** that attack its own cells and try to destroy them

basal body temperature temperature of the body fully at rest, such as first thing in the morning, before any activity

benign harmless, non-cancerous condition that will not spread to other parts of the body

bioflavonoids substances that have **antioxidant** benefits, are anti-inflammatory and help strengthen blood capillaries; found in fruits

blood pressure measure of how hard the circulating blood is pressing against the walls of the arteries

blood sugar blood glucose, which the body uses as a source of energy

bone turnover rate at which bone breaks down and builds up when the body replaces old bone with healthy new bone

bowels also called the intestines, the digestive system "tube" running from the stomach to the anus

breech fetal position in pregnancy, which results in the baby's buttocks or legs being born first, rather than the head

candida species of yeast (fungus), which can cause infections in the mouth, intestines, and vagina

capillaries smallest blood vessels in the body, which connect the arteries to the veins

cholesterol type of fat that forms part of all cell membranes and circulates in the blood; the starting point for the sex and stress hormones

chromosome coiled strands of DNA carrying genetic information, which is passed down the generations

circulatory system body system consisting of the heart and blood vessels, which transport blood around the body

colostrum sticky "pre-milk" full of **antibodies** with which a mother breastfeeds her baby until her milk starts to flow

colposcopy diagnostic test to investigate any abnormal cell changes in the cervix

congenital abnormality any abnormality that is present from birth

corpus luteum structure that forms on the ovary once the egg has been released from the follicle; produces **progesterone**

cortisol hormone produced by the adrenal glands in response to stress; releases sugar and fat into the bloodstream

diabetes disorder in which **blood-sugar** levels are too high, either because the body can't produce enough **insulin** or because it can't use it effectively

diuretic substance that causes the body to excrete urine

dysplasia abnormal cell changes that can occur in the cervix or the lining of the uterus

endocrine system group of glands in the body that produces hormones directly into the bloodstream

essential fats fats that have to come from the diet because the body can't make them, for example omega-3, -6 and -9; also known as essential fatty acids

essential oils aromatic oils extracted from leaves, flowers, and fruits; called "essential" because they carry the "essence" (the scent) of the plant

estradiol the strongest form of **estrogen**, produced in the ovaries

estriol form of **estrogen** made in the liver by converting **estradiol** and **estrone**; excreted through the urine; highest levels occur in pregnancy

estrone form of **estrogen** produced by the adrenal glands, and the main form produced after the menopause

estrogen umbrella term for the three different types of estrogen: **estradiol**, **estriol**, and **estrone**

estrogen dominance having an imbalance of the female hormones with too much **estrogen** compared to **progesterone**

follicle (ovarian) sac-like structure in the ovary, in which the egg matures ready for ovulation

follicle-stimulating hormone (FSH) hormone released by the **pituitary gland**; stimulates the **follicles** in the ovary to mature eggs

follicular phase first half of the menstrual cycle, before ovulation

free radicals highly reactive chemicals, which can accelerate aging, heart disease, and cancer

galactagogues herbs that can help a mother produce a good supply of milk when breastfeeding

goitrogen food that can block the absorption of iodine from the blood and worsen an underactive thyroid gland

gonadotrophin-releasing hormone (GnRH) hormone produced by the hypothalamus that triggers the **pituitary gland** to make **LH** and **FSH**

homocysteine toxic substance produced naturally by the body during the breakdown of methionine, a sulphur-containing amino acid; should be excreted by the body

hyperglycemia high **blood-sugar** (glucose) levels, caused by the body not producing enough **insulin** or by **insulin resistance**; symptom of diabetes

hyperthyroidism condition caused by the thyroid gland being overactive and producing too much thyroid hormone

hypoglycemia low **blood-sugar** (glucose) levels caused by insufficient fuel reaching the brain; symptoms include shaking, hunger, and sweating

hypothyroidism condition caused by the thyroid gland being underactive and producing too little thyroid hormone

insulin hormone produced by the pancreas to regulate **blood sugar** (glucose)

insulin resistance term for when the body is producing enough or even too much **insulin**, but can't use it effectively

laparoscopy surgical procedure performed under general anaesthetic in which a viewing tube (a laparoscope) is inserted below the navel

luteal phase second half of the menstrual cycle, after ovulation

luteinizing hormone (LH) hormone that triggers ovulation; released by the **pituitary gland**

lymphatic system network of channels carrying lymph, a clear fluid, around the body, helping to protect the body from disease and to expel toxins

malignant cancer, where normal healthy cells have mutated with uncontrolled growth and invade other healthy tissue

mastectomy surgical removal of all or part of the breast as a result of cancer

meridians in Traditional Chinese Medicine, pathways along which the vital force *qi* flows, connecting the acupuncture points

methylxanthine substance found in caffeine that may cause symptoms of fibrocystic breast disease in the body

natural killer cell type of white blood cell, which attacks cells that are dividing abnormally

neurotransmitters chemical messengers produced in the brain that transmit signals to other cells

ovarian reserve number of eggs remaining in the ovary; measure of fertility

ovum egg that is released from the **follicle** on an ovary at ovulation

phagocytes white blood cells that engulf and destroy bacteria and viruses

pituitary gland found at the base of the brain; releases the hormones **FSH**, **LH**, **TSH**, and **ACTH** (see box, p.17)

polyps tongue-like projections that can grow in the cervix, intestines, and uterus

premature menopause medical classification for a menopause that occurs before the age of 40

probiotic supplement containing beneficial bacteria that helps control the growth of unhealthy bacteria in the digestive system

progesterone female hormone that prepares the uterus for pregnancy; secreted primarily by the **corpeus luteum**

progestin US term for the synthetic version of the hormone **progesterone** produced by the ovaries

progestogen UK term for the synthetic version of the hormone **progesterone** produced by the ovaries

prolactin hormone secreted by the **pituitary gland**, primarily associated with breastfeeding; too much prolactin can stop ovulation

prostaglandins hormone-like substances in the body that help control blood clotting and inflammation

receptors (hormone) gateways into cells that respond to hormones—for example, estrogen receptors in the breast are stimulated by **estrogen**

reproductive hormones all the different hormones that are released to help conception

sacrum triangular-shaped bone located at the base of the spine and attached to the pelvis

saturated fat fat from animal or vegetable sources that contains chains of saturated rather than unsaturated fatty acids; solid at room temperature

serotonin calming, mood-enhancing **neurotransmitter** in the brain; the aim of antidepressant drugs is to keep serotonin at a good level

sex-hormone binding globulin (SHBG) protein that binds sex hormones, such as **estrogen** and **testosterone**; produced by the liver

testosterone "male" hormone that women produce in the ovaries and the adrenal glands; thought to help with sex drive and muscle strength

thyroxine hormone produced by the thyroid gland to regulate metabolism and hence can control weight

tincture medicinal solution or liquid remedy in which herbs and plant extracts are preserved in alcohol

trimester period of three months; term used to divide the time of pregnancy into three parts: the first, second, and third trimesters

trisomy where three chromosomes are in a group instead of the normal pair

tryptophan amino acid that is converted into **serotonin**, a calming **neurotransmitter** in the brain

urethra tube (present in both sexes) that carries urine from the bladder to be excreted; has a reproductive function in men as a channel for semen

urinary tract tube and organs involved in the production, storage, and excretion of urine

white blood cells immune system cells, which fight off invading bacteria and viruses; also called leucocytes

xenoestrogen "foreign **estrogen**," an environmental hazard that comes from the plastic and the pesticide industries

Bibliography

CHAPTER 1: INTRODUCING YOUR BODY

Bernstein, L. *Journal of the National Cancer Institute*, vol. 86 (1994), p.18

Davidson, R. J. et al, "Alternations in brain and immune function by mindfulness meditation," *Psychosomatic Medicine*, vol. 65 (2003), pp.564–70

Felson, D. et al, "Alcohol consumption and hip fractures: The Framingham study," *American Journal of Epidemiology*, vol. 128 (1988), pp.1102–10

Feskanich, D. et al, *JAMA*, vol. 288 (2002), pp.2300–06

Henriksen, T. B. et al, "Alcohol consumption at the time of conception and spontaneous abortion," *American Journal of Epidemiology*, vol. 160 (2004), pp.661–7

Jensen, T. K. et al, "Does moderate alcohol consumption affect fertility?" *BMJ*, vol. 317 (1998), pp.505–10

Lahmann, P. H. et al, *Cancer Epidemiol Biomarkers Prev*, vol. 16 (2007), pp.36–42

Solomon, Karen G. et al, "Long or highly irregular menstrual cycles as a marker for risk of type 2 diabetes mellitus," *JAMA*, vol. 286 (2001), pp.2421–6

Wagner, H. in Beal J. L. and Reinhard E. (eds.) *Natural Products as Medicinal Agents*, Hippokrates-Verlag, Stuttgart (1981)

CHAPTER 2: GENERAL BODY SYSTEMS

Abraham, G. E. and Lubran, M. M. "Serum and red cell magnesium levels in patients with premenstrual tension," *American Journal of Clinical Nutrition*, vol. 34 (1981), pp.2364–6

Adetumbi, M. et al, "Allium sativum (garlic) inhibits lipid synthesis by candida albicans," *Antimicrob Agents and Chemother*, vol. 30 (1986), pp.499–501

Adlercreutz, H. et al, "Dietary phytoestrogens and cancer: in vitro and in vivo studies," *Journal of Steroid Biochemistry and Molecular Biology*, vol. 41 (1992), pp.331–7

Al-Akoum, M. et al, "Synergistic cytotoxic effects of tamoxifen and black cohosh on MCF-7 and MDA-MB-231 human breast cancer cells: an in vitro study," *Can J Physiol Pharmacol*, vol. 85 (2007), pp.1153–9

Amin, A. et al, "Berberine sulfate: antimicrobial activity, bioassay, and mode of action," *Canadian Journal of Microbiology*, vol. 15 (1969), pp.1067–76

Aronson, K. J. "Breast adipose tissue concentrations of polychlorinated biphenyls and other organochlorines, and breast cancer risk," *Cancer Epidemiol Biomarkers Prev*, vol. 9 (2000), pp.55–63

Atmaca, M. et al, *Hum Psychopharmacol*, vol. 18 (2003), pp.191–5

Basu, J. et al, "Smoking and the antioxidant ascorbic acid: plasma, leukocyte, and cervicovaginal cell concentrations in normal healthy women," *American Journal of Obstetrics and Gynecology*, vol. 163 (1990), pp.1948–52

Benvenga, S., Ruggeri, R.M, Russo, A. et al, "Usefulness of L-carnitine, a naturally occurring peripheral antagonist of thyroid hormone action, in iatrogenic hyperthyroidism: a randomized, double-blind, placebo-controlled clinical trial." *J Clin Endocrinol Metab* vol. 86 (2001), pp.3579–94

Berga, S. L. "Stress and amenorrhoea," *The Endocrinologist*, vol. 5 (1995), pp.416–21

Bernstein, L. "Physical exercise and reduced risk of breast cancer in young women," *Journal of the National Cancer Institute*, vol. 86 (1994), pp. 1403–8

Bianchi, G. et al, "Oxidative stress and anti-oxidant metabolites in patients with hyperthyroidism: effect of treatment," *Horm Metab Res*. vol. 31 (1999), pp.620–24

Bodinet, C. and Freudenstein, J. *Breast Cancer Res Treat*, vol. 76 (2002), pp.1–10

Bohnert K. J. and Hahn, G. "Phytotherapy in gynecology and obstetrics— *Vitex agnus castus*," *Erfahrungsheilkunde*, vol. 39 (1990), pp.494–502

Borras, M. et al, *J Recept Res*, vol. 12 (1992), 463–84

Boyd, E. M. F. et al, "The effect of a low-fat, high complex carbohydrate diet on symptoms of cyclical mastopathy," *The Lancet*, vol. 2 (1988), pp.128–32

Boyd, N. F. and McGuire, V. "The possible role of lipid peroxidation in breast cancer risk," *Free Radic Biol Med*, vol. 10 (1991), pp.185–90

Butler, E. B. and McKnight, E. "Vitamin E in the treatment of primary dysmenorrhea," *The Lancet*, vol. 1 (1955), p.844ff

Cahill, D. J. et al, Multiple follicular development associated with herbal medicine, *Hum Reprod (UK)*, vol. 9 (1994), pp.1469–70

Carvajal, A. *Breast Cancer Res Treat*, vol. 94 (2005), pp.171–83

Chen, C. C. et al, "Adverse life events and breast cancer: case-controlled study," *BMJ*, vol. 311, (1995), pp.1527–30

Chiaffarino, F. et al, "Diet and uterine myomas," *Obstet Gynecol*, vol. 94 (1999), pp.395–8

Chu, D. et al, *Clinical Immunology and immunopathology*, vol. 45 (1987), pp.48–57

Chuong, C. J. and Dawson, E. B. "Zinc and copper levels in premenstrual syndrome," *Fertility and Sterility*, vol. 62 (1994), pp.313–20

Clark A. M. et al, "Weight loss in obese infertile women results in improvement in reproductive outcome for all forms of fertility treatment," *Human Reproduction*, vol. 13 (1998), pp.1502–5

Clark A. M. et al, "Weight loss results in significant improvement in pregnancy and ovulation rates in anovulatory obese women," *Human Reproduction*, vol. 10 (1995), pp.2705–12

Coeuginet, E. and Kuhnast, R. "Recurrent candidiasis: Adjuvant immunotherapy with different formulations of echinacin," *Therapiewoche*, vol. 36 (1986), pp.3352–8

Deutch, B. "Menstrual pain in Danish women correlated with low n-3 polyunsaturated fatty acid intake," *European Journal of Clinical Nutrition*, vol. 49 (1995), pp.508–16

Dirican, M. and Tas, S. "Effects of vitamin E and vitamin C supplementation on plasma lipid peroxidation and on oxidation of apolipoprotein B-containing lipoproteins in experimental hyperthyroidism," *J Med Invest* vol. 46 (1999), pp.29–33

Dittmar, F. W. et al, "Premenstrual syndrome: Treatment with a phytopharmaceutical," *Therapiwoche Gynakol*, vol. 5, pp.60–68

Edman, J. et al, "Zinc status in women with recurrent vulvovaginal candidiasis," *American Journal of Obstetrics and Gynecology*, vol. 155 (1986), pp.1082–5

El Midaoui, A. and de Champlain, J. "Prevention of hypertension, insulin resistance, and oxidative stress by alpha-lipoic acid," *Hypertension*, vol. 39 (2002), pp.303–7

van Enwick, J. et al, "Dietary and serum carotenoids and cervical intraepithelial neoplasia," *International Journal of Cancer*, vol. 48 (1991), pp.34–8

Evans, G. W. and Pouchnik, D. J. "Composition and biological activity of chromium-pyridine carbosylate complexes," *Journal of Inorganic Biochemistry*, vol. 49 (1993), pp.177–87

Foreyt, J. P. and Poston, W. S. "Obesity: A never-ending cycle?" *International Journal of Fertility and Women's Medicine*, vol. 43 (1998), pp.111–16

van Gaal, L. et al, "Biomedical and clinical aspects of coenzyme Q10," vol. 4 (1984), p.369

Gardella, C. et al, "Managing genital herpes infections in pregnancy," *Cleve Clin J Med.* vol. 74 (2007), pp.217–24

Gerhausser, C. et al, "What is the active antiviral principle of thuja occidentalis L? " *Pharm Pharmacol Lett*, vol. 2 (1992), pp.127–30

Gerli, S. et al, "Effects on inositol on ovarian function and metabolic factors in women with PCOS: a randomized double-blind, placebo-controlled trial." *Eur Rev Med Pharmacol Sci* vol. 7 (2003), pp.151–9

Gokhale, L. B. "Curative treatment of primary (spasmodic) dysmenorrhea, *Indian Journal of Medical Research*, vol. 103 (1996), pp.227–231

Graham, J. *Evening Primrose Oil*, Thorsons (1984), pp.37–8

Grodstein, F. et al, "Relation of female infertility to consumption of caffeinated beverages," *American Journal of Epidemiology*, vol. 137 (1993), pp.1353–60

Haggans, C. J. et al, *Nutr Canc*, vol. 33 (1999), pp.188–95

Haggans, C. J. et al, *Cancer Epid Bio Prev*, vol. 9 (2000), pp.719–25

Hardy, M. L. "Women's Health Series: Herbs of special interest to women," *Journal of the American Pharmaceutical Association*, vol. 40 (2000), pp.234–42

Hatcher, R. et al, *Contraceptive Technology*, Irvinton Publishers, Inc. and Contraceptive Technology Communications, Inc., New York (1994)

Herbert, J. and Rosen, A. "Nutritional, socioeconomic, and reproductive factors in relation to female breast cancer mortality: findings from a cross-national study," *Cancer Detect Preven*, vol. 20 (1996), pp.234–44

Hilton, E. et al, "Ingestion of yogurt containing lactobacillus acidophilus as prophylaxis for candidal vaginitis," *Annals of Internal Medicine*, vol. 116, (1992), pp.353–7

Hilton, E. et al, "Lactobacillus GG vaginal suppositories and vaginitis," *J Clin Microbiol*, vol. 33 (1995), p.1433

Hoeger, K. M. et al, "A randomized, 48-week, placebo-controlled trial of intensive lifestyle modification and/or metformin therapy in overweight women with polycystic ovary syndrome: a pilot study," *Fertility and Sterility*, vol. 62 (2004), pp.421–9

"How can I get rid of cellulite?" *Johns Hopkins Med Lett Health After 50.* vol. 15 (2004), p.8

Howell, A. B. et al, "Inhibition of the adherence of P-fimbriated escherichia coli to uroepithelia-cell surfaces by proanthocyanidin extracts from cranberries," *New England Journal of Medicine*, vol. 339 (1998), pp.1085–6

Hu, G. et al, "A study on the clinical effect and immunological mechanism in the treatment of Hashimoto's thyroiditis by moxibustion," *Journal of Traditional Chinese Medicine*, vol. 13 (1993), pp.14–18

Huang, Z. et al, *American Journal of Epidemiology*, vol. 150 (1999), pp.1316–24

International Journal of Cancer vol. 100 (2002), pp.723–8

Iritani, N. and Nagi, S. "Effects of spinach and wakame on cholesterol turnover in the rat," *Atherosclerosis*, vol. 15 (1972), pp.87–92

Janiger, O. et al, "Cross cultural study of premenstrual symptoms," *Psychosomatics*, vol. 13 (1972), pp.226–35

Journal of Ethnopharmacology, vol. 38 (1993), pp.63–77

Kelly, R. W. et al, "The relationship between menstrual blood loss and prostaglandin production in the human: evidence for increased availability of arachidonic acid in women suffering from menorrhagia," *Prost Leuk Med*, vol. 16 (1984), pp.69–77

Kemmis, C. M. et al, *J Nutr*, vol. 136 (2006), pp.887–92

Kiddy D. S. et al, "Differences in clinical and endocrine features between obese and non-obese subjects with polycystic ovary syndrome: an analysis of 263 consecutive cases," *Clinical Endocrinology*, vol. 32 (1990), pp.213–220

Kiddy D. S. et al, "Improvement in endocrine and ovarian function during dietary treatment of obese women with polycystic ovary syndrome," *Clinical Endocrinology*, vol. 36 (1992), pp.105–11

Konrad, T. et al, "Alpha-lipoic acid treatment decreases serum lactate and pyruvate concentrations and improves glucose effectiveness in lean and obese patients with type 2 diabetes," *Diabetes Care*, vol. 22 (1999), pp.280–87

Kretzschmar, G. et al, "No estrogen-like effects of an isopropanolic extract of *Rhizoma cimicifugae racemosae* on uterus and vena cava of rats after 17 day treatment," *J Steroid Biochem Mol Biol*, vol. 97 (2005), pp.271–7

Lahmann P. H. et al, *Cancer Epidemiol Biomarkers Prev*, vol. 16 (2007), pp.36–42

Levy, J. et al, "Carotene and antioxidant vitamins in the prevention of oral cancer," *New York Academy of Sciences* (1992), pp.260–26

Lidefelt, K. J. et al, "Changes in periurethral microflora after antimicrobial drugs," *Archives of Disease in Children*, vol. 66 (1991), pp.683–5

Liske, E. et al, *Journal of Womens' Health and Gender-based Medicine*, vol. 11 (2002), pp.163–74

Lithgow, D. and Politzer, W. "Vitamin A in the treatment of menorrhagia," *South African Medical Journal*, vol. 51 (1977), pp.191–3

London, R. et al, "Mammary dysplasia: Endocrine parameters and tocopherol therapy," *Nutrition Research*, vol. 7 (1982), p.243

London, R. S. et al, "Efficacy of alpha-tocopherol in the treatment of premenstrual syndrome," *Journal of Reproductive Medicine*, vol. 32 (1987), pp.400–404

Losh, E. and Kayser, E. "Diagnosis and treatment of dyshormonal menstrual periods in the general practice," *Gynakol Praxis*, vol. 14 (1990), pp.489–95

Lyon, J. et al, "Smoking and carcinoma in situ of the uterine cervix," *American Journal of Public Health*, vol. 73 (1983), pp.558–62

Martinez, M. E. et al, *J Natl Cancer Inst*, vol. 98 (2006), pp.430–31

Mikhail, M. S. et al, "Decreased beta-carotene levels in exfoliated vaginal epithelia cells in women with vaginal candidiasis," *American Journal of Reproductive Immunology*, vol. 32 (1994), pp.221–5

Milewica, A. et al, "*Vitex agnus castus* extract in the treatment of luteal phase defects due to hyperprolactinemia. Results of a randomized placebo-controlled double-blind study," *Arzneim-Forsch Drug Res*, vol. 43 (1993), pp.752–6

Minton, J. P. et al, "Clinical and biochemical studies of methylxanthines-related fibrocystic breast disease," *Surgery*, vol. 90 (1981), pp.299–304

Mori et al, "The clinical effect of proteolytic enzyme containing bromelain and trypsin on urinary tract infection evaluated by double blind methods," *Acta Obstet Gynecol Jpn*, vol. 19 (1972), pp.147–53

Mowrey, D. B. *The Scientific Validation of Herbal Medicine*, Keats Publishing, New Canaan, Conneticut, USA (1986)

Neri, A. et al, "Bacterial vaginosis: drugs versus alternative treatment," *Obstetrical and Gynecological Survey (US)*, vol. 49 (1994), pp.809–13

Olivieri, O. et al, "Low selenium status in the elderly influences thyroid hormones," *Clinical Science*, vol. 89 (1995), pp.637–42

Orr, J. et al, "Nutritional status of patients with untreated cervical cancer, II, vitamin assessment," *American Journal of Obstetrics and Gynecology*, vol. 151 (1985), pp.632–5

Palmieri, C. et al, *J Clin Pathol*, vol. 59 (2006), pp.1334–6

Parazzini, F. et al, "Selected food intake and risk of endometriosis," *Human Reproduction*, vol. 19 (2004), pp.1755–9

Pena, E. "Melaleuca alternifolia oil: its use for trichomonal vaginitis and other vaginal infections," *Obstetrics and Gynecology*, vol. 19 (1962), pp.793–5

Petcu, P. et al, "Treatment of juvenile menorrhagia with *Alchemilla vulgaris* L fluid extract," *Clujul Med*, vol. 52 (1979), pp.266–70

Phipps, W. R. et al, "Effect of flaxseed ingestion on the menstrual cycle," *Journal Clin Endocrinol Metab*, vol. 77 (1993), p.1215ff

Probst, V. and Roth, O. "On a plant extract with a hormone-like effect," *Dtsch Me Wschr*, vol. 79 (1954), pp.127–34

Puolakka, J. et al, "Biochemical and clinical effects of treating the premenstrual syndrome with prostaglandin synthesis precursors," *Journal of Reproductive Medicine*, vol. 30 (1985), pp.149–53

Pye, J. K. et al, "Clinical experience of drug treatments for mastalgia," *The Lancet*, vol. 2 (1985), pp.373–7

Qi-bing, M. et al, "Advance in the pharmacological studies of *Radix angelica sinensis* (olic) diels (Chinese danggui)," *Chinese Medicine Journal*, vol. 104 (1991), pp.776–81

Ramaswamy, P. and Natarajan, R. "Vitamin B6 status in patients with cancer of the uterine cervix," *Nutrition and Cancer*, vol. 6 (1984), pp.176–80

Regan, L. et al, "Future pregnancy outcome in unexplained recurrent first trimester miscarriage," *Human Reproduction*, vol. 12 (1997), pp.387–9

Reid, G. et al, "Influence of three-day antimicrobial therapy and lactobacillus vaginal suppositories on recurrence of urinary tract infections," *Clinical Therapies*, vol. 14 (1992), pp.11–16

Rivlin, M. E. *Endometrial hyperplasia: Manual of Clinical Problems in Obstetrics and Gynecology*, eds. M.E. Rivlin and R.W. Martin, Little, Brown, and Company, Boston (1994), pp.433–7

Rossignol, A. M. and Bonnlander, H. "Prevalence and severity of the premenstrual syndrome. Effects of foods and beverages that are sweet or high in sugar content," *Journal of Reproductive Medicine*, vol. 36 (1991), pp.131–6

Saxena, S. P. et al, "DDT and its metabolites in leiomyomatous and normal human uterine tissue, *Arch Toxicol*, vol. 59 (1987), pp.453–5

Schairer, C. "Menopausal estrogen and estrogen–progestin replacement therapy and breast cancer risk," *JAMA*, vol. 283 (2000), pp.485–491

Schellenberg, R. "Treatment for the premenstrual syndrome with agnus castus fruit extract: prospective, randomized, placebo-controlled study," *BMJ*, vol. 322 (2001), pp.134–7

Schiffman, M. H. "Latest HPV findings: some clinical implications," *Contemporary Ob Gyn*, vol. 38 (1993), pp.27–40

Schwabe, J. W. R. and Rhodes, D. "Beyond zinc fingers: Steroid hormone receptors have a novel motif for DNA recognition," *Trends in Biochemical Science*, vol. 15 (1991), pp.291–6

Seifert, B. et al, "Magnesium: a new therapeutic alternative in primary dysmenorrhea," *Zentralbl Gynakol*, vol. 111 (1989), pp.755–60

Sharma, V. D. et al, "Antibacterial property of allium sativum linn.: in vivo and in vitro studies," *Indian Journal of Experimental Biology*, vol. 15 (1977), pp.466–8

Shigeta, Y. et al, "Effect of coenzyme Q10 treatment on blood sugar and ketone bodies of diabetics," *Journal of Vitaminology*, vol. 12 (1966), pp.293–8

Siddle, N. et al, "The effect of hysterectomy on the age of ovarian failure: Identification of a subgroup of women with premature loss of ovarian function, and literature review," *Fertility and Sterility*, vol. 47 (1987), pp.94–100

di Silverio, F. et al, "Evidence that serenoa repens extract displays antiestrogenic activity in prostatic tissue of benign prostatic hypertrophy," *Eur Urol*, vol. 21 (1992), pp.309–314

Simone, C. B. et al, *J Orthomol Med*, vol. 16 (2001), pp.83–90

Singer, S. R. and Grismaijer, S. *Dressed to Kill: the link between breast cancer and bras*, Avery Publishing Group, New York (1995)

Sirsi, M. "Antimicrobial action of vitamin C on M. tuberculosis and some other pathogenic organisms," *Indian J Med Sci*, vol. 6 (1952), pp.252–5

de Souza, M. C. et al, *Journal of Women's Health and Gender-based Medicine*, vol. 9 (1998), pp.131–9

Stalder, R. et al, "A carcinogenicity study of instant coffee in Swiss mice," *Food Chem Toxicol*, vol. 28 (1990), pp.829–37

Takaya, J. et al, *Mag Res*, vol. 17 (2004), pp.126–136

Tamborini, A. and Taurelle, R. "Value of standardized ginkgo biloba extract (EGB 761) in the management of congestive symptoms of premenstrual syndrome," *Rev Fr Gynecol Obstet*, vol. 88 (1993), pp.447–57

Taussig, S. J. and Batkin, S. "Bromelain, the enzyme complex of pineapple (Ananas comosus) and its clinical application," *Ethnopharmacol*, vol. 22 (1988), pp.191–203

Terry, P. et al, *JAMA*, vol. 285 (2001), pp.2975–7

Vallee, B. "Zinc," in C. L. Comar and C. S. Bonner (eds), *Mineral Metabolism*, Vol. IIB, Academic Press, New York (1965)

Walboomers, J. M. M. et al, "Human papillomavirus is a necessary cause of invasive cervical cancer worldwide," *J of Pathology*, vol. 189 (1999), pp.12–19

Walsh, C. T. et al, *Environmental Perspectives*, vol. 102 (1994), pp.44–46

Watson, N. R. et al, Treatment of severe premenstrual syndrome with estradiol patches and cyclical oral noresthisterone, *The Lancet*, vol. 8665 (1989), pp.730–32

Webb, J. "Nutritional effects of oral contraceptive use: a review," *Journal of Reproductive Medicine*, vol. 25 (1980), pp.150–56

Writing Group for the Women's Health Initiative Investigators, *JAMA*, vol. 288 (2002), pp.321–333

Wurtman, J. J. et al, "Effect of nutrient intake on premenstrual depression," *American Journal of Obstetrics and Gynecology*, vol. 161 (1989), pp.1228–34

Wyatt, K. M. "Efficacy of vitamin B6 in the treatment of premenstrual syndrome: systematic review," *BMJ*, vol. 318 (1999), pp.1375–81

Wyshak, G. et al, "Smoking and cysts of the ovary," *International Journal of Fertility*, vol. 33 (1988), pp.398–400

Yamamoto, I. et al, "Anti-tumor effects of seaweed," *Japanese J Exp Med*, vol. 44 (1974), pp.543–6

Yang Zha, L. L. "Relation of hypothyroidism and deficiency of kidney," *Inst of the Integr of TCM-WM Med*, Shanghai Medical University, Chung Kuo Chung Hsi I Chieh Ho Tsa Chih (China), vol. 13 (1993), pp.202–4,195

Zhang, S. M. et al, "Women's Health Study: Alcohol consumption and breast cancer risk," *American Journal of Epidemiology*, vol. 165 (2007), pp.66–77

Ziaei, S., Sakeri, M. and Kazemnejad, A. *BJOG* vol. 112 (2005), p.1164

CHAPTER 3: CONCEPTION, PREGNANCY, AND BIRTH

Barnea, E. R. and Tal, J. *J IVF Embryo Transfer*, vol. 8 (1991), pp.15–23

Bodnar, L. K. et al, "Periconceptual multivitamin use reduces the risk of preeclampsia," *Am J Epidemiol* vol. 13 (2006), pp.1229–37

Cantorna, M. T. et al, "Mounting evidence for vitamin D as an environmental factor affecting autoimmune disease prevalence," *Exp Biol Med* (Maywood) vol. 229 (2004), pp.1136–1142

Hayes, C. E. et al, "The immunological functions of the vitamin D endocrine system, " *Cell Mol Biol*, vol. 49, (2003), pp.277–300

Jensen, T. K. et al, *BMJ*, vol. 317 (1998), pp.505–10

Kinney, A. et al, "Smoking, alcohol, and caffeine in relation to ovarian age during the reproductive years," *Human Reproduction*, vol. 22 (2007), pp.1175–85

Munafo, M. et al, *Journal of Biosocial Science*, vol. 34 (2002), pp.65–73

Rossi, E. and Costa, M. *Lupus*, vol. 2 (1993), pp.319–23

CHAPTER 4: THROUGH MENOPAUSE

Feskanich, D. et al, *JAMA*, vol. 288 (2002), pp.2300–06

Finkler, R. "The effect of vitamin E in the menopause," *Journal of Clin Endocrin Metab*, vol. 9 (1949), pp.89–94

Wilcox, F. et al, "Estrogenic effects of plant foods in postmenopausal women," *BMJ*, vol. 301 (1990), pp.905–6

Index

Resources

The Dr. Marilyn Glenville, Ph.D., Clinic
14 St. Johns Road
Tunbridge Wells
Kent TN4 9NP United Kingdom

Tel: 0870 5329244 / Fax: 0870 5329255
Int. tel: +44 189 251 5905 / Fax: +44 189 251 5914
Email: health@marilynglenville.com
Website: www.marilynglenville.com

If you'd like a consultation (by telephone or in person), please contact my clinic directly. In the UK, the clinic is run both in St John's Wood, London, and in Tunbridge Wells, Kent.

Where to find good-quality supplements, herbs and other natural products
The Natural Health Practice (NHP)
Tel: 0845 8800915 Int. tel: +44 189 250 7598
Website: www.naturalhealthpractice.com

NHP is my supplier of choice.
Supplements: NHP carries only the supplements and other "all-natural" products that I approve of and recommend personally in my clinics. Their supplements are all in the correct form, at the right dosage levels, made with the highest quality ingredients, and free from all "nasties," such as GMOs, sugar, and preservatives. They are also non-allergenic.

Natural Beauty Products: NHP carries a range of natural skin, hair, bodycare, and household products. I have given these my Seal of Approval and graded them into Gold, Silver, Bronze, and Nearly Natural categories. You can now see at a glance which ones are all natural and 100 percent organic, all natural but not organic, and organic with permitted inorganic ingredients.

To make things as easy as possible for you, I have read all the labels on the NHP website, so you don't have to. You can order with confidence from NHP—as I do—and have your order delivered to your door, in the UK usually by the following day, and overseas usually within 10 days.

Picture credits

The publisher would like to thank the following people and photographic libraries for permission to reproduce their material. Every care has been taken to trace copyright holders. If we have omitted anyone, we apologize and will, if informed, make corrections to any future editions of this book:

p.2 Tim Smith/Flowerphotos.com; **5** Bryce Attwell/Flowerphotos.com; **10–11** Mina Chapman/Corbis; **35** Gregor Schuster/Getty Images; **37** Dennis Halliman/Getty Images; **38** John Fedele/Getty Images; **41** esthAlto/Matthieu Spohn/Getty Images; **45** Steven Dewall/Getty Images; **49** Adam Gault/Getty Images; **54–55** Alix Minde/Getty Images; **71** Flying Colours Ltd/Getty Images; **75** TH Foto-werberg/Science Photo Library; **76** Stockbyte/Getty Images; **81** Wildlife GmbH/Alamy; **86** Jan Tove Johansson/Getty Images; **91** Grace Carlon/Flowerphotos.com; **93** Imagerwerks/Getty Images; **104** Dianna Jazwinski/GAP Photos; **108** Bruno Petriglia/Science Photo Library; **113** Tim Smith/Flowerphotos.com; **116** Science Photo Library; **124** Carol Sharp/Flowerphotos.com; **134** Will Heap/Getty Images; **136** Dr E. Walker/Science Photo Library; **146** Geoff Kidd/Science Photo Library; **160** Alix Minde/Getty Images; **164** Maike Jessen/Photolibrary; **167** Maria Murray/Babyarchive.com; **192** Nancy Brown/Getty Images; **197** Foodcollection/Getty Images; **208** ImageSource/Getty Images; **215** Tetra Images/Getty Images;

220 Jupiterimages/Getty Images; **223** Madeline Spokes/Babyarchive.com; **231** Carol Sharp/Flowerphotos.com; **232** Bryce Attwell/Flowerphotos.com; **241** Steffen Hauser/botanikfoto/Alamy; **244–245** Sam Edwards/Getty Images; **247** Cavan Images, LLC/Getty Images; **257** Ryuhei Shindo/Corbis; **265** Siri Stafford/Getty Images; **270** Lisa Stirling/Getty Images; **281** Trevor Sims/Garden World Images; **294** George Doyle/Getty Images

Toby Scott & Simon Smith/Watkins Media Archive:
pp.7, 23, 27, 28, 60, 64, 84, 98, 139, 145, 150, 171, 185, 189, 194, 203, 226, 253, 258, 267, 269, 274, 276, 301, 310.

Graph and chart permissions:
p.183 Reprinted with the kind permission of George R. Attia, MD, MBA, University of Miami, Miller School of Medicine
p.191 Reprinted from "Effects of male age on fertility," Hassan MA and Killick SR, *Fertility and Sterility*, vol. 79, suppl. 3, pp.1520–27, Copyright © (2003), with permission from Elsevier
p.236 *New England Journal of Medicine*, vol. 351, pp.1927–9 "Advanced maternal age—how old is too old?," Linda J. Heffner, MD, PhD Copyright © (2004) Massachusetts Medical Society. All rights reserved.